Endovascular Therapy

PRINCIPLES OF PERIPHERAL INTERVENTIONS

Alan B. Lumsden, MD
Peter H. Lin, MD
Ruth L. Bush, MD
Changyi Chen, MD, PhD
Baylor College of Medicine, Houston, Texas

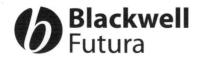

Blackwell
Futura

© 2006 by Blackwell Publishing
Blackwell Futura is an imprint of Blackwell Publishing

Blackwell Publishing, Inc., 350 Main Street, Malden, Massachusetts 02148-5020, USA
Blackwell Publishing Ltd, 9600 Garsington Road, Oxford OX4 2DQ, UK
Blackwell Science Asia Pty Ltd, 550 Swanston Street, Carlton, Victoria 3053, Australia

First published 2006

ISBN-13: 978-1-4051-24232
ISBN-10: 1-4051-24237

Library of Congress Cataloging-in-Publication Data

   Endovascular therapy : principles of peripheral interventions/edited by Alan B. Lumsden ... [et al.].
      p. ; cm.
   Includes bibliographical references and index.
   ISBN-13: 978-1-4051-2423-2 (hardcover : alk. paper)
   ISBN-10: 1-4051-2423-7 (hardcover : alk. paper)
1. Blood-vessels–Endoscopic surgery. 2. Peripheral vascular diseases–Endoscopic surgery.
[DNLM: 1. Arterial Occlusive Diseases–surgery. 2. Peripheral Vascular Diseases–surgery.
3. Angioplasty–methods. 4. Angioscopy–methods. 5. Stents. WG 500 E5665 2006] I. Lumsden, Alan B.

RD598.5.E56 2006
617.4′130597–dc22

                                                                                2005026041

A catalogue record for this title is available from the British Library

Acquisitions: Steve Korn
Production: Simone Dudziak
Set in 9.5/12pt Palatino
by Newgen Imaging Systems (P) Ltd, Chennai, India
Printed and bound by Replika Press PVT. Ltd, India

For further information on Blackwell Publishing, visit our website:
www.blackwellcardiology.com

The publisher's policy is to use permanent paper from mills that operate a sustainable forestry policy, and which has been manufactured from pulp processed using acid-free and elementary chlorine-free practices. Furthermore, the publisher ensures that the text paper and cover board used have met acceptable environmental accreditation standards.

Notice: The indications and dosages of all drugs in this book have been recommended in the medical literature and conform to the practices of the general community. The medications described do not necessarily have specific approval by the Food and Drug Administration for use in the diseases and dosages for which they are recommended. The package insert for each drug should be consulted for use and dosage as approved by the FDA. Because standards for usage change, it is advisable to keep abreast of revised recommendations, particularly those concerning new drugs.

Contents

Colour plates are found between pp. 80–81

Editors

Alan B. Lumsden, MD Professor of Surgery; and Chief, Division of Vascular Surgery and Endovascular Therapy, Michael E. DeBakey Department of Surgery, Baylor College of Medicine Houston, Texas

Peter H. Lin, MD Associate Professor of Surgery, Chief of Vascular Surgery, Michael E. DeBakey Veterans Affairs Medical Center, Division of Vascular Surgery and Endovascular Therapy, Michael E. DeBakey Department of Surgery, Baylor College of Medicine Houston, Texas

Ruth L. Bush, MD Assistant Professor of Surgery; and Director, Vascular Surgery Fellowship Program, Division of Vascular Surgery and Endovascular Therapy, Michael E. DeBakey Department of Surgery, Baylor College of Medicine Houston, Texas

Changyi Chen, MD, PhD Professor of Surgery & Molecular and Cellular Biology; and Director, Molecular Surgeon Research Center, Vice Chairman, Surgical Research, Division of Vascular Surgery and Endovascular Therapy, Michael E. DeBakey Department of Surgery, Baylor College of Medicine Houston, Texas

List of Contributors

Ulises Baltazar, MD
Division of Vascular Surgery
Department of Surgery
East Tennessee State University
Johnson City, Tennessee

Kristen L. Biggs, MD
Section of Vascular Surgery
Department of Surgery
Wilford Hall USAF Medical Center
Lackland Air Force Base, Texas

W. Todd Bohannon, MD
Division of Vascular Surgery
Department of Surgery
Scott & White Hospital and Clinic
Texas A & M University Health Science
    Center
Temple, Texas

Ruth L. Bush, MD
Division of Vascular Surgery and Endovascular
    Therapy
Michael E. DeBakey Department of Surgery
Baylor College of Medicine
Houston, Texas

Changyi Chen, MD, PhD
Division of Vascular Surgery and Endovascular
    Therapy
Michael E. DeBakey Department of Surgery
Baylor College of Medicine
Houston, Texas

Andy C. Chiou, MD, MPH
Section of Endovascular Surgery
Department of Surgery
University of Illinois College of Medicine
Peoria, Illinois

Mitchell Cox, MD
Uniformed Services University of the Health
    Sciences
Vascular Surgery Clinic
Walter Reed Army Medical Center
Washington, DC

Patrick E. Duffy, MD
Division of Vascular Surgery and Endovascular
    Therapy
Michael E. DeBakey Department of Surgery
Baylor College of Medicine
Houston, Texas

James P. Gregg, MD
Division of Vascular Surgery and Endovascular
    Therapy
Michael E. DeBakey Department of Surgery
Baylor College of Medicine
Houston, Texas

Marlon A. Guerrero, MD
Division of Vascular Surgery and Endovascular
    Therapy
Michael E. DeBakey Department of Surgery
Baylor College of Medicine
Houston, Texas

E. John Harris, Jr., MD
Division of Vascular Surgery
Department of Surgery
Stanford University School of Medicine
Stanford, California

Esteban A. Henao, MD
Division of Vascular Surgery and Endovascular
    Therapy
Michael E. DeBakey Department of Surgery
Baylor College of Medicine
Houston, Texas

Colleen M. Johnson, MD
Division of Vascular Surgery
University of Missouri
Health Sciences Center
Columbia, Missouri

Panagiotis Kougias, MD
Division of Vascular Surgery and Endovascular
    Therapy
Michael E. DeBakey Department of Surgery
Baylor College of Medicine
Houston, Texas

Russell Lam, MD
Division of Vascular Surgery
Department of Surgery
Cornell University Weil Medical College
New York, New York

W. Anthony Lee, MD
Division of Vascular Surgery & Endovascular
   Therapy
University of Florida
Gainesville, Florida

Peter H. Lin, MD
Division of Vascular Surgery and Endovascular
   Therapy
Michael E. DeBakey Department of Surgery
Baylor College of Medicine
Houston, Texas

Alan B. Lumsden, MD
Division of Vascular Surgery and Endovascular
   Therapy
Michael E. DeBakey Department of Surgery
Baylor College of Medicine
Houston, Texas

Daniel J. Martin, MD
Division of Vascular Surgery
Department of Surgery
University of Florida
Gainesville, Florida

Ross Milner, MD
Division of Vascular Surgery
Department of Surgery
Emory University School of Medicine
Atlanta, Georgia

Imran Mohiuddin, MD
Division of Vascular Surgery and Endovascular
   Therapy
Michael E. DeBakey Department of Surgery
Baylor College of Medicine
Houston, Texas

Leila Mureebe, MD, FACS
Division of Vascular Surgery
Columbia University Medical Center
New York Presbyterian Hospital
New York, New York

Joseph J. Naoum, MD
Division of Vascular Surgery
Department of General Surgery
The University of Texas Medical Branch
Galveston, Texas

Liz Nguyen, MD
Division of Vascular Surgery and Endovascular
   Therapy
Michael E. DeBakey Department of Surgery
Baylor College of Medicine
Houston, Texas

Mai Pham, MD
Department of Cardiothoracic and Vascular
   Surgery
University of Texas Health Science Center at
   Houston
Houston, Texas

Eric Peden, MD
Division of Vascular Surgery and Endovascular
   Therapy
Michael E. DeBakey Department of Surgery
Baylor College of Medicine
Houston, Texas

Gordon M. Riha, BS
Division of Vascular Surgery and Endovascular
   Therapy
Michael E. DeBakey Department of Surgery
Baylor College of Medicine
Houston, Texas

Rakesh Safaya, MD
Division of Vascular Surgery and Endovascular
   Therapy
Michael E. DeBakey Department of Surgery
Baylor College of Medicine
Houston, Texas

Eric J. Silberfein, MD
Division of Vascular Surgery and Endovascular
   Therapy
Michael E. DeBakey Department of Surgery
Baylor College of Medicine
Houston, Texas

Michael B. Silva, Jr., MD
Department of Vascular Surgery
Cleveland Clinic Foundation
Cleveland, Ohio

Wei Zhou, MD
Division of Vascular Surgery and Endovascular
   Therapy
Michael E. DeBakey Department of Surgery
Baylor College of Medicine
Houston, Texas

Foreword

A little more than a half-century has elapsed since the first "homemade" Dacron graft was first used successfully to restore continuity following resection of an aneurysm of the abdominal aorta. This, along with a number of other essential advancements in our basic understanding of the anatomic-pathologic aspects of aneurismal and occlusive diseases of the aorta and major arteries and innovative technologic surgical procedures to restore circulation, led to the establishment of highly successful therapy for most vascular diseases that previously meant only suffering and death. Concomitant with these advances was the development of newer and more precise diagnostic procedures, including particularly ultrasound, computerized axial tomography (CAT) scans, and magnetic resonance imaging (MRI), all of which have led to the advent of a new specialty in medicine – vascular surgery.

In many respects, these sophisticated scientific and technologic advances set the stage within the past two decades for the highly innovative development of endovascular therapy. Once this concept was recognized, an increasing number of investigators from a variety of disciplines, ranging from surgery, cardiology, and radiology to bioengineering and industrial technicians, focused their interest and energies on implementing this concept with rapidly improving clinical results. As a consequence, endovascular therapy has now replaced a number of open surgical procedures and expanded the therapy of some patients, who would otherwise be eliminated because of the unacceptable risk of operation, as, for example, an elderly patient with a ruptured aneurysm of the abdominal aorta and poor cardiac, pulmonary, or renal function.

This textbook on endovascular therapy is not only timely, but also valuable in providing current knowledge of this expanding field. The authors, all of whom are not only highly experienced but also contributors to this advancing form of vascular therapy, have provided a succinct but comprehensive text that will be useful not only to those working in this specialty, but to all physicians and surgeons concerned with vascular disease.

Michael E. DeBakey, MD
Chancellor Emeritus
Olga Keith Wiess and Distinguished Service Professor
Michael E. DeBakey Department of Surgery
Director, DeBakey Heart Center
Baylor College of Medicine
Houston, Texas

Preface

The treatment of vascular disease has evolved significantly over the past two decades with a greater emphasis on catheter-based interventions. This evolution has been energized by various factors, including the widespread acceptance of minimally invasive therapy, miniaturization of endovascular devices, and enhanced healthcare cost-effectiveness due in part to increased outpatient treatment. Vascular physicians and patients alike have largely embraced this minimally invasive therapy with enthusiasm due to reduced procedural-related discomfort and faster convalescence, when compared to the traditional operations. The continual evolution of catheter-based technologies has created a need for updating and educating physicians from varying specialty disciplines with regards to the new treatment paradigm. Equally important, this has placed an increased demand on students and residents to learn not only the fundamental knowledge of vascular disease but also modern therapeutic modality.

Because endovascular therapy has become an integral component of the overall care in vascular disease management, an understanding of the fundamental knowledge regarding the vascular pathology and modern catheter-based interventions for vascular diseases will undoubtedly enhance the ability of physicians to provide quality care to their vascular patients. Toward that effort, we have embarked on the development of this book to achieve two objectives. The first is to provide a general overview of the vascular diseases based on their respective circulatory anatomy. This is particularly geared toward medical students, residents, or healthcare providers with limited background knowledge in vascular intervention. The second is to provide a practical reference of catheter-based therapeutic modalities for vascular physicians specializing in peripheral intervention.

Since endovascular interventions can be performed by physicians from different specialty disciplines, this book is written to provide a general understanding of the clinical manifestations, treatment indications, and diagnostic evaluations for healthcare providers dedicated in the treatment of vascular disease. In addition, a basic knowledge of the pathophysiology of vascular disease, interventional techniques, and endovascular modalities of various disease categories is provided. Emphasis is also placed on the relevant complications associated with the wide spectrum of endovascular interventions. It is our hope that this book of *Endovascular Therapy: Principles of Peripheral Interventions* will provide both a comprehensive and practical reference for healthcare practitioners, regardless of their training background or specialty disciplines, in their clinical practice of endovascular therapy.

Alan B. Lumsden, MD
Peter H. Lin, MD
Ruth L. Bush, MD
Changyi Chen, MD, PhD

Acknowledgments

The creation of this book would not have been possible without the efforts and support from many people. To Dr. Michael E. DeBakey, we appreciate your support in our commitment to create this first endovascular textbook from the Baylor College of Medicine. To the contributors, we are indebted to the precious time and quality work you have provided to all the chapters. And lastly to our families, Terry, Donal, Sarah, Cynthia, Pete, Cathy, Aaron, Amber, and Bill, thank you for your tolerance and support to make this project a reality.

ABL, PHL,
RLB, CC

CHAPTER 1

General principles of endovascular therapy

Imran Mohiuddin, Panagiotis Kougias, Ross Milner

Cardiovascular disease remains a major cause of mortality in the developed world since the beginning of the twenty-first century. Although surgical revascularization has played a predominant role in the management of patients with vascular disease, the modern treatment paradigms have evolved significantly with increased emphasis of catheter-based percutaneous interventions over the past two decades. The increasing role of this minimally invasive vascular intervention is fueled by various factors, including rapid advances in imaging technology, reduced morbidity, and mortality in endovascular interventions, as well as faster convalescence following percutaneous therapy when compared to traditional operations. There is little doubt that with continued device development and refined image-guided technology, endovascular intervention will provide improved clinical outcomes and play an even greater role in the treatment of vascular disease. In this chapter, a framework is provided for a brief history of endovascular therapy along with an overview of commonly used endovascular devices. The fundamental techniques of percutaneous access is also discussed.

Brief history of endovascular therapy

Evolution of diagnostic imaging

The discovery of the X-ray imaging system by Charles Röentgen in 1895, marked one of the most remarkable milestones in the history of medicine. Within months after its discovery, X-rays were used by battlefield surgeons to locate and remove bullet fragments.[1] This imaging modality quickly gained acceptance from physicians around the world in providing valuable diagnostic information in the care of their patients. As a natural evolution of this discovery, X-rays were soon adapted to evaluate the vascular system in conjunction with the use of a contrast material. In 1910, Frank performed the first venography in rabbits and dogs by injecting a solution of bismuth and oil intravenously and following its flow fluoroscopically.[2] Heuser is credited (in 1919) for performing the first contrast study in humans by injecting a solution of potassium iodide into the dorsal vein of a child and following the flow of the substance to the heart.[3] The use of such materials was initially quite toxic. This led to the development of safe contrast media, for example water soluble iodine-based organic contrast called Selectran-Neutral by Binz in 1929.[4] Concurrently, newer injection methods were also being developed. In 1927, Moniz was the first to perform direct arterial injections, and he used this technique to inject sodium iodide into the internal carotid arteries.[5] This direct approach was initially used to image the heart and thoracic aorta but was soon abandoned due to its hazards.

Castellanos used an indirect method of injection whereby a contrast agent was injected into a vein in the arm and, after a delay, the aorta was visualized.[6] Due to dilution of the agent in the heart and lungs, the aorta could be visualized only 75% of the time. For a better study of these vessels, Werner Forssmann, a resident surgeon in Berlin in 1929, ran a urethral catheter through his own basilic vein to visualize his right ventricle. This earned him the Nobel prize in 1956.[7] Also in 1929, dos Santos et al. described a technique of visualizing the aorta using a direct puncture technique by translumbar injection of a contrast medium directly into the abdominal aorta.[8] The modern aortogram via a femoral approach was first performed by Farinas in 1941,[9] a technique that was quickly adapted by physicians around the world. With the advent of guidewires in the early 1950s, selective angiography with catheter-directed injection was developed further. In 1962, Guzman and colleagues reported a large series of patients who underwent coronary angiography using selective coronary catheterizations.[10] Since then, the application of guidewires, catheters, and introducer sheaths has become a standard approach when performing diagnostic angiography.

Evolution of therapeutic interventions

Ivar Seldinger, a Swedish radiologist, was the first physician to describe a unique method of establishing arterial access using a guidewire technique in 1953, which heralded an evolution from diagnostic to therapeutic angiography.[11] A decade later, Fogarty detailed the use of a balloon-tipped catheter to extract thrombus.[12] Building on this, Dotter and Judkin in 1964 described a method of dilating an arterial occlusion using a rigid Teflon catheter to improve the arterial circulation.[13] In the field of venous intervention, catheter-based vena caval filters were introduced by Greenfield in 1973, and have revolutionized the current approach in the prevention of pulmonary embolism.[14] The technique of balloon angioplasty was introduced by Gruntzig, who performed the first coronary artery intervention in 1974.[15] To this day, this remains the most commonly performed endovascular procedure in clinical practice. The application of the balloon angioplasty catheter subsequently led to the development of the first intravascular balloon-expandable stent by Palmaz et al. in 1985.[16] Several years later, Parodi, an Argentinean vascular surgeon, combined both a Dacron graft and balloon-expandable stent technology to create a stent-graft, which was successfully used to exclude an abdominal aortic aneurysm from the systemic circulation.[17] Technology in this field is rapidly evolving and more complex modular stents with thermal memory are in use today. There has also been an explosion in catheter-based technology, enabling access for the interventionalist to treat occlusive disease and increasingly, aneurysmal disease in nearly every vascular bed. Further development of this minimally invasive intervention is currently focused on combining a pharmacological agent with the current stent platform to create drug-eluting stents to improve the clinical outcome of endovascular therapy.

Basic vascular access

Percutaneous access can be achieved by a single- or double-wall puncture technique. In the former approach, a beveled needle is introduced, and a guidewire is passed after confirmation of arterial or venous access by visual inspection of back bleeding with or without the use of direct pressure measurement and inspection of arterial or venous waveforms. As a routine, we typically gain vascular access using a 21-gauge micropuncture needle and a 0.018-in. wire. The double-wall technique requires the use of a blunt needle with an inner cannula. The needle is inserted through the vessel, and then the inner cannula is removed, the introducer needle withdrawn until back bleeding is obtained, and a wire introduced. Although percutaneous access can be routinely achieved in nearly all patients, those with scarred access sites from prior interventions or patients with decreased pulses due to occlusive disease represent a specially challenging subset that may benefit from ultrasound guidance with Doppler insonation or B-mode visualization of the target vessel. Indeed, access site needles have been developed with integrated Doppler probes.

Retrograde femoral access

Percutaneous retrograde femoral puncture is the most commonly used arterial access technique. Both groins are prepped and draped in a sterile fashion. Visualization of the femoral head using fluoroscopy is recommended. In the majority of patients, the common femoral artery can be found over the medial third of the head of the femur (Figure 1.1). Another advantage of accessing the artery in this location is that the femoral head will serve as a hard surface to compress the artery against, after the completion of the procedure if manual compression is needed to achieve hemostasis. An 18-gauge angiographic needle is then advanced at a 45° angle through the skin until pulsatile back bleeding is encountered. As with all needle access, the bevel of the needle should point upward. Going through and through the artery should be avoided, as this can lead to problematic bleeding. Depending upon the body habitus, the artery may lie anywhere from 2–5 cm below the level of the skin. If venous entry is noted, it is useful to remember that the artery lies lateral to the vein. It is also important to remember that there is approximately 3 cm of common femoral artery that lies between the inferior ligament and the femoral bifurcation. Once brisk back bleeding is noted, a standard Bentson wire is passed through the needle into the artery for at least 20 cm. It is recommended

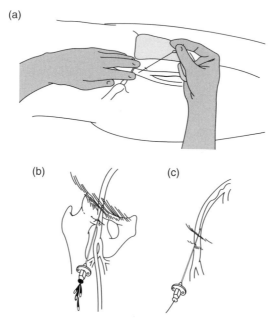

Figure 1.1 Retrograde femoral artery access. (a) The common femoral artery can usually be found medially 2–3 cm below the inguinal ligament. (b) Once the needle enters the common femoral artery, brisk back bleeding is seen. (c) The Bentson guidewire is next advanced through the needle under fluoroscopic guidance to establish the arterial access.

that this maneuver is performed under fluoroscopy to confirm that the wire is going into the aorta. Once the wire is in place, the introducer sheath with its dilator can be easily passed into the artery. If there is any doubt about the path of the wire, a small amount of contrast can be injected through the needle to delineate the needle location.

Arterial entry higher than the level of the femoral head can prove to be difficult in achieving hemostasis, and retroperitoneal hematoma often develops. Entry into the femoral artery far below the inguinal ligament can lead to entry into the superficial or profunda femoral arteries. Catheterization of either of these arteries can result in post-op hematoma and pseudoaneurysm development.

Antegrade femoral access

Antegrade femoral puncture is more challenging than retrograde but can be invaluable in problematic infrainguinal lesions. We recommend that the operator stand on the side that permits forehand approach of the needle (Figure 1.2). The needle is advanced at an angle of 45° to the skin until pulsatile back bleeding is noted. With this approach, it is even more important to avoid low punctures, as this would limit the working room to selectively catheterize the superficial femoral artery. With obese patients, it is often necessary to have

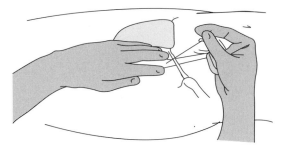

Figure 1.2 Antegrade femoral artery access. The needle is inserted just below the inguinal ligament in the common femoral artery whereby the guidewire is inserted in the ipsilateral superficial femoral artery.

an assistant retract the pannus cephalad out of the way. Once back bleeding is noted, the Bentson wire is placed, followed by a sheath. If there is little room between the site of entry of the wire and the femoral bifurcation, a sheathless technique may need to be employed. In order to selectively catheterize the superficial femoral artery, an angled catheter may help in directing the wire down the correct artery. If the guidewire begins to buckle, it should be withdrawn and retried using a different angle.

Difficult access

There are several techniques that can be employed to access the pulseless yet patent femoral artery. The common femoral artery almost always passes over the medial head of the femur, and attempts in this area will prove to be the most successful. Accessing the femoral artery via the contralateral side and placing a catheter over the bifurcation can be used to inject contrast and visualize the ipsilateral artery. Many patients have vessels that are calcified. Using magnification views, these calcifications can be used as a guide to determine the location of the femoral artery to which the needle can be inserted. Finally, a handheld ultrasound device can be used to determine the location of the noncompressible femoral artery with respect to the compressible femoral vein.

Crossing the aortic bifurcation

Crossing over the aortic bifurcation to gain access to the contralateral iliac artery is an indispensable technique in ileofemoral arterial interventions. This selective catheterization technique produces angiograms of significantly improved quality because of localized contrast injection. The first task is to determine the location of the aortic bifurcation. This can be done by either performing an aortogram for use as a road map or by using the L4 vertebrate and the iliac crest as a landmark. Calcifications in the arteries can help in establishing orientation. The catheter type can prove to be decisive in gaining access across the aortic bifurcation. We routinely use the Contra catheter, as this saves a step when an aortogram is also performed. The catheter is parked near where the bifurcation is suspected, and a glidewire is advanced. If initial attempts are

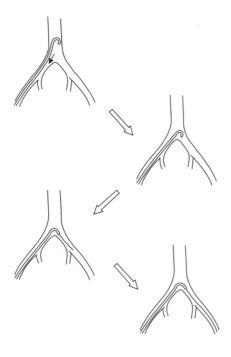

Figure 1.3 Gaining access across the aortic bifurcation. A curved catheter is inserted in a retrograde fashion from a femoral artery approach and is positioned across the aortic bifurcation. A guidewire is next advanced over the catheter to gain access in the contralateral common iliac artery.

unsuccessful, the catheter and wire can be rotated. Alternatively, the catheter can be advanced 1–2 cm up into the aorta, which helps the guidewire select the contralateral common iliac artery. Once the artery is selected, the catheter is pulled back down and securely positioned across the bifurcation (Figure 1.3). Alternative catheters for this approach may be the Cobra or C2 catheter. Once inside the contralateral iliac, the wire is advanced past the inguinal ligament in order to securely position the catheter in the iliofemoral arterial segment. Subsequently, catheters and sheaths can be advanced with ease. There are several specially shaped sheaths available that facilitate in crossing-over.

Brachial puncture

Occasionally when the distal aorta or bilateral ileofemoral axis are inaccessible, the brachial artery becomes a very useful access site. The left brachial artery is the preferred upper extremity access of choice, as this avoids the origin of the carotid artery and thus reduces the chance of a cerebrovascular accident due to catheter-related thrombus embolization. The arm is abducted and prepared on a radiolucent arm board. The most common location for puncture is just proximal to the antecubital crease, and this location reduces the incidence of nerve injuries (Figure 1.4). Once sterility has been established, a micropuncture kit is used to access the artery. The micropuncture sheath can then be exchanged for a 6 Fr sheath. Once at the aortic arch, an angled catheter can be used to deflect the wire down the aorta.

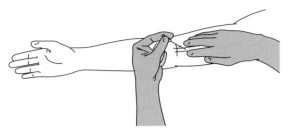

Figure 1.4 Brachial artery approach. A Seldinger needle is inserted in a retrograde fashion in the brachial artery just above the antecubital fossa, whereby the guidewire is next inserted in the brachial artery.

Table 1.1 Comparison of mobile C-arm and fixed angiosuite imaging system.

Imaging system	Mobile C-arm unit	Fixed angiosuite unit
Reliability	Adequate	Superior
Radiation exposure	More	Less
Availability	Can be moved to different locations because of its portability	Restricted to one location
Likelihood to overheat with prolonged usage	High	Low
Special construction	None	Needed
Cost	up to $20,000 US	up to $2 million US

Image-guided endovascular intervention

Choosing an imaging system

Excellent imaging is the key to endovascular therapies regardless of whether the intervention is performed in an imaging suite or an operating room. Fluoroscopy is the modality used for digital subtraction angiography. Fluoroscopy functions via an image intensifier that receives, concentrates, and brightens an X-ray image to produce an electronic image that can be displayed on a screen. The larger size of an image intensifier usually allows for better quality imaging. A standard imaging suite image intensifier is 15 in. in diameter, whereas a standard image intensifier on a portable C-arm is 12 in. in diameter. Both of these systems allow control of the irradiation by the use of a foot pedal. The advantages and disadvantages of each system are highlighted in Table 1.1. Although the versatility and durability of an angiosuite are better than a mobile C-arm unit, both are adequate for performing the majority of endovascular procedures. For most surgeons, performing an endovascular intervention in the operating room using a mobile C-arm unit is a common strategy to build an endovascular practice. The portability of a C-arm unit enables surgeons to perform catheter-based interventions in any operating room, an environment that is intimately familiar to most surgeons in contrast to an angiosuite in the radiology or cardiology service. Moreover, the cost of a C-arm unit is only a fraction of the price of an angiosuite, which is easier to acquire in hospitals with budgetary constraints. There are however several limitations, however, associated with a C-arm fluoroscopic equipment. Despite the significant technical improvements in the current model of C-arm systems, the image quality remains slightly inferior to that obtained from the angiosuite. This is due to several factors including higher focal spot size, fixed distance between the X-ray tube, and the power output of a C-arm image intensifier.[18,19]. A common concern about the mobile C-arm unit is its propensity to overheat. When this happens, the unit must be shut down and allowed to cool, which can be severely limiting. In contrast to a mobile fluoroscopic unit, an angiosuite is typically more robust with less likelihood of overheating. In addition, all the necessary imaging equipments, such as image intensifier, fluoroscopic table, and power injector are typically electronically integrated in an angiosuite. Consequently, activating the image intensifier dims the room lights, initiates the imaging sequence, and times the injector activation. Another benefit of the angiosuite is that most are directly linked to a hospital picture archiving and communication system (PACS), which facilitates viewing. Lastly, images captured from an angiosuite can be used to create rotational angiography or three-dimensional reconstruction for further image analysis.

Both portable C-arm and an angiosuite imaging unit have specialized functions that are commonly used during interventions. Magnified views are obtained when focusing on a limited area such as the aortic bifurcation for kissing stent deployment. Another feature is the road map technique. This allows for a representation of the arterial tree by contrast angiography on one digital screen with real-time fluoroscopy on another. Fluoroscopic images can be adjusted in different oblique angles to enhance the accuracy of visualizing certain vascular anatomy, such as the internal iliac arteries or the aortic arch. The most commonly used fluoroscopic angle is anteroposterior (AP) projection. In contrast, examples of the oblique views include the right anterior oblique (RAO) and left anterior oblique (LAO) angles. When visualizing the internal iliac arteries, for example, an oblique angle allows the origin of this vessel to be visualized so that it does not overlap with the common iliac artery. This is especially important with iliac arterial interventions to prevent stenting across the origin of the internal iliac artery. Additional views such as craniocaudal correction can also be obtained. This is particularly useful for correcting angulation in difficult aortic necks during endovascular aneurysm repair. Commonly used orientations of the image intensifier in diagnostic angiography are listed in Table 1.2.

Table 1.2 Commonly used image intensifier orientations in arterial angiography and its contrast injection rates and volume.

Procedure	Orientation	Injection rate (cc/s)	Injection volume (cc)
Abdominal aortogram	AP	20	30
Arch aortogram	LAO 30–50° Chin up Shoulders down	30	50
Descending thoracic aortogram	LAO 15–30°	30	50
Selective carotid angiogram	AP and lateral Face rotated to opposite side	4	8
Cerebral angiogram	AP @10° craniocaudal, lateral	4	8
Mesenteric or renal angiogram	Full lateral, pig catheter in aorta	20	30
Renal selective angiogram	10–20° oblique to ipsilateral side	7	12
Selective run off via CIA	AP	8	40
Dual run off via aorta	AP	10	60
iliac bifurcation	Contralateral 20° AO	—	
Common femoral angiogram	Ipsilateral 20° AO	—	—
Subclavian angiogram	AP	7	25
Inferior vena cavagram	AP	20	30
Common femoral venogram	AP	8	25
Superior vena cavagram	AP	10	30

Imaging table

The imaging table is an integral part of the endovascular suite. Although it is possible to perform an endovascular procedure in an operating room using a conventional operating room table, there are many drawbacks: variability in the cushioning and underlying metals provides for a nonuniform path for the radiation. For endovascular procedures, the primary requirement of the imaging table is that it must be radiolucent. In general, there are two types of radiolucent tables; fixed and movable. Fixed tables are constructed of a nonmetallic carbon-fiber supported usually at only one end. This allows for unobstructed access for the C-arm because there are no structural elements underneath the table. These tables are relatively fragile and do not support patients in excess of 300 lbs. Movable tables allow for versatile positioning of the patient in the horizontal plane. They come with a set of bedside controls that also permit selection of the radiographic settings including gantry rotation, image intensifier location, collimation, and table height.

Power injector

There are two methods for delivering contrast: hand injection with a syringe and electronically calibrated precise power injection. For most small vessel and selective angiography, hand injection is adequate. However, for optimal opacification of high-flow blood vessels like the aorta, the use of a power injector is mandatory. Conversely, the power injector is also useful in small vessels when the contrast must be injected at a fixed slow rate. The power injector permits the operator to determine the rate of injection, total volume of injection, and pressure of the injection. Table 1.2 briefly outlines commonly used injection rates and contrast volume for diagnostic arteriographic studies.

Basics of radiation safety

Radiation exposure

Radiation safety is important in endovascular surgery not only because of regulations but also due to patient and personnel considerations. There are several federal, state, and local guidelines that are available for review. Significant levels of radiation exposure pose serious health hazards to medical personnel if standard safety guidelines are not followed. The general guiding philosophy is ALARA (as low as reasonably achievable).[20] This protective philosophy mandates that all interventionalists must compare the benefits to the risks of radiation exposure. With regards to exposure, there are three key principles: monitoring time, scatter, and distance of exposure.

With longer and more complex endovascular procedures, it becomes imperative to use the personal dosimeter device or badge. An external dosimeter badge must be placed over any radiation protective garments on the collar near the thyroid. A second badge is recommended to be worn underneath the protective garments at the waist level. This second badge becomes mandatory in pregnant women. The effective dose equivalent is then calculated from a weighted average of the two badges and is used to calculate exposure risk.

The duration of exposure is directly proportional to the received radiation dose. In this way, personnel exposure is linked to patient exposure. Reduction of personnel exposure can be effectively accomplished by reducing the "beam-on" time by judicious use of the exposure switch to ensure that radiation exposure is occurring only when the fluoroscopist is actively viewing the image and optimizing the number of images used in an exposure sequence.

Road mapping, pulse-mode fluoroscopy, and image hold and transfer can also help limit the time of exposure. Use of a control booth whenever possible (as in lower extremity run off) will also help to minimize radiation exposure time.

Another very important consideration is the scatter phenomenon. Although the majority of the radiation beam is absorbed by the patient, there is scatter radiation that is emitted from the patient in all directions. This scatter can be a major source of hazard for angiosuite personnel. Emission of radiation follows the inverse-square law whereby the radiation intensity decreases proportionately as the square of the distance from a point source.[20] Because increasing the distance decreases the radiation field intensity, it is always prudent to back away from the source when proximity is not required. Keeping the image intensifier as close to the patient as possible helps to maintain low fluoroscopic beam intensity and also allows the image intensifier to serve as a scatter barrier between the patient and the operator. One final point is that use of magnification modes further increases beam intensity, scatter, and heat production and should be used judiciously.

Radiation shielding

Shielding involves the use of protective barriers. The best type of shielding protects the whole body of an individual. Barriers may be fixed, moveable, or worn by the individual. The control room is an example of a structurally fixed barrier. Mobile barriers may be rolled into position inside angiosuites to protect nurses and anesthesia personnel who do not need to be near the patient for extended periods of time. Alternatively, ceiling-mounted transparent barriers may also be used to protect the upper body of the interventionalist. Flexible protective clothing such as aprons, skirts, and vests should always be used when working in an unprotected zone. The typical protective clothing consists of 0.50 mm lead impregnated rubber. Ninety-five percent of scatter is directed towards the head and neck, and the use of a thyroid shield is strongly recommended. In addition, leaded eyeglasses are available that can absorb 70% of scatter exposure to the lens. Personnel who have frequent back exposure should wear wrap-around protective garments (others may wish to wear them for comfort).

Every angiosuite should have a protocol in place to monitor the integrity of its protective garments. Folding and rolling of lead garments should be avoided, as this will lead to cracking. At the minimum, annual X-ray evaluation of the protective clothing should be practiced to evaluate for cracks. Drop off lead garments with shoulder and waist Velcro is available which allows for removal without breaking scrub.

Common devices used in endovascular interventions

Guidewires

Guidewires are used to introduce, position, and exchange catheters. A guidewire generally has a flexible and stiff end. In general, only the flexible end of the guidewire is placed in the vessel. All guidewires are composed of a stiff inner core and an outer tightly coiled spring, which allows a catheter to track over the guidewire. There are five essential characteristics of guidewires: size, length, stiffness, coating, and tip configuration.

Guidewires come in different maximum transverse diameters ranging from 0.011 to 0.038 in. For most aortoilliac procedures, a 0.035 wire is most commonly used while the smaller diameter wires are reserved for selective small vessel angiography such as infrageniculate or carotid lesions. The 0.035 Bentson wire is often used as the initial guidewire to obtain access to the groin vessels for most interventions.

In addition to diameter size, guidewires come in varying lengths usually ranging from 180 to 260 cm in length. Increasing the length of the wire always makes it more difficult to handle and increases the risk of contamination. While performing a procedure, it is important to maintain the guidewire across the lesion until the arteriogram has been satisfactorily completed. A good rule of thumb to follow is that the guidewire should be twice the length of the longest catheter being used. This allows for easy catheter exchanges while maintaining the guidewire across the lesion.

The stiffness of the guidewire is also an important characteristic. Stiff wires allow for passage of large aortic stent-graft devices without kinking. They are also useful when trying to perform sheath or catheter exchanges around a tortuous artery. An example of a stiff guidewire is the Amplatz wire. For initial access, standard guidewires are coated with a nonhydrophilic coating composed of Teflon and heparin to lubricate the surface and reduce the thrombogenicity of the guidewire. The heparin coating lasts for about 10 min. Hydrophilic coated guidewires, such as the Glidewire, have become invaluable tools for assisting in difficult catheterizations. The coating is primed by bathing the guidewire in saline solution. The slippery nature of this guidewire along with its torque capability significantly facilitate difficult catheterizations. There are several disadvantages of hydrophilic coated guidewires that need to be remembered. These wires must be constantly rewetted in order to maintain their lubricated surface. Glidewires are often very slippery and difficult to handle with gloved hands, and one must be careful to monitor the tip of the wire while performing catheter exchanges.

Guidewires come in various tip configurations. Most tips of guidewires are soft. Many angiographers use the J-tip wire as the initial access guidewire, as it is associated with the lowest risk of dissection. We use the Bentson wire, which has a soft floppy tip that is straight in its packaged form but forms a functional large J-tip when being advanced through a vessel. Angled tip wires like the angled Glidewire can be steered to manipulate a catheter across a tight stenosis or to select a specific branch of a vessel. The Rosen wire has a soft curled end that makes it ideal for renal artery stenting. The soft curl of this wire prevents it from perforating small renal branch vessels.

Catheters

Catheters come in all different shapes and sizes and are sized according to their outer diameters. A plethora of catheters have been designed for specific arterial beds and designated by configuration, which are discussed in the last chapter of this book. Most catheters must be advanced over a wire to limit intimal injury. Catheters are generally differentiated based on whether they are nonselective or selective. An example of a nonselective catheter is the pigtail catheter. This type of catheter has multiple side and end holes that allow for a large cloud of contrast agent to be infused over a short period of time. They are most commonly used for viewing of high-flow vessels like the abdominal aorta. The other type of catheter is the selective catheter, which usually has only a single hole at the tip and is used to select certain vascular systems. Specific types of these selective catheters are described in the last chapter of this book. When using these catheters, care must be taken to avoid intimal injury by direct catheter tip advancement or by forceful injection of contrast material. The shape of catheters dictates their function. A commonly used selective catheter is the Bernstein catheter, which has a gentle angled tip and can be used to select many arterial branches.

Most other nonselective catheters have unique functions by design. In order to cannulate the contralateral iliac artery, we often use the Contra catheter. An alternate catheter for crossing over the aortic bifurcation is the C-2. For arch vessels, we recommend the use of Simmons-2 or JB-2. For bovine arches, a H-1 catheter is quite useful. These catheters must be reformed either in the ascending aorta or subclavian artery prior to using them to select a vessel. For renal and visceral vessels, we recommend the use of the renal double curve (RDC) catheter. This catheter can be advanced proximally and then slowly brought back down with a gentle rotation. It will generally land in a renal or visceral orifice. Once having been placed inside the ostia, a Glidewire can be slowly advanced across the lesion. A special category of catheters are the hydrophilic coated catheters like the Glidecath and Slip-Cath. They can be used for crossing tight lesions and can be advanced independent of a guidewire.

Introducer sheath, guiding sheaths, and guiding catheters

Vascular sheaths allow for easy exchange and introduction of catheters and guidewires. They have a hemostatic valve that prevents blood reflux and air embolism. Furthermore, they protect the vessel entry point from intimal injury and should be used whenever multiple guidewire exchanges are anticipated. Sizing of sheaths is based on their internal diameter: a 7 Fr sheath will accept up to a 7 Fr catheter. Sheaths come in multiple lengths. In addition, the side port of the sheath can be used to inject contrast or measure arterial pressure. All sheaths are packaged with dilators. Dilators serve as an obturator for entry of the sheath and also help to progressively enlarge the track once guidewire entry has been established. As with all sheaths, once placed they must be flushed with heparinized saline through the side port in order to prevent thrombosis.

Guiding catheters and sheaths can be used to facilitate passage of a smaller endovascular device through a tortuous curve. They are particularly useful in the renal and carotid system or contralateral iliac system. The distal portion of some guiding sheaths comes in a specialized shape like the renal curve sheath. Guiding sheaths are also particularly useful for intermittently assessing the results of angioplasty. The side port allows for puffing of contrast distally while the guidewire is still across the lesion.

Balloon catheters

Once the diseased arterial bed has been selected with the appropriate catheter and wire, the presence of the anticipated lesion needs to be confirmed, and where appropriate, its hemodynamic significance determined. An arteriogram is obtained by hand injection of contrast agent through the selective catheter, and a "road map" is acquired that creates a virtual image of the effected arterial segment through which repeated passes of catheters, wires, or stents can be visualized.

The contrast load is always minimized and tailored to the specific patient according to the intervention being performed. For patients with an elevated serum creatinine level (≥ 1.4 mg/dL), preintervention hydration, minimization of contrast load, and/or use of fenoldopam have been advocated to limit the nephrotoxic effects of the contrast agent.[21] Fenoldopam is administered as a continuous infusion at a rate of 0.01–1.6 mg/kg/min. A steady-state concentration is usually reached within 20 min. Other options for lesion localization when the baseline serum creatinine exceeds 2 mg/dL include use of gadolinium, CO_2 contrast, or intravascular ultrasound. Of note, the total administered volume of gadolinium should not exceed 0.2–0.4 mmol/kg, which is equivalent to 30–60 mL in a 75-kg person.

There is no consensus as to whether an intervention should be based on a pressure gradient difference measured by an intraarterial catheter. We suggest that a mean pressure gradient greater than 10 mm Hg is sufficiently significant to require treatment. If no difference is detected in the resting state, then 100 mg of nitroglycerin can be infused intra-arterially to mimic the increased demand that occurs with walking. The gradient can be checked after the infusion is complete.

For a given lesion, a balloon catheter is selected on the basis of balloon diameter (millimeters) and length (centimeters), as well as the length of the catheter shaft, which is dictated by lesion location and the chosen access site. Characteristically, angioplasty balloons are produced from a noncompliant plastic, such as polyethylene, which facilitates high-pressure inflation to a predetermined maximum shape and size. Pressure required for inflation may vary widely from 4 to 16 atm and is dependent upon the compliance of the vascular lesion to be dilated. Higher pressures are typically required for relatively stiff venous stenoses. The ability to respond to an inflation pressure without balloon disruption is dictated by the material properties of a given balloon, and as a consequence, is also a factor in selection of an appropriate balloon

Table 1.3 Commonly used angioplasty balloon
diameter size.

Arterial lesions	Commonly used balloon diameter (mm)
Abdominal aorta	8–16
Common illiac artery	6–10
External illiac artery	6–8
Superficial femoral artery	4–7
Popliteal artery	3–6
Tibial artery	2–4
Renal artery	4–7
Subclavian artery	5–8
Dialysis graft	4–6

catheter. Balloons that are composed of a compliant plastic, such as Silastic, have a much greater range of potential final diameters, with continued balloon expansion dictated as a function of the inflated volume. Embolectomy balloons fall in this category, as well as occlusion balloons that may be used to seat an aortic stent graft or temporarily facilitate proximal aortic occlusion in the presence of a ruptured aneurysm. Both balloon types are capable of inadvertently perforating a vessel wall. Cutting balloon technology has been primarily utilized in the coronary circulation. A recent report from England demonstrated the short-term efficacy of a 6-mm cutting balloon in the periphery.[15] Further studies of cutting balloons for applications in peripheral arterial disease are underway.

Selection of the appropriate balloon size is primarily dictated by the diameter of the normal vessel in which a given lesion is located. Table 1.3 summarizes the typical diameter of angioplasty balloons used in peripheral arterial interventions. With experience, balloon selection can be made on the basis of the appearance of the arteriogram, but more accurate measurement techniques exist, including use of integrated image-based software programs referenced to a fluoroscopically visualized catheter of known French size. Alternatively, intravascular ultrasound[16] also provides a very accurate means for defining vessel size, and marker catheters that contain radiopaque marks at known intervals can also be used for a more accurate assessment of vessel diameter. Balloon shaft lengths are commonly 75 cm or 120 cm, and depending on the system, can be coaxial or monorail and designed to be inserted over 0.014-in., 0.018-in., or 0.035-in. wires.

The balloon inflating solution is usually a mixture of saline and contrast solution. Whereas most balloons are best imaged using a 50–50 mix, larger aortic balloons can be easily visualized using 20–30% (v/v) of contrast agent, which decreases the viscosity of the solution and allows the balloon to be more rapidly inflated or deflated. To accurately pre-position an angioplasty catheter before inflation, balloons are designed with a radiopaque marker at each end of the cylindrical portion of the balloon. However, balloons may be designed with differing degrees of taper, and a significant "shoulder" may protrude past these marks. In this regard, when treating a lesion that lies near a branch point, it is important to account for balloon taper and limit inadvertent extension of the terminal portion of the balloon into a smaller branch vessel with attendant risk of vessel rupture or dissection.

Stents

Vascular stents are commonly used after an inadequate angioplasty with dissection or elastic recoil of an arterial stenosis. They serve to buttress collapsible vessels and help prevent atherosclerotic restenosis. Eventually, all intravascular stents have smooth muscle migration that leads to the formation of a neointima.[22] Appropriate indications for primary stenting of a lesion without an initial trial of angioplasty alone are evolving in manners that are dependent on the extent and site of the lesion. Stents are manufactured from a variety of metals including stainless steel, tantalum, cobalt-based alloy, and nitinol. Vascular stents are classified into two basic categories: balloon-expandable stents and self-expanding stents.

Self-expanding stents are deployed by retracting a restraining sheath and usually consist of Elgiloy (a cobalt, chromium, nickel alloy) or Nitinol (a shape memory alloy composed of nickel and titanium), the latter of which will contract and assume a heat-treated shape above a transition temperature that depends upon the composition of the alloy. Self-expanding stents will expand to a final diameter that is determined by stent geometry, hoop strength, and vessel size. In particular, if the vessel diameter is significantly less than that of the stent, final stent length may be longer than the anticipated unconstrained length. The self-expanding stent is mounted on a central shaft and is placed inside an outer sheath. It relies on a mechanical springlike action to achieve expansion. With deployment of these stents, there is some degree of foreshortening that has to be taken into account when choosing the area of deployment. In this way, self-expanding stents are more difficult to place with absolute precision. There are several advantages. Self-expanding stents generally comes in longer length than balloon-expandable stents and are therefore used to treat long and tortuous lesions. Their ability to continually expand after delivery allows them to accommodate adjacent vessels of different size. This makes these stents ideal for placement in the internal carotid artery. After the delivery system is inserted into the lesion, the stent is expanded to its predetermined diameter by withdrawing the sheath, while the end of the device is maintained in position. These stents are always oversized by 1–2 mm relative to the largest diameter of normal vessel adjacent to the lesion in order to prevent immediate migration.

Balloon-expandable stents are usually composed of stainless steel, mounted on an angioplasty balloon, and deployed by balloon inflation. They can be manually placed on a chosen balloon catheter or obtained premounted on a balloon catheter. The capacity of a balloon expandable stent to shorten in length during deployment depends on both stent geometry and the final diameter to which the balloon is expanded. These stents are more rigid and are associated with a shorter time to complete endothelialization. They are often of limited flexibility and have a higher degree of crush resistance when compared to self-expanding ones. This makes them ideal for short-segment lesions, especially those that involve the ostia such as proximal common iliac or renal artery stenosis.

The most exciting area of development in stents is the evolution of drug-eluting stents. These stents are usually composed of nitinol and have various anti-inflammatory drugs bonded to them. Over time, the stents release the drug into the surrounding arterial wall and help prevent restenosis. Numerous randomized-controlled trials have proven their benefit in coronary arteries.[23,24] Examples and descriptions of various drug-eluting stents for endovascular intervention are discussed elsewhere in this book.

Stent grafts

The combination of a metal stent covered with fabric gave birth to the first stent grafts. Covered stents have been designed with either a surrounding polytetrafluoroethylene or polyester fabric and have been used predominantly for treatment of traumatic vascular lesions, including arterial disruption and arteriovenous fistulas. However, these devices may well find a growing role in the treatment of iliac or femoral arterial occlusive disease as well as popliteal aneurysms.

Endovascular aneurysm repair using the concept of stent grafts was initiated by Parodi et al. in 1991.[17] Since that time, a large number of endografts have been inserted under the auspice of clinical trials at first, and now as Food and Drug Administration-approved devices. The AneuRx (Medtronic AVE, Santa Rosa, CA), Ancure (Guidant Corp., Menlo Park, CA), Excluder (W.L.Gore & Associates, Flagstaff, AZ), PowerLink (Endologix Inc., Irvine, CA), and Zenith (Cook Inc., Bloomington, IN) devices have all been approved for clinical use in the United States as of 2005. All of these devices require that patients have an infrarenal aneurysm with at least a 1-cm neck and not greater than 60° of angulation. For those patients with associated common iliac artery aneurysmal disease, endovascular treatment can be achieved by initial coil embolization of the ipsilateral hypogastric artery with extension of the endovascular device into the external iliac artery. Clinical trials are underway with devices that will expand indications to aneurysms involving the visceral segment of the abdominal aorta. Aortic endografts for treatment of thoracic aortic disease are not yet available. However, experience with experimental devices is rapidly accumulating. Early studies have demonstrated short-term efficacy of thoracic aortic devices in the treatment of descending thoracic aneurysms, traumatic aortic transections, and aortic dissections.[25–27] A larger experience with these devices exists in both Europe and Asia, and trials are underway in the United States with several devices.

References

1 Elke M. One century of diagnostic imaging in medicine. *Experientia* 1995; **51**:665–80.
2 Frank AA. Kreislaufstudien am Rontgenschirm. *Munich Med Wochenschr* 1910; **57**:1950.
3 Heuser C. Pieloradiografia con ioduro potasico y las injecciones intravenosas de iodura potasico en radiografia. *Sem Med* 1919; **26**:424–26.
4 Binz D. Die Wiedergrabe con Nieren und Harnwegen ina Rontgenbildedurch. Jodpyridon-deprivate. *Angew Chem* 1929; **43**:452–25.
5 Moniz E. L'encephalographie arterielle, son importance dans la localisation des tumeurs cerebrales. *Rev Neurol (Paris)* 1927; **2**:72–90.
6 Castellanos P. La Angiocardiografia radioopaca. *Arch Soc Estud Clin* 1939; **31**:523.
7 Forssman N. Ueber Kontrastdarstellung der hohlen des lebenden rechten Herzen und der Lungenschlagader. *Munich Med Wochenschr* 1931; **78**:489–92.
8 dos Santos R, Lamas A, Caldas J. L'arteriographic des membres, de l'aorta et de ses branches abdominales. *Bull Mem Soc Natl Chir* 1929; **55**:587–88.
9 Farinas P. A new technique for the examination of the abdominal aorta and its branches. *AJR* 1941; **46**:641–33.
10 Guzman SV, Swenson E, Jones M. Intercoronary reflex. Demonstration by coronary angiography. *Circ Res* 1962; **10**:739–45.
11 Seldinger SI. Catheter replacement of the needle in percutaneous arteriography; a new technique. *Acta Radiol* 1953; **39**:368–76.
12 Fogarty TJ, Cranley JJ. Catheter technic for arterial embolectomy. *Ann Surg* 1963; **161**:325–30.
13 Dotter CT, Judkins MP. Transluminal treatment of arteriosclerotic obstruction. Description of a new technic and a preliminary report of its application. *Circulation* 1964; **30**:654–70.
14 Greenfield LJ, McCurdy JR, Brown PP, Elkins RC. A new intracaval filter permitting continued flow and resolution of emboli. *Surgery* 1973; **73**:599–606.
15 Gruntzig A, Hopff H. [Percutaneous recanalization after chronic arterial occlusion with a new dilator-catheter (modification of the Dotter technique) (author's transl)]. *Dtsch Med Wochenschr* 1974; **99**:2502–10, 2511.
16 Palmaz JC, Sibbitt RR, Reuter SR, Tio FO, Rice WJ. Expandable intraluminal graft: a preliminary study. Work in progress. *Radiology* 1985; **156**:73–77.
17 Parodi JC, Palmaz JC, Barone HD. Transfemoral intraluminal graft implantation for abdominal aortic aneurysms. *Ann Vasc Surg* 1991; **5**:491–99.
18 Hodgson K, Mattos, MA, Sumner, DS. Angiography in the operating room: equipment, catheter skills and safety issue. In: Yao J, Pearce, WH, eds. *Techniques in Vascular Surgery.* Appleton & Lange, Samford, CT, 1997:25–45.
19 Mansour MA. The new operating room environment. *Surg Clin North Am* 1999, **79**:477–87.
20 Brateman L. Radiation safety considerations for diagnostic radiology personnel. *Radiographics* 1999; **19**:1037–55.
21 Stone GW, McCullough PA, Tumlin JA, *et al.* Fenoldopam mesylate for the prevention of contrast-induced nephropathy: a randomized controlled trial. *JAMA* 2003; **290**:2284–91.
22 Indolfi C, Mongiardo A, Curcio A, Torella D. Molecular mechanisms of in-stent restenosis and approach to therapy with eluting stents. *Trends Cardiovasc Med* 2003; **13**:142–48.
23 Fattori R, Piva T. Drug-eluting stents in vascular intervention. *Lancet* 2003; **361**:247–49.
24 Woods TC, Marks AR. Drug-eluting stents. *Annu Rev Med* 2004; **55**:169–78.

25 Criado FJ, Clark NS, Barnatan MF. Stent graft repair in the aortic arch and descending thoracic aorta: a 4-year experience. *J Vasc Surg* 2002; **36**:1121–8.

26 Ouriel K, Greenberg RK. Endovascular treatment of thoracic aortic aneurysms. *J Card Surg* 2003; **18**:455–63.

27 Bush RL, Lin PH, Lumsden AB. Endovascular treatment of the thoracic aorta. *Vasc Endovascular Surg* 2003; **37**:399–405.

CHAPTER 2

Basic science of endovascular therapy

Panagiotis Kougias, Liz Nguyen, Changyi Chen

Atherosclerosis is the most common cause of arterial occlusive disease, which is a highly prevalent condition in western societies. This disease process represents the leading overall cause of mortality, due in part to the consequence of myocardial infarction or stroke. Atherosclerosis is a complex cellular process that affects the elastic and muscular arteries. The process is both systemic and focal, with clear predilections for certain arterial segments and relative sparing of others. This chapter discusses the process of atherosclerotic plaque formation and the restenosis following interventions. Specifically, cellular events that occur as the result of endovascular interventions are discussed. This chapter also details endovascular strategies using drug-eluting technology as a means to attenuate restenosis.

Pathogenesis of atherosclerotic lesion

Atherosclerotic lesions progress through a series of well-recognized pathologic processes before clinical manifestations develop. A classic definition of an atherosclerotic plaque describes the lesion as "a variable combination of changes in the intima of arteries consisting of focal accumulation of lipids, complex carbohydrates, blood and blood products, fibrous tissue, and calcium deposits."[1] However, the process is much more complex and involves various cellular and molecular events. Early events in the development of the atherosclerotic lesion include low density lipoprotein (LDL) accumulation in the arterial wall and monocyte binding to the endothelium where they become tissue macrophages. This triggers a number of functional and morphological changes that take place in the endothelium and the media and ultimately lead to the development of the atherosclerotic plaque. Figure 2.1 provides a general overview of arthrogenic process in an arterial wall. The critical elements responsible for atherosclerotic plaque formation are discussed below.

LDL accumulation. This may occur because of (1) alterations in the permeability of the intima; (2) increases in the interstitial space in the intima; (3) poor metabolism of LDL by vascular cells; (4) impeded transport of LDL from the intima to the media; (5) increased plasma/LDL concentrations; or (6) specific binding of LDL to connective tissue components, particularly proteoglycans in the arterial intima.[2]

(a)

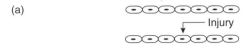

Injury

Atherogenic plaque formation is typically initiated by endothelial injury caused by infection, mechanical stress, lipids, or immunologic toxins.

(b)

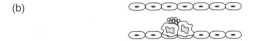

Monocytes and platelets next adhere to the injury site, which trigger the release of growth factors.

(c)

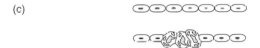

Monocytes then migrate through endothelial cells to form fatty streaks, which stimulate smooth muscle cell proliferation.

(d)

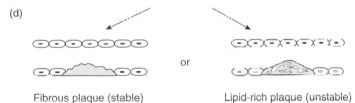

or

Fibrous plaque (stable)   Lipid-rich plaque (unstable)

Figure 2.1 Overview of atherogenic plaque formation in an artery following an injury response.

Monocytes. They bind to the endothelial lining with their subsequent migration into the subintimal layer to become tissue macrophages. Experimentally, fatty streaks are populated mainly by monocyte-derived macrophages.[3] These lipid-filled cells mainly become the foam cells characterizing fatty streaks and other lesions. LDL must be altered in some manner, as by oxidation or acetylation, to be taken up by the macrophages to form foam cells. Oxidized LDL (OXLDL) is a powerful chemoattractant for monocytes and its presence leads to a vicious cycle of further macrophage accumulation. It also induces gene products ordinarily unexpressed in normal vascular tissue, for example, tissue factor (TF), which initiates the coagulation cascade. Macrophages produce cytokines including monocyte chemotactic protein-1 (MCP-1), macrophage colony stimulating factor (MCSF), tumor necrosis factor (TNF), platelet-derived growth factor (PDGF), transforming growth factor-13 (TGF-13), and interleukin-1 (IL-1), therefore further favoring the development of a local inflammatory response.[4]

Endothelium. Endothelial cells (EC) tend to orient away from the direction of blood flow, become polyhedral or rounded, express cilia, and demonstrate a decrease in microfilament bundles. In atherosclerosis there is increased proliferation and cell death with retraction and exposure of subendothelial foam cells. The endothelium becomes more permeable to macromolecules, and it exhibits increased mural thrombus formation and TF expression. Leukocyte adherence increases with the expression of a vascular cell adhesion molecule 1 (VCAM-1). Endothelium-derived relaxing factor and prostacyclin release are decreased with enhanced vasoconstriction.[5]

Media. Experimentally, smooth muscle cells (SMCs) show increased proliferation with increased rough endoplasmic reticulum, phenotypic change, and increased production of altered intracellular and extracellular matrix, which includes types I and III collagen, dermatan sulfate, proteoglycan, and stromolysens.[1] The SMCs produce cytokines including MCSF, TNF, and MCP-1. The myocytes accumulate native and modified lipoproteins both by native receptor pathways and by nonspecific phagocytosis. These cells also express increased lipoprotein lipase activity and experimentally display a scavenger receptor similar to that of foam cells.

Cellular events in response to endovascular interventions

Biological response to balloon angioplasty

The objective of the balloon angioplasty is to exert a dilating force on the endoluminal surface of a vessel at the desired location. This causes desquamation of ECs and histologic damage proportional to the diameter of the balloon and the duration of the inflation. Balloon angioplasty results in a complex biological response in the vessel wall that is similar to generalized wound healing. The biological mechanism of balloon angioplasty in restoring luminal diameter was initially thought to be the result of compression of atherosclerotic lesion followed by remodeling of the plaque. In this scenario, longitudinal fracture of the plaque and stretching of the media and adventitia both increase the cross-sectional area of the diseased vessel. However, this process is responsible for only a fraction of the luminal restoration, since plaque compression does not add appreciably to the newly restored luminal diameter. The predominant effect of balloon angioplasty in enlarging vessel lumen is by stretching the elastic components of the arterial wall. Inelastic portion of the plaque fracture or tear results in a definite but discrete arterial wall dissection. In eccentric lesions, the less diseased part of the artery may distend due to balloon angioplasty, which may lead to minimal degree of dissection. However, histologically evident arterial dissection is nearly present in all diseased vessels following balloon angioplasty procedures.[6] Postangioplasty angiograms almost invariably demonstrate areas of dissection and plaque separation that tends to be unpredictable. The injury to the endothelium exposes the subendothelial space and attracts platelets and fibrin that cover the damaged surfaces. The oxidative stress that follows angioplasty favors the invasion

(a)

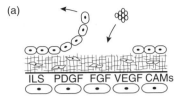

ILS PDGF FGF VEGF CAMs

• Renewal of endothelium
• Platelet aggregation
• Stimulation of inflammatory response

(b)

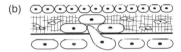

• Smooth muscle cell migration and
  proliferation
• Secretion of extracellular matrix

(c)

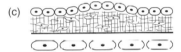

Figure 2.2 Cellular events in vessel wall following balloon angioplasty.

• Re-endothelialization
• Extracellular matrix organization

of neutrophils, macrophages, and T-lymphocytes. At the same time, vascular SMCs become mobile and migrate close to the site of injury. Figure 2.2 depicts the cellular events or healing response following balloon angioplasty procedure. All these events favor the local migration and proliferation of the SMC as a healing response, which may ultimately lead to restenosis, or intimal hyperplasia. Most angioplasty-induced dissections will ultimately heal within a month.

Biological response to intraluminal stenting

Studies using scanning electron microscopy have shown that within 15 min following stent implantation, there is an accumulation of red blood cells and platelets on the stent surface.[7] At 24 h, this cellular layer is replaced by a layer of fibrin strands oriented in the direction of blood flow as the positive electrical

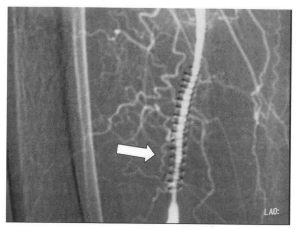

Figure 2.3 Severe angiographic restenosis (arrow) is seen within a superficial femoral artery stent 4 months following implantation.

potential of the metallic struts attracts the negatively charged circulating proteins on the stent surface. In the third and fourth weeks after stent insertion, SMC proliferation and endothelialization resulted in a neointimal layer of approximately 1 mm in thickness. Stent diameter in relation to vessel diameter plays an important part in determining the final thickness of this layer. Finally, several months after stent placement, the formation of the neointimal vessel begins (Figure 2.3). At 3–6 years, the fibromuscular tissue layer covering the stent surface is almost completely replaced by collagen. Stents placed into the venous system exhibit a faster rate of endothelialization than do intra-arterial stents.[8]

Stents are metallic objects, and as such, they elicit a foreign body reaction soon after deployment. Several factors determine the thrombogenicity of a stent.[9] The electrical charge of most metals and alloys used for intravascular devices is electropositive in electrolytic solutions, whereas all biologic intravascular substances are negatively charged. Soon after the intra-arterial stent deployment, the positive electrical potential of the metallic struts attracts the negatively charged circulating proteins to form a thin layer of fibrinogen strands on the stent surface. The proteins neutralize the stent surface and decrease thrombogenicity.

Surface tension is another property that influences biological stent interactions. The critical surface tension of a solid surface must be between 20 and 30 dyne/cm to be thromboresistant.[10] The initial layer of proteins that cover the metal within seconds of implantation helps reduce surface tension and thrombogenicity.

The technique of stent implantation itself may affect thrombogenicity and the rate of endothelialization. Ideally, stents should be deployed in such a way that the metal struts are embedded deep enough into the vessel wall to produce troughs where the struts are embedded, surrounded by intima that projects through the meshwork of the stent and provides the source for new EC formation. The achievement of this ideal deployment is dependent on multiple factors: the ratio of the diameter of the stent to that of the blood vessel, the depth of penetration of the struts into the vessel wall, thickness of the struts, and the composition and integrity of the intimal surface. If the struts are not properly embedded, the entire stented surface becomes covered with thrombus, preventing early endothelialization and thus predisposing to complete thrombosis and restenosis. Stent struts will be embedded adequately if the final stent diameter is 10–15% larger than the diameter of the adjacent vessel.

Biologic response to stent-graft implantation

Animal studies demonstrated that a uniformly aligned cellular neointima can occur in 1 month along the luminal surface of polyester stent grafts following implantation in the sheep aorta.[11] It remains unclear regarding the precise cellular events of the neointimal formation or whether this healing response can occur along the entire surface following implantation. Histological analyses have identified mixed cellular origins of the surface neointima beyond endothelium.[12] Additional cellular events analogous to a foreign body reaction are also seen, which include the thrombus formation organized around the graft. Following stent-graft implantation, the media of the underlying artery wall is partially replaced by collagen, perhaps due to the pressure from the stent-graft. In a canine model, endothelialization was more rapid when polytetrafluoroethylene (PTFE) grafts were placed inside the vessel, even if the artery was first denuded with a balloon catheter.[13] As in open vascular grafts, there is an endothelium in growth about 2–3 cm from the adjacent vessel. Endothelialization may occur in fabric grafts used to treat abdominal aortic aneurysms. One such device removed after 7 months from a patient who died of unrelated causes revealed healing with incorporation of the graft. There was endothelial ingrowth onto the proximal portion of the graft, with a neointima composed of a collagenous matrix, histiocytes, and myofibroblasts. Endovascular grafts placed to treat aneurysms may heal differently from those placed to prevent restenosis in atherosclerotic lesions. Stent grafts in aneurysmal sacs are surrounded by thrombus that finally undergoes organization and contraction causing deformation of the vessel.[14]

Fever often occurs after stent-graft placement for the treatment of abdominal aortic aneurysms. This likely represents a systemic response to the inflammatory foreign body reaction. A similar response has not been noted with standard open placement of similar prosthetic devices, likely because it is masked by all the other changes that accompany an open surgical procedure. Dacron stent grafts placed in sheep arteries cause a marked inflammatory response and vascular wall thickening, which can be seen on MRI and microscopic examination.[15]

Table 2.1 Biological factors that affect arterial wall remodeling.

Factors that cause arterial dilation	Factors that cause arterial constriction
Nitric oxide	Endothelin-1
Prostacyclin	Dyslipidemia
Endothelium-derived	Fibrinogen
hyperpolarizing factor	Hypertension
Exercise	Cigarette smoking

Restenosis following endovascular interventions

Vessel remodeling

Remodeling refers to a pattern of chronic – over weeks or months – changes of the structure of the vessel wall that follows injury. After angioplasty there appears to be a close relationship between luminal surface area and remodeling, with a parallel increase in vessel size as intimal thickening occurs. In restenosis, the amount of remodeling appears to be less for any given degree of intimal thickness. The factors linked to remodeling after angioplasty include hemodynamic changes in blood pressure, flow rates, patterns of sheer stress, and changes in extracellular matrix composition.[16] Vasoactive molecules (such as nitric oxide and prostacyclin) made by the endothelium in response to changes in shear stress cause SMCs to either contract or relax, with corresponding changes in vessel diameter. Flow changes that are chronic, result in chronic changes in wall structure. In addition, production, deposition, or organization of collagen is impaired under the influence of growth factors, cytokines, and matrix metalloproteinases with resultant increased extracellular matrix deposition. Table 2.1 lists common biological factors that influence vessel wall remodeling.

Neointimal hyperplasia

The pathologic changes observed during the healing process following endovascular interventions (such as balloon angioplasty or stenting) can result in the formation of a neointima that leads to a partial obliteration of the vascular lumen. This process, also known as neointimal hyperplasia, represents a chronic structural change in the blood vessel that leads to formation of a thickened fibrocellular layer between the endothelium and the inner elastic lamina of the arterial wall.[11] It often appears as a response to blood vessel injury and can become hemodynamically important in situations of luminal narrowing, reduced blood flow, or thrombotic occlusion.[17]

Neointimal hyperplasia is a significant clinical problem that threatens every known vascular reconstructive procedure and is responsible for 20–50% of the clinical failures of all vascular interventions. Within 3 weeks to 6 months after what seemed to be a successful dilation, percutaneous transluminal coronary angioplasty can be followed by restenosis in 25–50% of primary lesions.[2] The development of neointimal hyperplasia in patients who undergo carotid endarterectomy has been well documented, with restenosis appearing in 10–30% of those patients during the first year. Neointimal hyperplasia is also the primary etiology in approximately one-third of the failures that occur during the first 12–18 months following vein graft operations.[7]

Cellular and molecular mechanisms of neointimal hyperplasia

The precise mechanisms that initiate the formation of neointimal hyperplasia remain unclear. Much of our understanding in the field has been gained from studies performed in animal models. In general, the development of neointimal hyperplasia after vascular injury involves three phases: medial SMC proliferation (first wave), medial SMC migration into the intima (second wave), and intimal SMC proliferation and extracellular matrix production (third wave). The final result is vessel wall thickening and luminal narrowing.

Endothelial response

Endothelial injury can be a consequence of biochemical substances (e.g. cholesterol, nicotine, homocysteine), hemodynamic alterations (e.g. low shear stress, turbulent flow), oxidative stress (e.g. free radical generation), and surgical interventions (e.g. angioplasty, endarterectomy, or bypass grafting). After injury, the subendothelium that contains collagen and other thrombogenic molecules is exposed. Platelets adhere to the injured surface, and this binding is mediated through von Willebrand factor and the cell adhesion molecule P-selectin. Here they aggregate and release cytokines such as PDGF, transforming growth factor β, and endothelial growth factor, which are potent mitogens and chemotactic agents for vascular SMCs. Platelets also release vasoactive molecules such as serotonin and adenosine diphosphate, which contribute to increased vascular tone and luminal narrowing. They also display aberrant gene expression including upregulation of adhesion molecules such as intercellular adhesion molecule-1 (ICAM-1) and vascular cell adhesion molecule-1 (VCAM-1).[18] Significant free radicals are also generated by reperfusion following endovascular intervention, which can further activate neutrophils and red blood cells resulting in the release of additional inflammatory cytokines (Figure 2.4). Significant thrombus does not immediately form. The surface becomes completely nonthrombogenic by 24–48 h owing to adsorption of plasma proteins such as albumin, which inactivate the injured surface. In contrast to normal ECs, the injured or regenerated ECs grow as a sheet with close cell-to-cell contacts. Furthermore, these ECs are no longer aligned with blood flow and are both polygonal in shape and irregular in size, with the cytoplasm budding toward the lumen.[19]

Medial SMC response

After vascular injury has occurred, the activation of SMCs is associated with a shift from a so-called contractile to the synthetic phenotype, initiating a

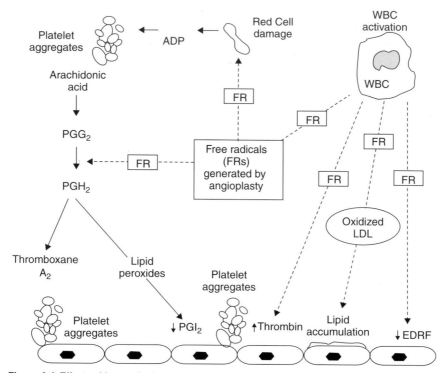

Figure 2.4 Effects of free radicals on vessel wall due to perfusion injury following endovascular interventions.

sequence of proliferation, migration, and synthesis of extracellular matrix.[20,21] SMC proliferation begins immediately after the initial injury and may last for weeks or months. In the rat carotid artery, about 20% of SMCs enter the cell cycle after balloon injury. Between 0 and 24 h, genes involved in the progression from the resting state (Go) to the S phase are induced in cells that will proliferate. SMC proliferation is greatest in the first 2 weeks after injury. It begins within 24 h, peaking as high as 70% at 48–72 h, and returns to quiescent levels by 12 weeks. At 4 days, SMCs begin to migrate from the media, across the damaged internal elastic lamina, and into the intima, a phenomenon mediated by PDGF. During the first 2 weeks, intimal mass increases due to SMC migration across the internal elastic lamina and proliferation of cells in the intima. Intimal mass continues to grow between 2 and 12 weeks, mainly by continued deposition of matrix components – elastin, collagen, and glycoproteins – by the SMCs. The increased production of extracellular matrix by neointimal SMCs is a very significant mechanism of neointimal expansion and lumen narrowing during the later stage of neointimal hyperplasia formation, with the extracellular matrix component usually constituting about 80–90% of neointimal volume. Administration of heparin in the first 24 h after vessel injury inhibits the proliferative response in this rodent model, with a significant decrease in intimal thickening.[22] Prolonged administration of heparin has no further effect. Additional growth factors that may play a role in the medial changes include basic fibroblast growth factor (bFGF), epidermal growth factor (EGF), transforming growth factor (TGF), vascular endothelial growth factor (VEGF), insulin growth factor type 1 (IGF-1), angiotensin II, and endothelins. In addition, a wide variety of hemodynamic events, including high- and low-flow velocities, high and low shear stress, and mechanical compliance mismatch have all been implicated in vascular remodeling or the development of neointimal hyperplasia. These forces may either damage the ECs or alter the gene expression and interaction between components of the vessel wall and elements of circulating blood.

Clinical strategy for restenosis

Because of the clinical sequelae of restenosis following endovascular interventions, a wide variety of strategies to prevent neointimal hyperplasia have been proposed as a means to decrease restenosis and improve clinical outcomes. One clinical strategy in particular that has demonstrated a significant efficacy relates to delivering intraluminal stents, which elute pharmacological agents designed to inhibit neointimal hyperplasia. These various pharmacologic strategies as well as the concept of drug-eluting stents to attenuate neointimal hyperplasia are discussed below.

Pharmacologic approach
Antiplatelet drugs
Low dose Aspirin has documented efficacy for prevention of rethrombosis in the early phase of balloon angioplasty and should be administered 2 h before the procedure and indefinitely thereafter. If side effects make treatment with Aspirin problematic, an equivalent agent (e.g. clopidrogel or ticlopidine – inhibit ADP induced platelet aggregation) can be given. Combination of Aspirin with Ticlopidine (phosphodiesterase inhibitor) appears to be superior to Aspirin alone; however, Ticlopidine is associated with neutropenic side effects. The platelet receptors IIb–IIIa bind fibrinogen and promote platelet aggregation. IIb–IIIa site antagonists (e.g. abciximab) have been proved to be efficacious in coronary vessels, whereas studies in peripheral vessels are under way.[23]

Anticoagulants
Periprocedural administration of heparin is important because (1) it reduces the risk of thrombosis and (2) heparin has anti-SMC proliferative activity. No data demonstrate any long-term benefit of unfractionated heparin or low molecular weight heparin on the restenosis rate, however. The direct thrombin inhibitors hirudin and bivalirudin show a significant reduction in the rate of major cardiac events in the first 96 h after percutaneous coronary balloon angioplasty compared to heparin, but no effect on the rate of restenosis. Use of

warfarin does not seem to be justified in prevention of either acute thrombosis or long-term restenosis; warfarin has a high risk side effect profile and is less effective than heparin.

Essential fatty acids

Eicosapentanoic acid and docosahexanoic acid produce antiplatelet vasodilator effect via production of prostacyclin (PGI_3) that has function similar to PGI_2. Essential fatty acids (EFA) produce thromboxane (TXA_3) that has a much less thrombogenic potential compared to TXA_2. In addition, EFA may attenuate free radical generation and modify the body's inflammatory response to tissue injury. Studies published to date show a clear but moderate benefit in reduction of restenosis with the use of EFAs.

Antiproliferative drugs

These agents include angiotensin-converting enzyme (ACE) inhibitors, antagonists of growth factors (e.g. turbinafine or trapidil), angiopeptin (e.g. simvastatin analog), cytostatic agents (e.g. etoposide or colchicines) cGMP analogs and NO donors. Agents that block the cell cycle are also of interest (sirolimus). Some experience has been gained with the use of these drugs in animals; however studies in humans have not reproduced promising results.

Gene therapy

Gene therapy involves overexpression of genes that are considered protective or blockade of genes that are involved in the pathogenesis of the intimal hyperplasia. Gene blockade can be achieved through the use of nucleic acids known as antisense oligodeoxynucleotides (ODN).[24] Initial results from studies in animal models appear promising.

Radiation therapy

Initial results from animal and small uncontrolled human trials delivering radiation with either intraluminal or external beam radiation are encouraging. Short-term side toxicity appears to be limited, but the long-term side effects have not been well defined yet. Photodynamic therapy utilizes the cytotoxic properties of light-excitable photosensitizers to destroy SMCs that would otherwise be involved in the proliferative neointimal lesion. These photosensitizers, which have no adverse effects in the absence of light, become cytotoxic when activated by an appropriate wavelength of light.[25]

Endovascular strategy for restenosis
Drug elution technology

Over the past decade, the advances in endovascular therapy have led to improved outcomes for patients with atherosclerotic vascular disease. Many of these results have been attributed to the advances obtained from experiences in the treatment of coronary artery disease with endovascular stenting. However, one of the continued problems with endovascular therapy has been in-stent restenosis after stent deployment. The pathology of stent failure results from the basic biology of intimal hyperplasia and lumen narrowing over time. The rate of in-stent restenosis has been reported to be anywhere in the range from 15 to 60% depending on the location of stent deployment.[26] Pharmacologic inhibition of the pathologic process of intimal hyperplasia and lumen narrowing has met with limited success. It has been theorized that systemic delivery of medications has failed due to the low concentrations of the medication at the stent site. The differing systemic pharmacokinetics of each medication also plays a critical role in bioavailability. Furthermore, many antiproliferative drugs possess a very narrow therapeutic window and to achieve the desired level may be difficult with unwanted side effects. The only drug that has shown any benefit has been abciximab, a platelet IIb/IIIa receptor antagonist. To overcome the complications of in-stent restenosis, the novel idea of the drug-eluting stent has been slowly developed over the past decade. The drug-eluting stent allows for release of a concentrated medication directly onto the injured endothelium. The basis of the drug-eluting stent is based on a number of engineering principles, which harness the scaffolding properties of the stent and the pharmacokinetics of individual medication to deliver an antiproliferative medication to a local site in sufficient concentration to have a biologic effect.

Drug-eluting stent design principles

Drug-eluting stents are composed of a three-dimensional complex that is composed of the stent backbone, the delivery system of the drug, and the drug itself. The stent-based drug delivery system can be accomplished using a number of methods.

The most common method for drug delivery is through application of thin layers of a drug-polymer solution to the stent surface. The key component of using any biopolymer is that the polymer is a noninflammatory inert component. Furthermore, the polymer must be a nonthrombogenic compound and possess the necessary characteristics to withstand the mechanical forces of stent deployment and placement. Other considerations for use of polymer-based elution solution are predictable drug kinetics and ideal logistical requirements of the polymer solution (i.e. drug shelf life, expense, and solution stability). Currently used matrix polymers consist of silicone, polyurethane, polyethylene glycol, and polyethylene vinyl chloride. Newer biopolymers maintain the noninflammatory characteristics of current generation polymers; however, they are biodegradable and possess improved drug release kinetics. These newer generation biopolymers dissolve into inert compounds such as CO_2 and water.

An alternative approach for drug delivery is direct application of the drug to a bare stent or incorporation of the drug into microscopic fenestration in the stent. To apply this system to stent design and drug delivery necessitates a drug that will remain in the tissue for a prolonged period of time due to the rapid bolus dosing nature of drug release in this design system. This approach is currently being used for the paclitaxel-eluting stents. The benefit of this method is that it eliminates the possibility of a polymer-induced inflammatory reaction and simplifies device manufacturing and testing. However, the absence of a polymer allows for unpredictable drug delivery. Unfortunately, without a polymer to aid in drug delivery, 40% of the drug can be lost during stent placement, and after placement, the remainder of the drug will completely elute in 1–2 weeks. A final method for drug delivery is to create a polymeric sheath, which encases the stent. The sheath's positioning is between the stent and the vessel wall, thereby serving as a large-volume drug reservoir to prevent neointimal proliferation.

Drug-eluting stent systems: current and future systems

To design the optimal stent, the stent design needs to contain a number of fundamental characteristics. For optimal performance and patency, the stent should provide a scaffold that maintains lumen patency and serves as a reservoir for drug delivery. Currently, there are two stent systems that are Food and Drug Administration approved for use in the United States. These two systems are the CYPHER system (Cordis/Johnson and Johnson, Miami Lakes, FL) and the TAXUS system (Boston Scientific, Natick, MA). The CYPHER system is a sirolimus-based system while the TAXUS system is a paclitaxel-based system. Both the CYPHER system and TAXUS system have demonstrated significant benefit (i.e. restenosis rate, reoperation, myocardial infarction) in using the drug-eluting stent versus the bare metal stent. The CYPHER and TAXUS system are based on the use of a nonerodible polymeric coating containing the drug of choice. The TAXUS system was compared to stents that were only coated with paclitaxel and no polymer. Their results demonstrated that the TAXUS group had decreased rates of long-term restenosis, thereby supporting the idea that the use of a polymeric coating is necessary for efficient and sustained drug delivery. The next generation of drug-eluting stents will incorporate a number of improvements discovered by the earlier trials. One of the changes that has been proposed is to change the underlying stainless steel alloy to an advanced cobalt-based alloy. Use of a cobalt-based alloy surpasses the limitations of stainless steel stents. This stronger alloy makes it possible to develop thinner struts, which allows for improved flexibility plus optimal vessel support. Other design modifications have been to use a bioabsorbable polymeric coating for drug delivery. The benefit of the bioabsorbable coating is that the polymer is restricted to the outer surface of the stent at the interface between the stent and vessel wall. The outer surface coating prevents exposing the drug to blood flow in the arterial lumen. Furthermore, the biodegradability of the polymer allows for complete elimination of the drug in a finite period of time, therefore allowing for sustained and measured drug delivery. The use of a biodegradable polymer eliminates the possibility of drug retention and long-term adverse events.

Table 2.2 Potential pharmacological agents and mechanisms of action for stent-based clinical application.

Antiproliferative/ antineoplastic	Anti-inflammatory/ immunomodulators	Migration inhibitor/ ECM-modulators	Promote healing and stimulate re-endothelialization
Paclitaxel	Sirolimus	Probucol	VEGF
Methotrexate	Everolimus	Batimastat	Estrogen
ABT-578	Biolimus A9	Halofuginone	BCP671
Actinomycin	Dexamethasone	Prolyl hydroxylase	Estradiols
Statins	Tacrolimus	inhibitor	Nitric oxide donors
Angiopeptin	M-prednisolone	C-proteinase	EPC antibodies
Mitomycine	Interferon g-1b	inhibitors	Biorest
C MYC antisense	Leflunomide		
2-chloro-deoxyadonosine	Mizorbine		
PCNA ribozyme	Cyclosporino		
	Tranilast		

Drug eluting agents

Currently, there are a number of different drugs that are used in drug-eluting stents. The basic function of the drugs used in these stents is to create an antiproliferative environment around the stent in order to prevent luminal stenosis and neointimal hyperplasia. In particular, the drug should preferentially interfere with the migration and proliferation of vascular SMCs. In addition, the drug should have a reasonably long half-life of at least 4 weeks postprocedure since this is the time during which the greatest endothelial injury and reactivity to stent placement occurs. A list of potential drug-eluting agents which can be used to inhibit neointimal hyperplasia is noted in Table 2.2.

Sirolimus. Sirolimus (Rapamycin) is an antiproliferative/immunosuppressive medication, which was originally discovered in *Streptomyces hygroscopicus*. Sirolimus has been the basic drug from which a number of analogs have been created. These medications are further discussed in this section. Sirolimus is a hydrophobic drug, and this property allows it to directly cross the cell membrane. After entry into the cytosol, sirolimus binds to an immunophilin molecule named the FK binding protein (FKBP)-12. The sirolimus and FKBP complex then binds to and inhibits the activation of the mammalian target of rapamycin (mTOR), a key regulatory kinase. This inhibition suppresses cytokine-driven T-cell proliferation, inhibiting the progression from the G1 to the S phase of the cell cycle. The hydrophobic properties allow for higher mean tissue concentration, and the diffused drug maintains a closer relation to the proliferating intima.[27] These pharmacologic characteristics make it an ideal agent for placement in endovascular stents. The results from sirolimus drug-eluting stents in coronary arteries have been encouraging. The Ravel study, which was a large randomized comparison of sirolimus drug-eluting stents versus a standard uncoated stent, showed a 26% restenosis rate (>50% stenosis of the lumen) in the uncoated stent group versus 0% in the sirolimus group.[28] The use of a standard uncoated stent also correlated with a significant increase in the rate of cardiac complications when compared to the treatment group. Due to this study, sirolimus-coated stents have also been tested in patients with peripheral vascular disease. The results from these studies have been less impressive than in endovascular therapy for coronary arterial disease. The results only showed trends towards increased stent diameter in the drug-eluting stent group and no difference in restenosis rates.

Paclitaxel. Paclitaxel (Taxol) is an antineoplastic agent, which has been widely used in the treatment of solid tumor malignancies. It belongs to a class of drugs called diterpenoids. Paclitaxel functions by inhibiting microtubule depolymerization during cellular mitosis. Microtubules are polymers that are assembled from tubulin dimers. They function as the major component of the mitotic spindle apparatus and also play a role in cellular conformity and migration.[29] This effect on the microtubule system prevents the dynamic reorganization of the tubules, thereby preventing the action necessary for cellular mitosis. Furthermore, the lipophilic nature of paclitaxel allows for rapid crossing of the drug across the cell membrane. Paclitaxel has been found to prevent the proliferation and migration of vascular SMC *in vitro*, and this observation initiated its testing for use in drug-eluting stents. Paclitaxel has been mainly tested in the TAXUS system. In the large TAXUS studies, the drug-eluting stent arm was found to have a decreased restenosis rate when paclitaxel was used in conjunction with a polymer-based delivery system.

Everolimus. Everolimus is a derivative of sirolimus and has a similar mechanism of action, exerting potent inhibition of growth factor-induced proliferation of lymphocytes, as well as other hematopoietic and nonhematopoietic cells of mesenchymal origin. Each agent complexes with the FK506 binding protein 12 to inhibit cyclin-dependent kinases, thereby blocking cell cycle progression from the G1 phase to the S phase. In particular, Il-2 and Il-15 driven proliferation is inhibited. Compared to sirolimus, everolimus absorbs into local tissue more rapidly and possesses longer cellular residence time and activity. The first trial to evaluate the effect of everolimus was conducted in 27 patients with *de novo* coronary artery lesions.[30] In this preliminary study with only short-term data, the investigators found that everolimus was safe, and the results were comparable to those of the standard nondrug eluting stent. Moreover, these studies revealed a remarkable reduction of neointimal proliferation with everolimus-eluting stent implantation versus procedures utilizing bare metal stents.

ABT-578. ABT-578 is a synthetic analog of sirolimus; however, ABT-578 differs at position 42 in the drug molecule where there is a substitution of a tetrazole ring. ABT-578 also binds to the FKBP-12 and forms a trimeric complex with the protein kinase mTOR, thereby preventing progression of the cell cycle. ABT-578 was considered to be beneficial for arresting the process of neointimal hyperplasia after stenting and angioplasty. Due to these pharmacologic properties, a 100 patient trial was initiated in patients with native *de novo* coronary lesions. The trial was entitled the ENDEAVOR trial and has recently completed the initial phases.[31] The accumulated data has demonstrated that the system is safe, and usage is feasible in patients with coronary lesions. The drug will progress into further studies in direct comparisons with more well established drug-eluting stents.

Biolimus A9. Biolimus A9 is a macrocyclic lactone with a chemical modification at position 40 of the rapamycin ring. Similar to sirolimus, biolimus exerts its cellular effect by binding to the FKBP-12 to inhibit the downstream signaling cascade, which is necessary for T-cell and SMC proliferation. Experimental studies have shown that when administered in the vascular lumen, biolimus A9 is a potent immunosuppressive and anti-inflammatory agent that elutes more rapidly from the resorbable polylactic acid (PLA) polymer as compared to sirolimus-eluting stents. Furthermore, due to the modification at position 40, biolimus A9 crosses the vessel wall more rapidly than its analog, sirolimus. Currently, there is an ongoing trial to evaluate the safety and efficacy of biolimus A9.

Actinomycin D. Actinomycin D is an inhibitor of DNA-dependent RNA synthesis and exerts a potent effect on inhibiting cell proliferation. It binds specifically to the GC region of DNA and prevents the transcription of DNA to RNA as well as inhibiting DNA repair. Current work has centered around one study that described the effect of actinomycin D versus bare metal stents. The results from this study were discouraging and found no difference between the two arms in any of the variables measured.[32] Other problems with actinomycin D are that the drug has a very narrow therapeutic window. Due to its water soluble nature, the pharmacokinetics of the drug are extremely unpredictable, thereby preventing any accurate prediction of drug release and duration of action. The narrow therapeutic window can lead to an increased range of side effects such as local tissue damage, which can result in necrosis of the vessel wall. Due to these problems, the enthusiasm for use of actinomycin D in drug-eluting stents is waning.

Complications of drug-eluting stents
The use of drug-eluting stents has been a recent phenomenon, and thus, there has been no long-term data on the complications of the drug-eluting stents. Potential toxic effects include weakening of the vessel wall due to the medication. These effects have not been seen in any of the recent trials but continue to remain a possibility. Another possible complication can result from the polymer that remains in the stent after the drug has been completely released. The possibility of restenosis due to the presence of a foreign material is a legitimate concern; however, at the 3-year follow-up, the CYPHER stent trials have shown no such complication.[33]

Future of drug-eluting medications

In regards to the future of drug development, the idea of a single drug concept may need to be changed. Ongoing areas of research are evaluating the possibility of delivery of two drugs that work by differing pathways. The use of cell cycle inhibitors in conjunction with a vasoprotective or healing agent may significantly decrease the pathologic response and vessel injury after stent deployment. In drug development, the identification of drugs with enhanced long-term effect and a wide therapeutic window with low toxicity would be ideal for drug-eluting stents. Further work on stent design would be the optimization of a polymer reservoir that will decrease the inflammatory response and allow for predictable kinetics in drug delivery. Finally, the idea of genetic modification by use of cellular gene therapy to decrease the local neointimal and endothelial response to stent placement is an area of intense future research.

References

1 Mitchell ME, Sidawy AN. The pathophysiology of atherosclerosis. *Semin Vasc Surg* 1998; **11**:134–41.

2 Scott J. The pathogenesis of atherosclerosis and new opportunities for treatment and prevention. *J Neural Transm Suppl* 2002; **63**:1–17.

3 Choy PC, Siow YL, Mymin D, O K. Lipids and atherosclerosis. *Biochem Cell Biol* 2004; **82**:212–24.

4 Bhakdi S, Lackner KJ, Han SR, Torewski M, Husmann M. Beyond cholesterol: the enigma of atherosclerosis revisited. *Thromb Haemost* 2004; **91**:639–45.

5 Kher N, Marsh JD. Pathobiology of atherosclerosis – a brief review. *Semin Thromb Hemost* 2004; **30**:665–72.

6 Marijianowski MM, Crocker IR, Styles T, *et al.* Fibrocellular tissue responses to endovascular and external beam irradiation in the porcine model of restenosis. *Int J Radiat Oncol Biol Phys* 1999; **44**:633–41.

7 Lee MS, David EM, Makkar RR, Wilentz JR. Molecular and cellular basis of restenosis after percutaneous coronary intervention: the intertwining roles of platelets, leukocytes, and the coagulation-fibrinolysis system. *J Pathol* 2004; **203**:861–70.

8 Williams D. The god of small things: the biology of intimal hyperplasia. *Med Device Technol* 1999; **10**:8–11.

9 Parsson H, Norgren L, Ivancev K, Thorne J, Jonsson BA. Thrombogenicity of metallic vascular stents in arteries and veins – an experimental study in pigs. *Eur J Vasc Surg* 1990; **4**:617–23.

10 Hehrlein C, Zimmermann M, Metz J, Ensinger W, Kubler W. Influence of surface texture and charge on the biocompatibility of endovascular stents. *Coron Artery Dis* 1995; **6**:581–86.

11 Schurmann K, Vorwerk D, Kulisch A, *et al.* Neointimal hyperplasia in low-profile Nitinol stents, Palmaz stents, and Wallstents: a comparative experimental study. *Cardiovasc Intervent Radiol* 1996; **19**:248–54.

12 Schurmann K, Vorwerk D, Kulisch A, *et al.* Experimental arterial stent placement. Comparison of a new Nitinol stent and Wallstent. *Invest Radiol* 1995; **30**:412–20.

13 Virmani R, Kolodgie FD, Dake MD, *et al.* Histopathologic evaluation of an expanded polytetrafluoroethylene-nitinol stent endoprosthesis in canine iliofemoral arteries. *J Vasc Interv Radiol* 1999; **10**:445–56.

14 Benson AE, Palmaz JC, Tio FO, Sprague EA, Encarnacion CE, Josephs SC. Polytetrafluoroethylene-encapsulated stent-grafts: use in experimental abdominal aortic aneurysm. *J Vasc Interv Radiol* 1999; **10**:605–12.

15 Schürmann K, Vorwerk D, Bucker A, Neuerburg J. Perigraft inflammation due to Dacron-covered stent-grafts in sheep iliac arteries: correlation of MR imaging and histopathologic findings. *Cardiovasc Radiol* 1997; **204**:757–63.

16 Wilcox JN, Waksman R, King SB, Scott NA. The role of the adventitia in the arterial response to angioplasty: the effect of intravascular radiation. *Int J Radiat Oncol Biol Phys* 1996; **36**:789–96.

17 Ferns GA, Avades TY. The mechanisms of coronary restenosis: insights from experimental models. *Int J Exp Pathol* 2000; **81**:63–88.

18 Cotran RS, Mayadas-Norton T. Endothelial adhesion molecules in health and disease. *Pathol Biol* (Paris) 1998; **46**:164–70.

19 Pober JS. Immunobiology of human vascular endothelium. *Immunol Res* 1999; **19**:225–32.

20 Libby P, Li H. Vascular cell adhesion molecule-1 and smooth muscle cell activation during atherogenesis. *J Clin Invest* 1993; **92**:538–39.

21 Munro JM, Cotran RS. The pathogenesis of atherosclerosis: atherogenesis and inflammation. *Lab Invest* 1988; **58**:249–61.

22 Chia MC. The role of adhesion molecules in atherosclerosis. *Crit Rev Clin Lab Sci* 1998; **35**:573–602.

23 Ibbotson T, McGavin JK, Goa KL. Abciximab: an updated review of its therapeutic use in patients with ischemic heart disease undergoing percutaneous coronary revascularisation. *Drugs* 2003; **63**:1121–63.

24 Morishita R, Kaneda Y, Ogihara T. Therapeutic potential of oligonucleotide-based therapy in cardiovascular disease. *BioDrugs* 2003, **17**:383–89.

25 Nigri GR, Brini C, LaMuraglia GM, Vietri F. Photodynamic therapy in cardiac and vascular surgery. *G Chir* 2002; **23**:301–6.

26 Moreno R, Fernandez C, Alfonso F, *et al.* Coronary stenting versus balloon angioplasty in small vessels: a meta-analysis from 11 randomized studies. *J Am Coll Cardiol* 2004; **43**:1964–72.

27 Degertekin M, Regar E, Tanabe K, Lee CH, Serruys PW. Sirolimus eluting stent in the treatment of atherosclerosis coronary artery disease. *Minerva Cardioangiol* 2002; **50**:405–18.

28 Toutouzas K, Di Mario C, Falotico R, *et al.* Sirolimus-eluting stents: a review of experimental and clinical findings. *Z Kardiol* 2002; **91**: 49–57.

29 Hong MK, Kornowski R, Bramwell O, Ragheb AO, Leon MB. Paclitaxel-coated Gianturco-Roubin II (GR II) stents reduce neointimal hyperplasia in a porcine coronary in-stent restenosis model. *Coron Artery Dis* 2001; **12**:513–15.

30 Grube E, Buellesfeld L. Everolimus for stent-based intracoronary applications. *Rev Cardiovasc Med* 2004; **52**: S3–8.

31 Buellesfeld L, Grube E. ABT-578-eluting stents. The promising successor of sirolimus- and paclitaxel-eluting stent concepts? *Herz* 2004; **29**:167–70.

32 Serruys PW, Ormiston JA, Sianos G, *et al.* Actinomycin-eluting stent for coronary revascularization: a randomized feasibility and safety study: the ACTION trial. *J Am Coll Cardiol* 2004; **44**:1363–67.

33 Perin EC. Choosing a drug-eluting stent: a comparison between CYPHER and TAXUS. *Rev Cardiovasc Med* 2005; **6**:S13–21.

CHAPTER 3

Pharmacotherapy in endovascular interventions

Leila Mureebe, Colleen M. Johnson, Changyi Chen

Despite routine usage in percutaneous interventions, the indications, type and duration of anticoagulation remains largely dependent upon individual practitioners. In addition to the use of heparinized saline for flushes, anticoagulation is systemically utilized during many studies, including both diagnostic and therapeutic procedures. Although heparin remains the mostly used anticoagulant, newer anticoagulants and lessons from percutaneous coronary interventions (PCI) are rapidly influencing decisions regarding anticoagulation. Endovascular interventions in a blood vessel typically expose the subendothelial cellular components to circulating blood elements. This initiates the coagulation cascade due in part to the exposure of tissue factor to factor VII that activates the coagulation enzymatic reactions. Figure 3.1 summarizes the schematic process of the coagulation cascade. Pharmacological agents used to minimize the consequence of coagulation process are an essential component of an endovascular procedure, which are reviewed in this chapter.

In addition to the use of anticoagulants to prevent thrombus formation during endovascular procedures, physicians frequently encounter clinical situations of either pathological coagulation or, more commonly, thrombosis resulting in a pathological state. Under a normal circumstance, the activation of the coagulation cascade triggers an endogenous fibrinolytic system in the human body, which removes coagulants resulting in a homeostatic condition. However, this builtin or endogenous fibrinolytic cascade can be overwhelmed by a pathological coagulation process, which can result in thrombotic process with catastrophic clinical consequences. Thrombolytic agents, which can be delivered by catheter-directed administration to dissipate thrombus by means of the fibrinolytic cascade, are an important armamentarium for physicians to utilize in thrombus management. This chapter also reviews the clinical rationale and various thrombolytic agents in the management of thrombotic occlusion.

Rationale for anticoagulation in endovascular interventions

The possibility of a thromboembolic event due to vessel trauma can occur in an endovascular procedure. Such a thromboembolic risk is increased with

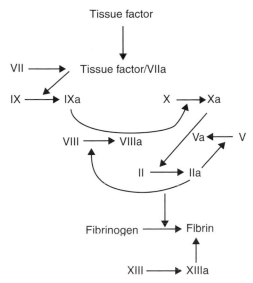

Figure 3.1 Current understanding of the coagulation cascade with tissue factor as the instigator of the enzymatic chain reaction.

procedural complexity, prolonged treatment duration, and decreased treatment vessel caliber.[1] In an open vascular operation, anticoagulation is utilized to prevent thrombosis caused in part by the placement of an occluding vascular clamp. The same tenet should be followed in an endovascular procedure. The creation of a temporary vessel occlusion, by means of an angioplasty balloon inflation or endograft deployment, should similarly mandate systemic anticoagulation to reduce the risk of thrombus formation. In addition, the presence of foreign body, such as guidewires, catheters, or introducer sheaths, also serves as a nidus for thrombus formation. The closer the outer diameter of a sheath approaches the inner diameter of the artery it enters, the higher the thrombotic risk due to stasis. In addition, many patients requiring endovascular therapies may have a hypercoagulable state. Researchers have found that up to 10% of patients undergoing peripheral vascular procedures were found to have a hypercoagulable state.[2] Moreover, others have reported that platelets of patients with peripheral vascular disease are overactive, which can predispose them to a prothrombotic condition.[3]

Despite all these indications, there is a lack of evidence-driven data to support the indications for anticoagulation, choice of anticoagulant, and duration of anticoagulant therapy required for optimal patient outcome. Most current understanding and practice is derived by extrapolating data from PCI to peripheral interventions. Anticoagulant agents can be broadly divided into two categories – antiplatelet agents and inhibitors of the coagulation cascade.

Antiplatelet agents

The most commonly used antiplatelet agent remains aspirin (acetylsalicylic acid, ASA). Aspirin irreversibly inhibits cyclooxygenase, blocking the synthesis of the platelet agonist prostacyclin.[4] The minimum dose of aspirin is 80–300 mg administered at least 2 h before PCI.[4,5] Although clinically effective, aspirin is a weak antiplatelet agent, and does not inhibit any of the other routes of platelet activation (thrombin, adenosine diphosphate, epinephrine, and serotonin).

Clopidogrel [Plavix, Bristol-Myers Squibb/Sanofi Pharmaceuticals Partnership, New York, NY] is an inhibitor of adenosine diphosphate (ADP), preventing the binding of this potent platelet agonist. Multiple studies have evaluated the benefit of combining ADP inhibition with cyclooxygenase inhibition.[6,7] Pretreatment with ADP inhibition prior to coronary stenting improves patency, and reduces periprocedural infarction. An aliquot 300 mg of clopidogrel is an effective dose. The optimal duration of this therapy after stenting is unclear.[8,9] It seems that a minimum of 1 month is required. As is also true of aspirin, the effect of clopidogrel is irreversible. For both drugs, there must be turnover of platelets in the absence of active drug in order to restore platelet function. This process generally takes at least 5 days.

Both aspirin and clopidogrel inhibit the activation and adhesion of platelets, both of which are early events. The final step in platelet aggregation is the cross-linking of platelets across fibrinogen, which allows the platelet phospholipid membrane to serve as a scaffold for larger reactions of the coagulation cascade. This occurs via interaction between fibrinogen and platelet surface receptors. The specific receptor is a dimer of glycoproteins IIa and IIIb (IIb/IIIa receptor, integrin IIb/IIIa, GP2b3a). The IIb/IIIa inhibition was a major step in improving outcomes from PCI. The first agent, abciximab [ReoPro, Centocor and Eli Lilly and Company, Malvern, PA and Indianapolis, IN] is a monoclonal antibody fragment that binds to the glycoprotein IIb/IIIa complex on the platelet membrane, preventing binding to fibrinogen. The drug is active within 2 h after infusion, but has a prolonged effect. The clinical effect is reduced at 6–12 h, but the blockade remains detectable for up to 14 days. Newer agents, such as eptifibatide [Integrillin, Millennium Pharmaceuticals, Inc., and Schering-Plough Corporation Cambridge, MA and Kenilworth, NJ] are more specific and are competitive inhibitors resulting in a shorter clinical effect (12 h for abciximab versus 2.5 h for eptifibatide). Abciximab is approved by the United States Federal Drug Administration (FDA) for administration in acute coronary syndromes as well as PCI, and eptifibatide is approved for use during PCI. Abciximab was found to reduce death rates, myocardial infarction, and need for urgent revascularization at 30 days, 3 months, and 6 years.[10] Similar finding was also confirmed in a large meta-analysis that assessed the beneficial role of abcximab in more than 3000 patients following acute myocardial infaction.[11] This improvement, however, comes with the cost of increased bleeding complications (odds ratio = 1.74).[11]

Coagulation cascade inhibitors

Heparin

Heparin was introduced into clinical use in 1935. It remains the most common anticoagulant in use today, and it is estimated that 30% of all patients admitted to a hospital receive some form of heparin. Heparin's anticoagulant effect occurs though acceleration of the action of endogenous antithrombin (AT). The most commonly used form is unfractionated heparin (UFH), which is a mixture of polysaccharide chains. Heparin complexes with AT and inactivates coagulation factors Xa, XIIa, XIa, and IXa. UFH is quickly available after intravenous (IV) administration (within 3 min) and its effect is easily assessed by way of the activated clotting time (ACT). Duration of action depends on the dose administered, but is roughly 60 min. The activated partial thromboplastin time (aPTT) is used to monitor longer-term therapy. Heparin has an antidote in protamine. Protamine (derived from salmon sperm) complexes with heparin in a 1 : 100 ratio (1 mg protamine : 100 U heparin) and prevents the binding of heparin to AT. The indirect activity of heparin represents a major drawback to its use. In addition, heparin is ineffective against existing thrombus, and has significant biologic variability. There are no firm recommendations regarding dosing of heparin for endovascular interventions. High-risk interventions (brachiocephalic vessels) may benefit from administration of 75–100 U heparin per kilogram body mass during balloon angioplasty, whereas straightforward aortoiliac interventions may only require doses of 25–50 U/kg.[1] However, lower doses may be safe. One study demonstrates safety and efficacy of roughly 50 U/kg for coronary interventions.[12] The implication of this study is that lower doses may be sufficient for small vessel interventions.

Low molecular weight heparins (LMWH) are shorter segments of depolymerized UFH. There are several available clinically, and they are differentiated by the specific fraction utilized in the preparation, and slight differences in anticoagulant strength. LMWH offer more anti-Xa activity the UFH and less anti-IIa activity. This theoretically leads to greater efficacy, and lower bleeding complications. In addition, LMWH are administered as a single SQ injection, and does not require monitoring to determine anticoagulant ability due to more predictable biologic activity. This however, is also its greatest problem, as there is no rapid method to assess anticoagulant adequacy. There are studies that show efficacy and safety of LMWH as the sole heparin administered for the purpose of PCI.[13,14]

A potential clinical concern with administration of all heparins relates to their immunogenicity. The heparin-induced thrombocytopenia syndrome (HIT) occurs in roughly 1–3% of all patients who receive heparin. Heparin complexes with endogenous platelet factor 4 to form a unique epitope that an IgG antibody (most commonly) develops. In the presence of exogenous heparin, this antibody binds to platelets, and leads to platelet cross-linking and generation of procoagulant microparticles and endothelial damage. Morbidity and mortality of HIT were recently assessed at 30% and 7%, respectively.[15] Therapy of HIT requires immediate cessation of all heparin, including flushes, and decision regarding need for further anticoagulation. Although LMWH is historically associated with a lower rate of antibody formation, once heparin-associated antiplatelet antibodies (HAAb) are present, 20–60% of patients with HAAb due to UFH will cross-react to LMWH.[16] Also, plasma from 34% of patients with HIT will aggregate platelets in the presence of LMWH. In addition to immunogenicity, UFH is associated with hemorrhagic complications. Due to the long history of heparin use, these complications may simply be more visible than with less frequently or more recently introduced anticoagulants. In a study that evaluate the heparin-related complications following peripheral vascular interventions, major bleeding occurred in 4.6% of 213 patients who received an average of 59.1 ± 20.0 U/kg of heparin.[17] Among those patients who developed bleeding complications, 7.6% required emergent procedure for repeat revascularization of the same vessel.[17]

Direct thrombin inhibitors

In contrast to the indirect inhibition of thrombin offered by heparin, direct thrombin inhibitors work directly on thrombin (Factor IIa). They are more specific, and offer activity against both soluble and thrombus-bound thrombin, in contrast to heparin, which has no activity against thrombus-bound thrombin. The prototype of this class of drugs is lepirudin [Refludan, Berlex Laboratories; Wayne, NJ]. Lepirudin is a recombinant derivative of hirudin, the anticoagulant present in the saliva of the medicinal leech (*Hirudo medicinalis*). Lepirudin is a bivalent thrombin inhibitor, binding at both the catalytic site of thrombin (preventing the conversion of fibrinogen to fibrin) as well as binding at the fibrinogen-binding site. Lepirudin is renally cleared, and its effect is markedly prolonged in patients with renal failure. There is no direct antidote for overdosage with lepirudin. These two facts limit its utility in patients with advanced renal insufficiency. The dose for patients with normal renal function is a bolus of 0.4 mg/kg followed by continuous infusion at 0.15 mg/kg/h, and the half-life is about 80 min. The anticoagulant effect is monitored by the aPTT. It may also be monitored at point-of-care via ecarin clotting time (ECT). Studies have found that lepirudin is a safe and effective anticoagulant for patients with HAAb.[18] Although some patients form antibodies against hirudin, of 23 patients prospectively studied 56% developed antibodies against hirudin as detected by enzyme-linked immunosubant assay (ELISA). However, since no patient demonstrated resistance or other effects attributable to the anti-hirudin antibodies, the clinical significance of these antibodies remains inconsequential.[19]

Argatroban (Glaxo SmithKline Pharmaceuticals) is a small (527 Da), synthetic, direct thrombin inhibitor derived from L-arginine. Unlike lepirudin, argatroban binds reversibly to the catalytic domain of thrombin. There is activity against both free and clot-bound thrombin, with no activity against factor

Xa or plasmin. In a study of anticoagulation for PCI using historical controls (HIT patients treated with heparin), argatroban resulted in improved clinical outcomes and no increase in hemorrhagic complications.[20] Argatroban is titrated to achieve an aPTT of 1.5 to 3 times control, and may be monitored at point-of-care via ACT. Argatroban undergoes hepatic metabolism and excretion. It is a reversible inhibitor, with a half-life of 40–50 min. This allows rapid normalization of coagulation after cessation of infusion. Since it is not renally cleared, it has a predictable effect in patients with end-stage renal disease. There is no specific antidote for argatroban, and administration should be discontinued if suspicion of overdosage or hemorrhagic complication exists. In the setting of PCI, argatroban is approved for use in patients with HIT and has been used at a dose of 25 g/kg/min after a 350 g/kg initial bolus and titrated to an ACT of 250–300 s. Results in these patients are comparable to historic heparin controls.[20]

Another direct thrombin inhibitor, bivalirudin, has been more extensively studied in PCI than the others, but not in placebo-controlled trials. Bivalirudin [Angiomax The Medicines Company, Parsippany, NJ, prior trade name – hirulog] has been studied in subtherapeutic doses (Thrombolysis In Myocardial Infarction trial 7 – TIMI 7), heparin controlled trials (HERO-2, TIMI 8). In a large meta-analysis of six studies looking at outcomes after myocardial infarction, which included 5674 patients, bivalirudin was associated with a significant reduction not only in the composite of death or infarction but also in major hemorrhage.[21] Hirulog and Early Reperfusion or Occlusion-II trial (HERO-II) evaluated early angiography in patients undergoing fibrinolysis and the HERO-2 trial specifically evaluated bivalirudin in PCI. Grade 3 flow was achieved in 48% of patients versus 35% of patients who received heparin. 17,073 patients were randomized to 2 arms. Bivalirudin failed to reduce mortality but did reduce the reinfarction rate.[22] The REPLACE (Randomized Evaluation in PCI Linking Angiomax to Reduced Clinical Outcomes)-2 trial compared bivalirudin with IIb/IIIa inhibition on a provisional basis to heparin with IIb/IIIa during PCI. The dose of bivalirudin in this study was 0.75 mg/kg bolus and 1.75 mg/kg/h infusion. Only 7.2% of patients in the bivalirudin group received IIb/IIIa inhibitors, and there were similar 30-day outcomes in both groups.[23]

Despite numerous clinical studies that documented the benefits of antiplatelet therapy in coronary interventions, there is a paucity of literature regarding the ideal anticoagulation regiments following peripheral interventions. Similarly, there are no firm consensus statements on dosage or preferred anticoagulation agent in any peripheral vascular system. If the data from the coronary circulation can be extrapolated to the peripheral circulation, platelet inhibition prior to intervention results in improved outcomes and platelet inhibition during the procedure with glycoprotein IIb/IIIa inhibitors results in an improvement over heparin alone. Other than platelet inhibition, direct thrombin inhibitors may offer further improvement by breaking the thrombin-platelet activation-thrombus cycle.

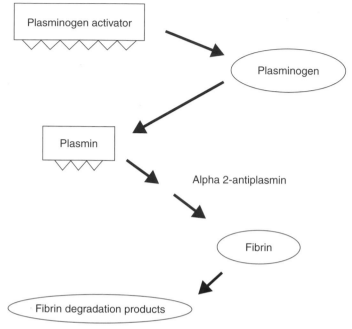

Figure 3.2 The fibrinolytic pathway.

Thrombosis and fibrinolytic system

Thrombotic process represents a normal hemostatic phenomenon that limits local hemorrhage from microscopic or macroscopic vascular injury. Physiologic thrombosis is counterbalanced by physiologic anticoagulation and physiologic fibrinolysis. Under normal physiologic environment, thrombus is removed from the injured vascular tissue once hemostasis is established by means of the fibrinolytic pathway. A basic fibrinolytic cascade is depicted in Figure 3.2. This pathway results in an end product of plasmin, which is a potent proteolytic enzyme with a broad spectrum of activity. Plasmin is formed by activation of the proenzyme, plasminogen by either plasma or tissue activators. Under pathological conditions, thrombus can propagate into otherwise normal vessels. Thrombus that has propagated where it is not needed can obstruct flow in critical vessels and can obliterate valves and other structures that are essential to normal hemodynamic function. Abnormal thrombosis can occur in any vessel at any location in the body. The principal clinical syndromes that result are acute myocardial infarction, deep vein thrombosis, pulmonary embolism, acute nonhemorrhagic stroke, acute peripheral arterial occlusion, and occlusion of indwelling catheters.

Tissue plasminogen activators are found in most tissues, except the liver and the placenta, where they are synthesized by endothelial cells and are found concentrated in the walls of blood vessels. The two best characterized are vascular activator (commonly known as tissue plasminogen activator or t-PA) and urokinase. There is great interest in using t-PA as a therapeutic agent for dissolving blood clots – the gene for t-PA has now been cloned and the expressed gene product is available for clinical trials. Plasminogen activator is also a product of macrophages. The level of tissue activator in the plasma is normally low, but can be increased by exercise and stress.

Thrombolytic therapy in peripheral circulation

The intravascular administration of thrombolytic agents originated in the 1960s with the IV treatment of pulmonary embolism. Thrombolysis by means of selective catheter infusion for vascular occlusion entered the mainstream during the 1970s.[24] Since then, techniques for thrombolysis have branched in several directions with the treatment of thrombus and/or thrombosis in the coronary arteries, peripheral vascular and visceral arteries, dialysis grafts, veins, and IV catheters. The fibrinolytic agents available today are serine proteases that work by converting plasminogen to the natural fibrinolytic agent plasmin. Plasmin lyses clot by breaking down the fibrinogen and fibrin contained in a clot. Urokinase-like plasminogen activators are produced in renal cells. They circulate in blood and are excreted in the urine. Their ability to catalyze the conversion of plasminogen to plasmin is affected only slightly by the presence or absence of local fibrin clot. Tissue-type plasminogen activators are found principally in vascular endothelial cells. Their activity is enhanced in the presence of fibrin, and they have been described as clot specific despite the fact that their activity in the general circulation is approximately equal to that of urokinase. The following sections discusses different thrombolytic agents, which have been used in clinical practice. Table 3.1 summarizes various FDA-approved or investigational thrombolytic agent.

Table 3.1 Overview of approved and investigational thrombolytic agents.

Thrombolytic agent			Approved indications					
Generic name	Abbreviated term	Trade name	MI	PE	DVT	AS	CC	AO
Streptokinase	SK	Steptase	X	X	X		X	X
Urokinase	UK	Abbokinase	X	X			X	
Anistreplase	APSAC	Eminase	X					
Alteplase	rt-t-PA	Activase	X	X		X		
Reteplase	r-PA	Retavase	X					
Prourokinase	pro-UK							
Recombinant urokinase	r-UK							
Staphylokinase	SAK							
Tenecteplase	TNK t-PA							
Lanoteplase	n-PA							
Saruplase	r-scu-PA							

MI, myocardial infarction; PE, pulmonary embolism; DVT, deep venous thrombosis; AS, acute stroke; CC, catheter clearance; AO, arterial occlusions.

Thrombolytic agents

Streptokinase

Streptokinase is produced by various strains of β-hemolytic streptococci of the Lancefield groups A, C, and G. Group C is preferred because of a lack of erythrogenic toxins. It was first isolated in 1933, and entered clinical use in the mid-1940s.[25] Streptokinase by itself is not a plasminogen activator, but it binds with free circulating plasminogen (or with plasmin) to form a complex that can convert additional plasminogen to plasmin. This enzyme indirectly activates plasminogen through mechanisms that are still being delineated to form a plasminogen-activating complex. Once the activator is formed, it functions through both fibrin-dependent and fibrin-independent mechanisms to activate plasminogen to plasmin. The activator complex not only cleaves unbound plasminogen, but plasminogen bound to streptokinase is also activated. Inactivation of streptokinase through antibody neutralization accounts for its initial half-life of 16 min. The antibodies may be overwhelmed by administering a large initial bolus of drug. The second half-life of streptokinase is approximately 83 min due to the complexing of streptokinase and neutralization by circulating antiplasmins. Since streptokinase is produced from streptococcal bacteria, it often causes febrile reactions and other allergic problems.

Immunogenicity is a problem with the use of streptokinase, which usually cannot be administered safely a second time within 6 months. This is because it is highly antigenic and results in high levels of antistreptococcal antibodies. Neutralizing antibodies can be isolated from patients with recent streptococcal infections and account for significant interpatient variability in thrombolytic potential of the drug. Attempts to overpower the immune response have been attempted by administering large initial bolus doses. This can, however, result in depletion of the necessary substrates to form the activator complex. Studies show that streptokinase result in higher rates of vein patency, and are associated with an increased incidence of hemorrhagic complications when compared to the use of UFH alone for the treatment of deep venous thrombosis.[26]

Since the late 1970s systemic administration of IV streptokinase has been largely abandoned. There are few head-to-head trial comparing various fibrinolytic agents. An open trial was conducted to compare the intraarterial administration of streptokinase to the combined intraarterial and IV administration of recombinant tissue plasminogen activator (rt-PA).[27] The initial rates of angiographic success were superior in the group receiving intra-arterial rt-PA than streptokinase (100% versus 80%; $p < 0.04$). The 30-day limb salvage rates were 80% in the intra-arterial rt-PA group, 60% in the streptokinase group, and 45% in the arm receiving IV rt-PA.[27]

Urokinase

Urokinase (UK), a trypsin-like protease that directly cleaves plasminogen to plasmin, was described in 1952.[28] Urokinase is extracted from human urine or long-term cultures of neonatal kidney cells. The lytic potential of urokinase may be enhanced by previous concomitant administration of plasminogen. It has a half-life of 15 min and is primarily metabolized in the liver. UK is a physiologic thrombolytic agent that is produced in renal parenchymal cells. Unlike streptokinase, UK directly cleaves plasminogen to produce plasmin. When purified from human urine, approximately 1500 L of urine are needed to yield enough urokinase to treat a single patient. A theoretic advantage over streptokinase is that UK is nonantigenic. This corresponds to a standardized dosing regimen and a more predictable patient response. It has no discernable fibrin-binding properties.[29] Despite these differences, to date no discernable difference between UK and streptokinase has been determined with regard to thrombolytic potential.[30,31] There has been a decreased incidence of bleeding associated with its administration (5–10%) compared with streptokinase (15–20%).[30]

Urokinase has been the agent of choice in the last decade, because of its possible results better than those of streptokinase. However, the perceived clinical superiority of UK over streptokinase has not been proven in any prospective comparative study. Similar to streptokinase, UK lacks fibrin specificity and induces a systemic lytic state. Its initially recommended dose for peripheral thrombolysis was low, but this has been abandoned in favor of higher doses. The current schemes involve infusion of 240,000 IU/h for 2 h or until restoration of antegrade flow. This is reduced to 120,000 IU/h for another 2 h and then 60,000 IU/h until lysis is complete. Questions were raised relating to the manufacturing process of UK in 1999, which resulted in its from clinical market in the United States that year. Although it was reintroduced back in 2002, this agent is currently not available in the United States due a production halt by the manufacturer since 2004.

The clinical efficacy of UK in peripheral arterial thrombosis has been investigated in numerous trials. The thrombolysis or peripheral arterial surgery (TOPAS) trial prospectively evaluated the use of recombinant UK versus surgery in the treatment of acute arterial occlusion.[32] There was a 75% amputation-free survival rate at 1 year in the arm treated with 4000 IU/min, compared to 65% in the surgical arm. The study also found the optimal infusion rate of urikase to be 4000 IU/min, at which concentration the lytic potential is maximized and the bleeding risk minimized.[33]

The surgery versus thrombolysis for ischemia of the lower extremity (STILE) trial encompassed a comparison of UK and rt-PA.[34] Patients assigned to thrombolysis were randomly allocated to receive one of the two agents versus primary operation. UK was administered as a 250,000 IU bolus followed by an infusion of 4000 IU/min for 4 h then 2000 IU/min for up to 36 h. rt-PA was administered as a continuous infusion without an initial bolus at 0.05–0.1 mg/kg/h for up to 12 h. Notably, the study excluded patients suffering from embolic occlusion. A second analysis of the STILE data evaluated patients treated who had occlusion of native arteries. There was a reduction in surgeries in those with femoropopliteal occlusions (58%) and in 51% of those with ileofemoral occlusions. At 1 year of follow-up, however, the rate of recurrent ischemia and major amputation was increased in those randomized to thrombolysis compared to the surgical arm. Factors associated with poor lytic outcomes were femoropopliteal occlusion, diabetes mellitus, and degree of ischemia. Despite a difference in rates of recurrent ischemia and amputation, mortality was not affected.[34]

Alteplase

Alteplase (t-PA, Activase) was the first recombinant tissue-type plasminogen activator and is identical to native tissue plasminogen activator. The presence of fibrinogen enhances its ability to activate plasmin. At the site of thrombus formation, both t-PA and plasminogen undergo conformational changes that enhance the conversion of plasminogen to plasmin with subsequent clot dissolution. *In vivo*, tissue-type plasminogen activator is synthesized and made available by cells of the vascular endothelium. Alteplase is a serine protease produced by recombinant DNA technology and chemically identical to human endogenous t-PA. It acts by stimulating fibrinolysis of blood thrombi. Alteplase promotes the binding of plasminogen to the fibrin thrombus in conjunction with the increased affinity of fibrin-bound t-PA for plasminogen and it facilitates the ordered adsorption of plasminogen and its activator to the fibrin surface. The half-life of t-PA is exceedingly short at 5 min and has a higher fibrin specificity than UK *in vitro*.

Alteplase is the most widely used thrombolytic agent in emergency situations. It is the lytic agent most often used for the treatment of coronary artery thrombosis, pulmonary embolism, and acute stroke. In theory, alteplase should be effective only at the surface of fibrin clot. In practice, however, a systemic lytic state is seen, with moderate amounts of circulating fibrin degradation products and a substantial systemic bleeding risk. The agent is not antigenic and almost is never associated with any allergic manifestations.

The clinical differences between t-PA and UK are incompletely understood. There have been extensive clinical experience and trials establishing the safety and efficacy of alteplase in the treatment of myocardial infarction, pulmonary embolism, and acute ischemic cerebral infarction.[35] This agent is emerging as the thrombolytic of primary consideration in the setting of peripheral arterial occlusion. Activase is now firmly established as the thrombolytic treatment of choice for the management of acute myocardial infarction. It is also indicated for acute massive pulmonary embolism and acute ischemic stroke.

t-PA has been used successfully with both IV and direct arterial infusion. The higher complication rate with t-PA than with UK may have been related to the use of a higher bioequivalent dose. No consensus exists regarding the ideal dosage of t-PA for peripheral vascular occlusion. More traditional reports suggest a dose of about 2 mg/h, while recent work has shown successful thrombolysis with a dose of 0.2 mg/h.[36] Relatively high rates of bleeding complications have been noted at this dose, particularly when concomitant heparin therapy is used. A recombinant form of t-PA, rt-PA, has been developed that has been approved for both myocardial infarction and massive pulmonary embolism. The GUSTO-I (Global use of Strategies to Open Occluded Coronary Arteries) trial evaluated the use of rt-PA compared with streptokinase in treating myocardial infarction. This demonstrated a slightly increased risk of intracranial hemorrhage with rt-PA, but an overall reduction in mortality.[37]

Reteplase

Reteplase (r-PA, Rapilysin, Retavase, Ecokinase; Boehringer Mannheim) is a single chain, nonglycosylated deletion mutant of alteplase. This is a second generation recombinant tissue-type plasminogen activator that seems to work more quickly and to have a lower bleeding risk than the first generation agent alteplase. This agent has a longer half-life of 18 min secondary to a reduced affinity for hepatocytes. The drug is produced in *Escherichia coli* by recombinant techniques. Reteplase does not bind fibrin as tightly as native tissue plasminogen activator, allowing the drug to diffuse more freely through the clot rather than binding only to the surface, the way tissue plasminogen activator does. This is thought to translate into decreased distant bleeding complications. It is inhibited by plasminogen-activator inhibitor similarly to alteplase. In high concentrations, reteplase does not compete with plasminogen for fibrin-binding sites, allowing plasminogen at the site of the clot to be transformed into clot-dissolving plasmin. These two modifications help explain the faster clot resolution seen in patients receiving reteplase than in those receiving alteplase. The modifications also resulted in a molecule with a faster plasma clearance and shorter half-life (about 11–19 min) than alteplase. Reteplase undergoes both renal and hepatic clearance. The shorter half-life makes the drug ideal for double-bolus dosing. The result is more convenient administration and faster thrombolysis with reteplase than with alteplase, which is given by a bolus followed by an IV infusion.

Reteplase has been used in several hundred cases of peripheral vascular occlusion, and early results appear promising. A multi-center randomized GUSTO-III trial which evaluated the use of reteplase for myocardial infarction demonstrated that there was an increase in coronary flow rates, but this did not translate into increased survival.[38]

Saruplase

This recombinant form of single chain UK-type plasminogen activator (r-scu-PA) or proUK (P-UK) is converted by plasmin into an active form of UK. Saruplase is a relatively new fibrinolytic agent that is currently undergoing clinical trials for a variety of indications. It is a relatively inactive precursor that must be converted to UK before it becomes active *in vivo*. Administration causes a decrease in plasminogen inhibitors α_2-antiplasmin and fibrinogen. It also increases the concentration of fibrin degradation products. P-UK has a much higher affinity for thrombus-bound Lys-plasminogen than Glu-plasminogen, resulting in a fibrin affinity similar to UK. This recombinant form of UK is very resistant to degradation by plasma inhibitors and ionized calcium. It's preference for Lys-plasminogen is thought to confer a longer half-life, estimated to be in the order of days. Its advantages over other plasminogen activators are that it is inactive in plasma and does not bind to or consume circulating inhibitors.[39] As with tissue-type plasminogen activator, saruplase is somewhat clot specific, since the presence of fibrin enhances the conversion of P-UK to active UK.

Anisoylated purified streptokinase activator complex

Anisoylated purified streptokinase activator complex (APSAC) is a complex of streptokinase and plasminogen that does not require free-circulating plasminogen to be effective. The half-life of APSAC in plasma is somewhere between 40 min and 90 min. It has many theoretical benefits over streptokinase but suffers antigenic problems similar to those of the parent compound.[40]

Anistreplase

Anistreplase is an equimolar complex of streptokinase and para-anisoylated human Lys-plasminogen (APSAC) in which the active site in the plasminogen moiety is reversibly blocked by acylation. It has a slightly longer half-life than streptokinase. The acylation makes it less susceptible to degradation. However, when studied in the coronary arteries, it was found to have little benefit over streptokinase, and has not been routinely used in peripheral interventions.[41]

Tenecteplase

Tenecteplase (Metalyse, Genentech) is another mutant t-PA with improved fibrin selectivity. There are two amino acid substitutions that translate into a longer half-life, enhanced resistance to plasminogen-activator inhibitor. A third substitution confers a slower clearance and a 200-fold greater resistance to plasminogen-activator inhibitor.[42]

References

1 Kandarpa K, Becker GJ, Hunink MG, et al. Transcatheter interventions for the treatment of peripheral atherosclerotic lesions: part I. *J Vasc Interv Radiol* 2001; **12**:683–95.
2 Donaldson MC, Weinberg DS, Belkin M, Whittemore AD, Mannick JA. Screening for hypercoagulable states in vascular surgical practice: a preliminary study. *J Vasc Surg* 1990; **11**:825–31.
3 Jagroop IA, Milionis HJ, Mikhailidis DP. Mechanism underlying increased platelet reactivity in patients with peripheral arterial disease. *Int Angiol* 1999; **18**:348–51.
4 Awtry EH, Loscalzo J. Aspirin. *Circulation* 2000; **101**:1206–18.
5 Smith SC, Jr., Dove JT, Jacobs AK, et al. ACC/AHA guidelines for percutaneous coronary intervention (revision of the 1993 PTCA guidelines) – executive summary: a report of the American College of Cardiology/American Heart Association task force on practice guidelines (Committee to revise the 1993 guidelines for percutaneous transluminal coronary angioplasty) endorsed by the Society for Cardiac Angiography and Interventions. *Circulation* 2001; **103**:3019–41.

6 Steinhubl SR, Lauer MS, Mukherjee DP, *et al*. The duration of pretreatment with ticlopidine prior to stenting is associated with the risk of procedure-related non-Q-wave myocardial infarctions. *J Am Coll Cardiol* 1998; **32**:1366–70.

7 Levine GN, Kern MJ, Berger PB, *et al*. Management of patients undergoing percutaneous coronary revascularization. *Ann Intern Med* 2003; **139**:123–36.

8 Claeys MJ. Antiplatelet therapy for elective coronary stenting: a moving target. *Semin Vasc Med* 2003; **3**:415–18.

9 Pekdemir H, Cin VG, Camsari A, *et al*. A comparison of 1-month and 6-month clopidogrel therapy on clinical and angiographic outcome after stent implantation. *Heart Vessels* 2003; **18**:123–29.

10 Topol EJ, Ferguson JJ, Weisman HF, *et al*. Long-term protection from myocardial ischemic events in a randomized trial of brief integrin beta3 blockade with percutaneous coronary intervention. EPIC Investigator Group. Evaluation of Platelet IIb/IIIa Inhibition for Prevention of Ischemic Complication. *JAMA* 1997; **278**:479–84.

11 Kandzari DE, Hasselblad V, Tcheng JE, *et al*. Improved clinical outcomes with abciximab therapy in acute myocardial infarction: a systematic overview of randomized clinical trials. *Am Heart J* 2004; **147**:457–62.

12 Caussin C, Fsihi A, Ohanessian A, Jacq L, Rahal S, Lancelin B. Direct stenting with 3000 i.u. heparin. *Int J Cardiovasc Intervent* 2003; **5**:206–10.

13 Montalescot G, Cohen M. Low molecular weight heparins in the cardiac catheterization laboratory. *J Thromb Thrombolysis* 1999; **7**:319–23.

14 Choussat R, Montalescot G, Collet JP, *et al*. A unique, low dose of intravenous enoxaparin in elective percutaneous coronary intervention. *J Am Coll Cardiol* 2002; **40**:1943–50.

15 Shuster TA, Silliman WR, Coats RD, Mureebe L, Silver D. Heparin-induced thrombocytopenia: twenty nine years later. *J Vasc Surg* 2003; **38**:1316–22.

16 Mureebe L, Silver D. Heparin-induced thrombocytopenia: pathophysiology and management. *Vasc Endovascular Surg* 2002; **36**:163–70.

17 Shammas NW, Lemke JH, Dippel EJ, *et al*. In-hospital complications of peripheral vascular interventions using unfractionated heparin as the primary anticoagulant. *J Invasive Cardiol* 2003; **15**:242–46.

18 Mudaliar JH, Liem TK, Nichols WK, Spadone DP, Silver D. Lepirudin is a safe and effective anticoagulant for patients with heparin-associated antiplatelet antibodies. *J Vasc Surg* 2001; **34**:17–20.

19 Song X, Huhle G, Wang L, Hoffmann U, Harenberg J. Generation of anti-hirudin antibodies in heparin-induced thrombocytopenic patients treated with r-hirudin. *Circulation* 1999; **100**:1528–32.

20 Lewis BE, Matthai WH, Jr., Cohen M, Moses JW, Hursting MJ, Leya F. Argatroban anticoagulation during percutaneous coronary intervention in patients with heparin-induced thrombocytopenia. *Catheter Cardiovasc Interv* 2002; **57**:177–84.

21 Kong DF, Topol EJ, Bittl JA, *et al*. Clinical outcomes of bivalirudin for ischemic heart disease. *Circulation* 1999; **100**:2049–53.

22 White HD, Aylward PE, Frey MJ, *et al*. Randomized, double-blind comparison of hirulog versus heparin in patients receiving streptokinase and aspirin for acute myocardial infarction (HERO). Hirulog Early Reperfusion/Occlusion (HERO) Trial Investigators. *Circulation* 1997; **96**:2155–61.

23 Lincoff AM, Bittl JA, Harrington RA, *et al*. Bivalirudin and provisional glycoprotein IIb/IIIa blockade compared with heparin and planned glycoprotein IIb/IIIa blockade during percutaneous coronary intervention: REPLACE-2 randomized trial. *JAMA* 2003; **289**:853–63.

24 Comerota AJ, Cohen GS. Thrombolytic therapy in peripheral arterial occlusive disease: mechanisms of action and drugs available. *Can J Surg* 1993; **36**:342–48.

25 Mueller K. [1st experiences with highly purified streptokinase in thrombolysis in surgery.]. *Bruns Beitr Klinischen Chir* 1961; **202**:340–49.

26 Rogers LQ, Lutcher CL. Streptokinase therapy for deep vein thrombosis: a comprehensive review of the English literature. *Am J Med* 1990; **88**:389–95.

27 Berridge DC, Gregson RH, Hopkinson BR, Makin GS. Randomized trial of intra-arterial recombinant tissue plasminogen activator, intravenous recombinant tissue plasminogen activator and intra-arterial streptokinase in peripheral arterial thrombolysis. *Br J Surg* 1991; **78**:988–95.

28 Sobel GW, Mohler SR, Jones NW. Urokinase: an activator of plasma fibrinolysin extracted from urine. *Am J Physiol* 1952; **171**:768–69.

29 Lijnen HR, Zamarron C, Blaber M, Winkler ME, Collen D. Activation of plasminogen by pro-urokinase. I. Mechanism. *J Biol Chem* 1986; **261**:1253–58.

30 van Breda A, Katzen BT, Deutsch AS. Urokinase versus streptokinase in local thrombolysis. *Radiology* 1987; **165**:109–11.

31 Belkin M, Belkin B, Bucknam CA, Straub JJ, Lowe R. Intra-arterial fibrinolytic therapy. Efficacy of streptokinase versus urokinase. *Arch Surg* 1986; **121**:769–73.

32 Ouriel K, Veith FJ, Sasahara AA. Thrombolysis or peripheral arterial surgery: phase I results. TOPAS Investigators. *J Vasc Surg* 1996; **23**:64–73; discussion 74–75.

33 Ouriel K, Veith FJ, Sasahara AA. A comparison of recombinant urokinase with vascular surgery as initial treatment for acute arterial occlusion of the legs. Thrombolysis or Peripheral Arterial Surgery (TOPAS) Investigators. *N Engl J Med* 1998; **338**:1105–11.

34 Results of a prospective randomized trial evaluating surgery versus thrombolysis for ischemia of the lower extremity. The STILE trial. *Ann Surg* 1994; **220**:251–66; discussion 266–68.

35 Shen W, Zhang R, Zhang J, Zhang D, Zhang X, Zheng A. A comparative study on the effects of low dose of tPA and different regimens of intravenous urokinase in acute myocardial infarction. *Chin Med J (Engl)* 1999; **112**:18–21.

36 Cundiff DK. Thrombolysis for acute myocardial infarction: drug review. *MedGenMed* 2002; **4**:1.

37 An international randomized trial comparing four thrombolytic therapies for acute myocardial infarction. The GUSTO investigators. *N Engl J Med* 1993; **329**:673–82.

38 Stringer KA. TIMI grade flow, mortality, and the GUSTO-III trial. *Pharmacotherapy* 1998; **18**:699–705.

39 Bar FW, Meyer J, Vermeer F, *et al.* Comparison of saruplase and alteplase in acute myocardial infarction. SESAM Study Group. The Study in Europe with Saruplase and Alteplase in Myocardial Infarction. *Am J Cardiol* 1997; **79**:727–32.

40 Bell WR. Present-day thrombolytic therapy: therapeutic agents – pharmacokinetics and pharmacodynamics. *Rev Cardiovasc Med* 2002; **3** Suppl 2:S34–44.

41 McNeill AJ, Roberts MJ, Wilson CM, *et al.* Anistreplase in early acute myocardial infarction and the one-year follow-up. *Int J Cardiol* 1991; **31**:39–49.

42 Rabasseda X. Tenecteplase (TNK tissue plasminogen activator): A new fibrinolytic for the acute treatment of myocardial infarction. *Drugs Today (Barc)* 2001; **37**:749–60.

CHAPTER 4

Complications of endovascular therapy

Gordon M. Riha, Changyi Chen, Ruth L. Bush

As technology and knowledge progress, the frequency of complications resulting from endovascular therapy has declined, but unfortunately, these complications have not been eliminated. Despite foresight and preparation, complications will occur, and vascular surgeons must be prepared for a range of situations, which may transpire during the course of or following endovascular therapy. This broad milieu of complications, as with conventional surgery, is often due to one of two overlying general aspects. The first involves case selection of patients with underlying morbidities, an element of surgery that will become increasingly common with the aging population. The second general aspect concerns deficient technique or lack of endovascular experience. Innovative technologies and techniques assure that a learning curve will always exist for endovascular therapy, and thus, continuing education is a necessity as therapy evolves. As with conventional surgery, the existence and corresponding management of these general aspects should be dealt with on a case-by-case basis.

Unlike conventional surgery, unique complications specific to endovascular procedures demand insight into recognition and management strategies for the interventional radiologist or vascular surgeon carrying out these therapies. A malleable definition of a complication is used in this chapter as an adverse effect directly related to the therapy that occurs during or up to 30 days after the indicated endovascular procedure. Although the definition and the scope of endovascular procedures continue to expand, certain general complications exist that are applicable to all endovascular techniques. Studies have shown that complications following endovascular procedure can range from 1.5–9%.[1-3] Given the increased utility of endovascular intervention in the clinical setting, it is conceivable that the incidence of complication might rise as more catheter-based therapeutic procedures are performed. Thus, this chapter will provide a broad overview of these general complications relating to endovascular therapy and will elucidate strategies for its prevention and management. Thorough coverage of complications specific to certain endovascular procedures will be handled in depth within the respective chapters.

Table 4.1 Acceptable threshold complication rate for quality assurance following groin puncture and angiography as recommended by the Society of Interventional Radiology.

Complications	Acceptable threshold (%)
Hematoma	3
Arterial occlusion	0.5
Pseudoaneurysm	0.5
Arteriovenous fistula	0.1
Catheter-induced complications	–
Arterial dissection	2
Subintimal injection	1
Cerebral angiography	–
All neurologic complications	4
Permanent neurologic complications	1
Contrast reactions	–
All reactions	3
Major reactions	0.5
Contrast-induced renal failure	10

Complications related to the access site

Complications at the access site are the most common adverse consequences of endovascular therapy. Peripheral vascular complications include hematoma, pseudoaneurysms, arteriovenous fistula (AVF), acute arterial occlusions, cholesterol emboli, and infections. Following cardiac diagnostic catheterization, the incidence of groin complications is 0.05–0.7%.[4,5] In contrast, complications following percutaneous transluminal angioplasty occurred at a much higher incidence, which ranged from 0.7–9.0%.[5,6] Data collection of these adverse occurrences and a complication rate audit should take place within respective institutions that administer endovascular therapy. Acceptable threshold incidences for these complications have been described by the Society for Interventional Radiology, which is summarized in Table 4.1.[1]

Groin hematoma

Groin hematoma, remains one of the more common complication following endovascular procedures, and it can vary from being trivial to potentially life threatening (Figure 4.1). Susceptibility to groin hematoma is related to a number of factors including utilization of anticoagulants, patient comorbidities and condition (obesity, hypertension, and restlessness), physician's experience, size of device introduction, and type of procedure being performed. The patient with a hematoma under observation should be cautioned about these developments. Eventually, the discoloration will extend into the leg below the knee and does not represent new bleeding. The extent of a hematoma and presence or absence of retroperitoneal extension is best determined by CT scanning (Figure 4.2).

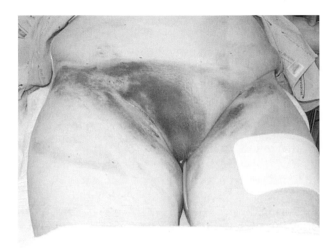

Figure 4.1 A tense thigh hematoma that has been observed, which is represented by the extensive groin ecchymosis.

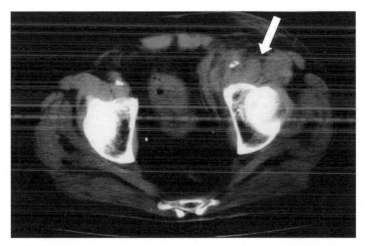

Figure 4.2 CT scan showing left groin hematoma around the femoral vessels and in the subcutaneous tissues (arrow).

Symptoms of a groin hematoma may vary from mild groin discomfort to severe pain, massive swelling, and potential necrosis of the overlying skin from pressure of the hematoma. Initially, there is minimal ecchymosis, with discoloration developing over time. As the patient ambulates, the ecchymosis may extend down the thigh, transforming into a more yellowish appearance. The patient with a hematoma under observation should be cautioned about these changes. In addition, sudden onset of massive bleeding can also occur, and complaints of lower extremity or groin coolness, numbness, or pain should be evaluated immediately.

Indications for groin exploration and hematoma evacuation include severe pain, progressive enlargement, skin compromise, or evidence of femoral nerve compression. After a standard longitudinal groin incision, dissection down to the level of the artery, not just the fascial planes, must be assured before placing one or two interrupted repair sutures. Cephalad dissection for proximal control may be necessary in instances of amplified bleeding. There is a high incidence of wound infection following hematoma evacuation.

Prevention of groin hematoma formation can be viewed as both a patient and technique-based undertaking. The coagulation status of the patient should be known at the time of the procedure and sheath withdrawal, with judicious use of heparin during the procedure. Hypertension control and assurance of immobilization postprocedurally for 6–8 h are also often overlooked as preventative measures. Within the scope of the endovascular procedure itself, proper techniques of establishing femoral arterial access can reduce the incidence of groin hematoma. A study that examined the anatomic correlation between pelvic radiographic landmark and groin complications found that needle access at 1 cm lateral to the most medial cortex of femoral head and proper maintenance of 30–45° angle of puncture can reduce the likelihood of groin hematoma formation.[7]

Arteriovenous fistula

The most common cause of AVF is inadvertent puncture of the profunda femoris artery and the vein, which crosses between it and the superficial femoral artery (Figure 4.3). Fistulae are usually detected clinically by the presence of a palpable thrill in the groin or by an auscultating a continuous bruit. Duplex ultrasound confirms the presence of a fistula showing the characteristic systolic-diastolic flow pattern with arterialization of the venous signal. Kresowik in a prospective duplex examination of 144 patients undergoing

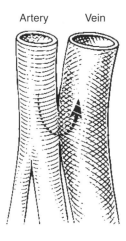

Artery   Vein

Figure 4.3 Diagrammatic depiction of an iatrogenic arteriovenous fistula.

coronary angioplasty noted a 2.8% incidence of AVF[8] Kent in contrast, using the detection of an audible bruit as a trigger for duplex scanning reported a 0.3% incidence, although this clearly will underestimate the true incidence.[9] Fistulae, usually do not close spontaneously, therefore operative repair is indicated when they are detected. Fistulae progressively enlarge with time, therefore expeditious intervention is warranted.

Risk factors for development of an AVF include: female gender, hypertension, left femoral puncture, and periprocedural anticoagulation. The increased incidence associated with left groin puncture may be due to the physician standing on the patients right side and the wrong angle of approach resulting in the arterial and venous puncture.[10]

Surgical repair is performed by dissection of the artery until the defect is identified by brisk arterial bleeding. The arterial bleeding is then controlled either by clamping or digital pressure. The venous bleeding is usually easily controlled with direct pressure, until repair can be effected. The defect in the artery is first repaired with interrupted Prolene sutures followed by repair of the vein. Usually, only one or two horizontal mattress sutures are required in each vessel. Recently, there have been reports using stent grafts to treat femoral AVF. Only those fistulae that are remote from the origin of the profunda femoris artery should be considered, so that the profunda orifice is not covered during deployment. Only very short term data currently exists for this approach. Consequently, it should remain a secondary option in patients for whom surgery would be challenging.[11] Several studies have reported the feasibility of endovascular repair of AVF caused by iatrogenic injury using stent grafts.[12,13] However, available literature does not support the routine use of covered stents in a femoral AVF, due to high risk of thrombosis caused by hip joint flexion.

Pseudoaneurysm

Pseudoaneurysms, following arterial puncture result from failure of the closure in the arterial puncture site, resulting in contained bleeding into the soft tissue around the artery (Figure 4.4). Pseudoaneurysms can occur in any vessel, although most frequently they develop in the femoral artery due to high or low femoral puncture, puncture of a femoral branch, or use of procedural anticoagulation. The presence of expansile pulsation and tenderness should raise a suspicion and lead to diagnosis by duplex scanning (Plate 1, facing p. 80). The duplex examination should note the size and likely source of the pseudoaneurysm. Furthermore, the neck of the pseudoaneurysm should be defined as to whether there is a single wide neck or a long tortuous narrow neck, which is likely to be treated successfully with ultrasound-guided compression. Some pseudoaneurysms are complex and appear to have multiple lobes while others are a single, simple cavity. Pseudoaneurysms can be difficult to detect if accompanied by a hematoma.

There are now a variety of approaches for treatment of pseudoaneurysms, and management should be based upon its size and whether it is associated

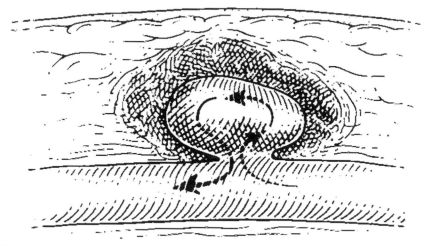

Figure 4.4 Diagrammatic depiction of a typical femoral pseudoaneurysm.

with threatened overlying skin viability, nerve compression, limb ischemia, or a large hematoma. If a pseudoaneurysm remain small, observation may be appropriate that is not associated with significant patient discomfort. Most small pseudoaneurysms will thrombose spontaneously within 2–4 weeks, but it is likely that concurrent anticoagulation will decrease the likelihood that spontaneous thrombosis will occur.

Surgical repair has been the mainstay of therapy for larger aneurysms with progressive enlargement or an association of groin pain, skin necrosis, or compression neuropathy. The femoral artery is exposed through a groin incision. Techniques vary, but some surgeons prefer to gain full control of the artery prior to exposing the puncture site. Sliding down the external oblique and identifying the femoral artery as it enters the thigh can help in obtaining proximal control. Rolling the inguinal ligament superiorly or dividing the external oblique fibers also permits exposure of the external iliac artery. Gaining proximal control is particularly important with a large hematoma or pseudoaneurysm. As an alternate approach, knowing that the arterial defect is usually only a 2–3 mm puncture site, other surgeons opt to enter the pseudoaneurysm directly while controlling the bleeding digitally and oversewing the puncture site with Prolene suture. As a surgical principle, it is important to ensure that the arterial wall is well exposed prior to repair with sutures. A common error is to misidentify a hole in the fascia as the arterial defect and place sutures within the fascia. This can lead to recurrent pseudoaneurysm formation or persistent bleeding.

Several less invasive approaches can be considered to avoid surgery, which includes utilizing a trial of ultrasound compression or thrombin injection before surgery. Ultrasound-guided compression of the neck of a smaller pseudoaneurysm can be effective if the neck is long and narrow. This neck is identified with ultrasound as a high velocity jet, and direct compression is applied with the transducer. Pressure is increased until the jet is obliterated. The mean time to thrombosis is 22 min, but some may require up to 120 min. This, however, may be associated with significant discomfort, and consequently, sedation and analgesia are always required. In addition, this is very labor intensive since it requires a dedicated technician to apply pressure. However, multiple studies have demonstrated success rates ranging from 76–98% when ultrasound compression was utilized.[14,15] Ultrasound-guided thrombin injection is an off-label use for thrombin, but it is very successful in inducing thrombosis of pseudoaneurysms, thereby avoiding surgery.[14,16,17]

Retroperitoneal hematoma

Perhaps the most feared complication of groin puncture, retroperitoneal hematoma (RPH), is an infrequent (0.15% incidence) but severe complication.[3] The term refers to blood contained within the retroperitoneum, but several patterns occur. An iliopsoas hematoma occurs when bleeding enters and is confined within the fascia of the iliopsoas muscle. The psoas muscle contains the lumbar plexus, and this pattern of hematoma may be more likely to be associated with a compression neuropathy. In contrast, the space between the peritoneum and retroperitoneal structures is potentially vast, and a hematoma in this location can contain huge quantities of blood, which may be very difficult to detect clinically. These hematomas can lead to dramatic elevation and compression of the ipsilateral kidney.

Any patient who has had groin puncture and develops lower abdominal or back pain should be suspected of having a RPH. Postcatheterization anticoagulation and high arterial puncture above the level of the inguinal ligament are major risk factors to consider.[2,3] Abdominal examination usually shows tenderness, but occasionally, palpable fullness may be detected. Thigh pain, numbness, or weakness in the quadriceps should also lead to the suspicion of RPH due to resulting femoral nerve compression. Early recognition is essential, and a falling hematocrit accompanied by the physical signs described above should direct the physician to investigate for RPH. There should be a low threshold for performing abdomino-pelvic CT scans to establish the definitive diagnosis in such patients (Figure 4.5). Management of RPH must be individualized: (1) anticoagulation should be stopped or minimized, (2) patients with neurological deficits in the ipsilateral extremity require urgent decompression of the hematoma, and (3) hematoma progression by serial CT necessitates surgical evacuation and repair of the arterial puncture site.

Axillary and brachial artery access-related injury

Access through the axillary and brachial arteries may be preferred for a variety of endovascular procedures, or it may be necessitated due to occlusive iliac disease. All of the complications that can occur with femoral artery catheterization, such as pseudoaneurysm, AVF formation, and vessel thrombosis, have similarly been noted as complicating axillary artery and brachial arterial

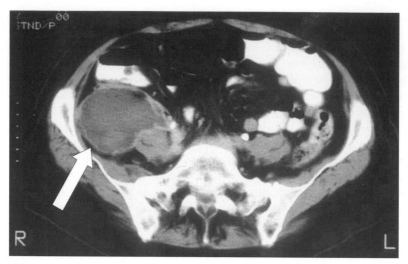

Figure 4.5 A large retroperitoneal hematoma is noted on the CT scan (arrow).

puncture. However, in particular, there is a higher incidence for neuropraxia involving the median nerve or other branches of the brachial plexus. The frequency of nerve injury to nerves of the brachial plexus is between 0.4 and 12.7%.[18,19] This is in stark contrast to a recent prospective study of cardiac catheterizations via the femoral artery where damage to the adjacent femoral nerve occurred in only 20 out of 9585 cases (0.2%).[20]

There are three potential mechanisms of nerve injury, and hematoma formation is likely the most common. The hematoma forms within a fascial compartment containing the neurovascular bundle, resulting in nerve compression. The second mechanism likely involves direct nerve damage caused by the needle, catheter, or introducer sheath. Lastly, nerve damage may be due to nerve ischemia caused by varying degrees of arterial thrombosis, which may be contributory in a minority of patients.

Time to symptom onset varies from immediate to 3 days, with an average of 12 h.[19,20] Pain at the puncture site is the most common symptom, and the pain may radiate down the arm. Muscle weakness accompanied by numbness indicates more severe symptoms and mandates immediate intervention. Swelling from a hematoma is inconsistent, as even a small hematoma in the right location can result in nerve compression. The size of the hematoma or the presence of ecchymosis does not correlate with either the severity of symptoms or the degree of nerve damage.

The treatment principles consist of both an awareness of the possibility of nerve compression following axillary or brachial artery puncture and mandatory evaluation of the hand postprocedure for pain, sensory, or motor dysfunction. Early surgical decompression is recommended for any patient in pain excess of that anticipated from arterial puncture or the presence of a motor/sensory deficit. The artery should be surgically exposed, any hematoma evacuated, and the puncture site repaired with Prolene sutures. The fascia of the neurovascular bundle must then be widely opened and any perineural hematoma evacuated. The deep fascia of the forearm is not closed, and only the subcutaneous fat and skin should be approximated. Functional outcomes from a missed nerve injury are poor, and although most patients report having some improvement, the majority describe persistent sensory or motor impairment, with a few patients developing disabling pain syndromes.

Miscellaneous complications related to access site

Occlusion at the access site may result from dissection, vasospasm, or thrombosis. Acute thrombosis of the femoral artery occurs infrequently and manifests as typical lower extremity ischemia. Exploration of the femoral artery usually reveals a large posterior plaque with thrombosis of the residual lumen. Femoral endarterectomy patch angioplasty and balloon catheter embolectomy of the external iliac and superficial femoral arteries are the most commonly required procedures. Distal embolization is more commonly due to the passage of catheters in an atherosclerotic vessels than the actual intervention itself. However, both of these instances can result in trash foot. Rarely catheter/wire passage can result in arterial perforation and more rarely mycotic pseudoaneurysm. Femoral endarteritis and mycotic femoral artery aneurysm has also been reported as a result of the use of percutaneous closure devices.[21,22] Although the incidence of this complication is low, obesity and diabetes mellitus have been shown to increase the risk of this complication.[21,22]

Compared to femoral artery access, thrombosis occurs much more frequently when gaining access through the upper extremity, especially the brachial artery. The relative smaller size of the brachial artery predisposes to thrombosis, and patients often exhibit hand coolness and pain with movement. A pulse deficit or symptoms of ischemia necessitate immediate surgical exploration, thrombectomy, and arterial repair. Infection at the puncture site is exceedingly rare. However, due in part to the increasing use of groin closure devices, the unusual complication of arterial infection has recently been reported.[23–25]

Complications related to endovascular interventions

As the spectrum of procedures performed by endovascular access has expanded, the size and variety of devices introduced into the vasculature has also increased. When a wire, catheter, or device is passed through a blood vessel, it may injure the vessel wall directly or augment the risk for dissection, perforation, rupture, or embolization during the process. Other complications related to the site of endovascular interventions can occur, which include vessel restenosis or luminal occlusion, or device infection from a hematogenous source. Problems related to specific interventions of various arterial systems will be discussed within the corresponding chapters elsewhere.

Dissection

Dissection can generally be divided into two categories based upon the site of the ensuing complication. The first involves subintimal dissection at the puncture site due to incomplete passage of the beveled needle into the arterial lumen, followed by initial positioning of guidewire into the vessel wall with subsequent tracking in an intramural position. Lack of blood return through the catheter and resistance to the passage of guidewire should raise a suspicion of dissection. Hand injection of 3–5 cc of a dye will confirm catheter position by the appearance of a spot of the dye, which fails to wash out. The catheter and wire should then be pulled back and redirected until blood return is obtained. When identified, these types of dissections are usually of no clinical consequence. The second or more serious type of complication involves iatrogenic subintimal dissection during the passage of devices after obtaining access to the vasculature (Figure 4.6). In particular, the tortuosity and high incidence of atherosclerotic disease in the iliac arteries predispose to dissection within these vessels. For example, the most common problem encountered with iliac angioplasty is subintimal passage of the guidewire, which can potentially track into the aortic wall. Observing the movement of the wire as it crosses a lesion can prevent this. Suspicion of subintimal passage is raised by failure to aspirate blood from the catheter, and hand injection of 2–3 cc of dye, as previously mentioned, will form a spot in the aortic wall that fails to wash out. The catheter and wire should then be retrieved and the lesion recrossed. Failure to

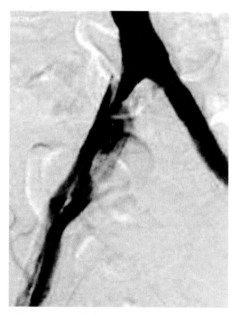

Figure 4.6 Severe dissection caused by balloon angioplasty of a calcified iliac artery.

recognize a subintimal location can lead to catastrophic problems if devices are then advanced over the subintimal wire.

Arterial perforation or rupture

During the course of endovascular therapy, perforation and rupture of an artery or other structure is uncommon, but one should be aware of the possibility and revise their respective technique to assure that neither occurs. Gentle manipulation of a stiff guidewire is of utmost importance, and the need for visualization cannot be overemphasized. When wires are passed blindly, they can enter side branches or even the supra-aortic trunks where they can lead to cerebrovascular accident. Even at the femoral access site, wires may deflect inferiorly down the SFA or profunda, or they may deflect superiorly up the circumflex iliac artery. Femoral arterial injury will result from attempts at sheath introduction when the wire is misplaced in these positions. Again, good fundamental technique involves imaging of the wire and control of the wire tip. In addition, it is possible for inadvertent perforation of organs to occur. For example, renal perforation and perinephric hematoma may arise if the wire enters a renal artery and is not visualized.

Due to the insertion and passage of comparatively large catheters and aortic stent grafts, arterial rupture is possible. The bleeding may only become apparent after catheter removal due to the tamponading effect of the catheter in place. After rupture occurs, patients should be dealt with on a case-by-case basis determined by the severity of the bleeding, with more severe hemorrhage requiring immediate surgical intervention. Rupture is particularly likely in patients with small, calcified iliac arteries, especially those with concomitant aortoiliac occlusive disease (Figure 4.7). Increasing awareness of this problem

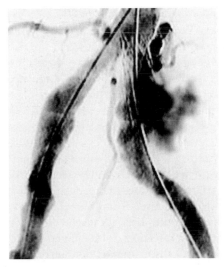

Figure 4.7 Rupture of an iliac artery due to stent placement.

has led to the development of alternative approaches such as insertion of an iliac conduit using a retroperitoneal approach to avoid such difficult iliac arteries.

Embolization

Passage of an endovascular device may dislodge an arterial mural thrombus or plaque and result in distal embolization, or thrombus formed contiguous to the catheter at the access site may be displaced. Distal embolization as a consequence of these two circumstances most likely occurs in the majority of endovascular procedures, but the emboli are usually small and inconsequential. Again, microembolization can occur following passage of any endovascular device. It is particularly likely to happen in patients with severe atheromatous disease, and stroke from catheter manipulation in an atheromatous aortic arch is well recognized. Catheters and wires should be kept out of the arch unless access is necessary for the procedure, and manipulation should be minimized. Another severe consequence is that larger emboli may produce trash foot or limb-threatening ischemia (Plate 2, facing p. 80). Management of these conditions is determined by the degree of ischemia and may range from catheter-directed thrombolysis to surgical embolectomy.

A rare, but serious, event following device passage is cholesterol embolization, which can result in visceral ischemia, renal failure, and cutaneous necrosis. Patient diagnosis is suggested by a typical livedo reticularis skin rash, elevated ESR, and abdominal pain, but conclusive documentation is attained by renal biopsy. In these cases, treatment is mainly supportive.

Device-related infection

Infection of endovascular devices has generally been rare. Given the large number of coronary procedures performed (including stent implantation), reports of infection in these devices are remarkably uncommon. Antibiotic prophylaxis recommendations have been published based upon a survey by the Society for Cardiovascular and Interventional Radiology,[1] but prophylaxis overall has been sporadic and its necessity questioned. However, the advent of aortic stent grafting has clearly been associated with increasing reports of device infection. Two mechanisms likely exist, including infection at the time of implantation and seeding of an implanted graft via bacteremia. Unlike aortic graft infections that are indolent, slowly progressive, and present years after implantation, infections of endografts are rapidly progressive and result in rapid conformational changes with rupture of the aneurysm. The patient shows all the classic sign of sepsis and the device has to be removed with aortic reconstruction performed using the standard techniques for aortic graft infection. There have also been increasing reports of infection in bare stents, which can occur if stents are placed in patients with long duration of catheter insertion, such as prolonged thrombolytic therapy. Stent infection results in septic arteritis within the wall of the host artery, which can lead to pseudoaneurysm formation and vessel rupture.[26,27]

Restenosis and Occlusion

Dissection, thrombosis, and misplacement of stent grafts can all give rise to occlusion of the arterial lumen of the vessel to which therapy is being directed or of an associated artery in the proximity. For instance, misplacement of an aortic stent graft can result in coverage of the renal arteries and lead to development of renal failure. Likewise, stent-graft occlusion of the inferior mesenteric artery or hypogastric arteries can lead to colon ischemia. Renal artery occlusion occurs infrequently, usually as a result of dissection. However, this complication threatens the viability of the kidney and mandates immediate intervention. This includes thrombolysis, stenting, and occasionally surgical bypass grafting.

A late complication after an endovascular procedure includes restenosis at the site of intervention. The clinical consequence of stent-related stenosis is largely influenced by the anatomical location of the intervention. For example, restenosis remains the Achilles heel of renal stenting, with rates reported as high as 20%.[28-30] This can result in return of hypertension or deterioration in renal function. Repeat angioplasty is required, and surgical bypass can be significantly more complicated if stents extend well beyond the ostia of the renal arteries.

Miscellaneous intervention site-related complications

Complications related to specific devices are beyond the scope of this chapter, but generally speaking, both mal-deployment and migration can occur during device placement. Once endovascular devices are in place, further complications and conditions are still possible. Endoleak, a condition whereby continuous blood flow persists outside the lumen of the stent graft but within the aneurysm sac, is also beyond the scope of this chapter but will be fully covered elsewhere.

Conclusion

Even while technology and knowledge continue to improve, the general complications discussed above will not disappear, and as surgery moves toward being more minimally invasive, the spectrum of procedures performed under an endovascular approach will undoubtedly continue to increase. Thus, training should emphasize these complications and strategies for management. However, the real responsibility for quality control falls upon those practicing endovascular therapies who should be familiar with these complications and take steps to lessen the probability that they will occur.

References

1 Singh H, Cardella JF, Cole PE, *et al.* Quality improvement guidelines for diagnostic arteriography. *J Vasc Interv Radiol* 2003; **14**:283–88.

2 Nasser TK, Mohler ER, 3rd, Wilensky RL, Hathaway DR. Peripheral vascular complications following coronary interventional procedures. *Clin Cardiol* 1995; **18**:609–14.

3 Fransson SG, Nylander E. Vascular injury following cardiac catheterization, coronary angiography, and coronary angioplasty. *Eur Heart J* 1994; **15**:232–35.

4 Fellmeth BD, Roberts AC, Bookstein JJ, *et al.* Postangiographic femoral artery injuries: nonsurgical repair with US-guided compression. *Radiology* 1991; **178**:671–75.

5 Levine GN, Kern MJ, Berger PB, *et al.* Management of patients undergoing percutaneous coronary revascularization. *Ann Intern Med* 2003; **139**:123–36.

6 Juran NB. Minimizing bleeding complications of percutaneous coronary intervention and glycoprotein IIb-IIIa antiplatelet therapy. *Am Heart J* 1999; **138**:297–306.

7 Rupp SB, Vogelzang RL, Nemcek AA, Jr., Yungbluth MM. Relationship of the inguinal ligament to pelvic radiographic landmarks: anatomic correlation and its role in femoral arteriography. *J Vasc Interv Radiol* 1993; **4**:409–13.

8 Kresowik TF, Khoury MD, Miller BV, *et al.* A prospective study of the incidence and natural history of femoral vascular complications after percutaneous transluminal coronary angioplasty. *J Vasc Surg* 1991; **13**:328–33; discussion 333–35.

9 Kent KC, McArdle CR, Kennedy B, Baim DS, Anninos E, Skillman JJ. A prospective study of the clinical outcome of femoral pseudoaneurysms and arteriovenous fistulas induced by arterial puncture. *J Vasc Surg* 1993; **17**:125–31; discussion 131–33.

10 Perings SM, Kelm M, Jax T, Strauer BE. A prospective study on incidence and risk factors of arteriovenous fistulae following transfemoral cardiac catheterization. *Int J Cardiol* 2003; **88**:223–28.

11 Baltacioglu F, Cimsit NC, Cil B, Cekirge S, Ispir S. Endovascular stent-graft applications in Iatrogenic vascular injuries. *Cardiovasc Intervent Radiol* 2003; **26**:434–39.

12 Uflacker R, Elliott BM. Percutaneous endoluminal stent-graft repair of an old traumatic femoral arteriovenous fistula. *Cardiovasc Intervent Radiol* 1996; **19**:120–22.

13 Criado E, Marston WA, Ligush J, Mauro MA, Keagy BA. Endovascular repair of peripheral aneurysms, pseudoaneurysms, and arteriovenous fistulas. *Ann Vasc Surg* 1997; **11**:256–63.

14 Gorge G, Kunz T, Kirstein M. A prospective study on ultrasound-guided compression therapy or thrombin injection for treatment of iatrogenic false aneurysms in patients receiving full-dose anti-platelet therapy. *Z Kardiol* 2003; **92**:564–70.

15 Morgan R, Belli AM. Current treatment methods for postcatheterization pseudoaneurysms. *J Vasc Interv Radiol* 2003; **14**:697–710.

16 Etemad-Rezai R, Peck DJ. Ultrasound-guided thrombin injection of femoral artery pseudoaneurysms. *Can Assoc Radiol J* 2003; **54**:118–20.

17 Weinmann EE, Chayen D, Kobzantzev ZV, Zaretsky M, Bass A. Treatment of postcatheterisation false aneurysms: ultrasound-guided compression versus ultrasound-guided thrombin injection. *Eur J Vasc Endovasc Surg* 2002; **23**:68–72.

18 Braun RM, Newman J, Thacher B. Injury to the brachial plexus as a result of diagnostic arteriography. *J Hand Surg [Am]* 1978; **3**:90–94.

19 Lyon BB, Hansen BA, Mygind T. Peripheral nerve injury as a complication of axillary arteriography. *Acta Neurol Scand* 1975; **51**:29–36.

20 Kent KC, Moscucci M, Gallagher SG, DiMattia ST, Skillman JJ. Neuropathy after cardiac catheterization: incidence, clinical patterns, and long-term outcome. *J Vasc Surg* 1994; **19**:1008–13; discussion 1013–14.

21 Tiesenhausen K, Tomka M, Allmayer T, *et al.* Femoral artery infection associated with a percutaneous arterial suture device. *Vasa* 2004; **33**:83–85.

22 Whitton Hollis H, Jr., Rehring TF. Femoral endarteritis associated with percutaneous suture closure: new technology, challenging complications. *J Vasc Surg* 2003; **38**:83–87.

23 Cherr GS, Travis JA, Ligush J, Jr., *et al.* Infection is an unusual but serious complication of a femoral artery catheterization site closure device. *Ann Vasc Surg* 2001; **15**:567–70.

24 Geary K, Landers JT, Fiore W, Riggs P. Management of infected femoral closure devices. *Cardiovasc Surg* 2002; **10**:161–63.

25 Pipkin W, Brophy C, Nesbit R, Mondy Iii JS. Early experience with infectious complications of percutaneous femoral artery closure devices. *J Vasc Surg* 2000; **32**:205–8.

26 Schachtrupp A, Chalabi K, Fischer U, Herse B. Septic endarteritis and fatal iliac wall rupture after endovascular stenting of the common iliac artery. *Cardiovasc Surg* 1999; **7**:183–86.

27 Deiparine MK, Ballard JL, Taylor FC, Chase DR. Endovascular stent infection. *J Vasc Surg* 1996; **23**:529–33.

28 Schwartz RS, Henry TD. Pathophysiology of coronary artery restenosis. *Rev Cardiovasc Med* 2002; **3**:S4–9.

29 Holmes DR, Jr. In-stent restenosis. *Rev Cardiovasc Med* 2001; **2**:115–19.

30 Dauerman HL. Approaches to restenosis: mechanical and pharmacological strategies. Overview. *Coron Artery Dis* 2004; **15**:303–5.

CHAPTER 5

Carotid bifurcation disease

Wei Zhou, Ruth L. Bush, Peter H. Lin, Alan B. Lumsden

Occlusive lesion at the origin of the internal carotid artery remains the most common cause of cerebrovascular accident, which is the third most common cause of death and accounts for 160,000 deaths annually in the United States.[1] Management of cerebrovascular accidence consumes $45 billion annually in this country. The morbidity caused by a cerebrovascular accident is more disabling than that encountered with other arterial ischemia, including myocardial infarction. Neurologic sequelae related to cerebrovascular accident including aphasia, paralysis, blindness, and weakness severely limit patient's ability to carry routine activity and invariably create an enormous burden on the health-care cost. As a result, prevention of cerebrovascular accident, particularly the treatment of extracranial carotid occlusive disease, will remain an important health-care issue in our society.

Epidemiology

Focal cerebral ischemic disease, or stroke, is responsible for 4.5 million deaths worldwide, with the majority occurring in nonindustrialized countries. The incidence of stroke is 0.2% per year in general population, but rises significantly with concurrent risk factors, age, sex, and ethnic background. Overall, the 20-year risk for a 45-year-old male is 3% but this increases to 25% for a 40-year risk.[1,2] The annual incidence of stroke doubles for each decade in patients greater than 55 years of age. The largest incidence of stroke is observed in patients greater than 80 years of age when the prevalence is 2%. Whereas a transient ischemic attack (TIA) is far more common in younger population, in the United States the prevalence of TIA in males aged between 65 and 69 years is 2.7%, which increases markedly to 3.6% for males aged between 75 and 79 years.

Pathogenesis of carotid disease

Approximately 80% of all strokes are caused by ischemic etiologies, while the remaining is caused by hemorrhagic disease. Patients with ischemic neurologic deficit can be further classified into anterior or hemispheric symptoms and posterior or vertebrobasilar symptoms. The predominant causes of hemisphere symptoms arise from the occlusive lesion of the extracranial carotid artery, which may cause internal carotid artery thrombosis, flow-related ischemic events, and/or cerebral embolization.

Atherosclerosis is the most common pathology affecting the carotid artery bifurcation. The tendency for atherosclerotic plaque to occur at the carotid bifurcation is related to a number of factors, including geometry, velocity profile, and shear stress. It has been demonstrated that plaque formation in the carotid artery bifurcation is increased within areas of low flow velocity and low shear stress and decreased in areas of high flow velocity and elevated shear stress. Postmortem specimens showed that atherosclerosis was particularly pronounced along the outer or lateral aspect of the proximal internal carotid artery and carotid bulb. This zone corresponds to areas of low velocity and low shear stress. Conversely, the medial or inner aspect of the cadaveric carotid bulb, which were associated with high blood flow velocity and high shear stress in the flow model, were relatively free of plaque formation.

The smooth muscle cell has an important role in the initial stages of plaque development. Smooth muscle cells migrate through the intima, proliferate within the media, and promote accumulation of cholesterol and other lipid molecules within the evolving lesion. Thereafter, the macrophage becomes a source of growth factor production that stimulates further smooth muscle cell proliferation and extracellular matrix production. Smooth muscle cells and macrophages initiate a secondary inflammatory cell reaction and are capable of ingesting lipid and of being transformed into vacuolated foam cells that are characteristic of atherosclerotic lesions.

In addition to these cellular components, the majority of carotid plaques have a necrotic core consisting of loose cellular debris and cholesterol crystals. The necrotic core is separated from the carotid lumen by a fibrous cap, which is composed of a rim of variable thickness comprising cellular components and extracellular matrix. The structural integrity of the fibrous cap is crucial to the final stage of plaque disruption and its clinical and pathological sequelae. It is now generally accepted that acute changes within the plaque with exposure of the deeper lipid contents predisposes towards thromboembolization.

Another feature, characteristic of advanced atherosclerotic plaques, is intraplaque hemorrhage that can occur in the absence of a disrupted fibrous cap. Symptomatic carotid disease is associated with increased neovascularization within the atherosclerotic plaque and fibrous cap. These vessels are larger and more irregular and may contribute to plaque instability and the onset of thromboembolic events.

Clinical presentation

Transient ischemic attack (TIA) is a focal loss of neurological function, lasting for less than 24 h. Crescendo TIAs refers to a syndrome comprising of repeated TIAs within a short period of time that is characterized by complete neurological recovery in between. At a minimum, the term should probably be reserved either for those with daily events or multiple-resolving attacks within

24 h. Hemodynamic TIAs represent focal cerebral events that are aggravated by exercise or hemodynamic stress and typically occur after short bursts of physical activity, post-prandially or after getting out of a hot bath. It is implied that these are due to severe extracranial disease and poor intracranial collateral recruitment. Reversible ischemic neurologic deficits (RIND) refer to an ischemic focal neurological symptoms lasting longer than 24 h but resolving within 3 weeks. When a neurologic deficit lasts longer than 3 weeks, it is considered a completed stroke. Stroke in evolution refers to progressive worsening of the neurological deficit, either linearly over a 24-h period, or interspersed with transient periods of stabilization and/or partial clinical improvement.

The patients who suffer cerebrovascular accidents typically present with three categories of symptoms including ocular symptoms, sensory/motor deficit, and/or higher cortical dysfunction. The common ocular symptoms associated with extracranial carotid include; amaurosis fugax (transient monocular blindness) and Hollenhorst plaques. Amaurosis fugax is a temporary loss of vision in one eye (likened to a shutter coming down), but which can also refer to "graying" of the vision. The blindness usually lasts for a few minutes and then resolves. Most (>90%) are due to embolic occlusion of the main artery or the upper/lower divisions. Monocular blindness progressing over a 20-min period suggests a migrainous etiology. Occasionally, the patient will recall no visual symptoms while the optician notes a yellowish plaque within the retinal vessels (the Hollenhorst plaque). These are frequently derived from cholesterol embolization from the carotid bifurcation and warrant further investigation. Additionally, several ocular symptoms may be caused by microembolization from the extracranial carotid diseases including monocular visual loss due to retinal artery/optic nerve ischemia, the ocular ischemia syndrome, and visual field deficits secondary to cortical infarction and ischemia of the optic tracts. Typical motor and/or sensory symptoms associated with cerebrovascular accidents are lateralized or focal neurological deficit. Ischemic events tend to have an abrupt onset with the severity of the insult being apparent from the onset and not usually associated with seizures or paresthesia. In contrast, they represent loss or diminution of neurological function. Furthermore, motor or sensory deficits can be unilateral or bilateral with the upper and lower limbs being variably affected depending on the site of the cerebral lesion. The combination of a motor and sensory deficit in the same body territory is suggestive of a cortical thrombo-embolic event as opposed to lacunar lesions secondary to small vessel disease of the penetrating arterioles. However, a small proportion of the latter may present with a sensorimotor stroke secondary to small vessel occlusion within the posterior limb of the internal capsule. Pure sensory and pure motor strokes and those strokes where the weakness affects one limb only or does not involve the face are more typically seen with lacunar as opposed to cortical infarction. A number of higher cortical functions, including speech and language disturbances, can be affected by thrombo-embolic phenomena from the carotid artery, with the most important clinical example for the dominant hemisphere being dysphasia/aphasia and visuospatial neglect being an example of nondominant hemisphere injury.

Diagnosis

The most important tool in the diagnosis of carotid artery disease is a careful history of the patient and complete neurological examination, which should localize the area of cerebral ischemia responsible for the neurologic deficit. The neurologic examination of the patient should be complemented by a complete physical examination to determine the presence of vascular occlusive disease in either the coronary or peripheral arteries as well as to define the other risk factors for stroke, such as acute arrhythmia. The diagnosis of carotid bifurcation disease is facilitated by the relatively superficial location of the carotid artery, rendering it accessible to auscultation and palpation. The cervical carotid pulse is usually normal in patients with carotid bifurcation disease, since the common carotid artery is the only palpable vessel in the neck and is rarely diseased. Carotid bifurcation bruits may be heard just anterior to the sternocleidomastoid muscle near the angle of the mandible. Bruits do not become audible until the stenosis is severe enough to reduce the luminal diameter by at least 50%. Bruits may be absent in extremely severe lesions because of the extreme reduction of flow across the stenosis.

The utility of noninvasive carotid imaging modalities has provided more accurate information regarding the nature and severity of the carotid artery lesion. Color-flow duplex scanning uses real-time B-mode ultrasound and color-enhanced pulsed Doppler flow measurements to determine the extent of the carotid stenosis with reliable sensitivity and specificity. Real-time B-mode imaging permits localization of the disease and determination of the presence or absence of calcification within the plaque. Determination of the extent of stenosis is based largely on velocity criteria. As the stenosis increasingly obliterates the lumen of the vessel, the velocity of blood must increase in the area of the stenosis so that the total volume of flow remains constant within the vessel. Thus, the velocity is correlated with the extent of carotid artery stenosis (Table 5.1). The internal carotid artery velocity profile is one of a low-resistance artery characterized by a significant period of carotid blood flow during diastole. In contrast, the external carotid artery reflects a signal typically found in a high-resistance artery, in which little blood flow occurs during diastole. Standard color-flow duplex scans cannot assess the cerebral arterial circulation beyond the first several centimeters of the internal carotid artery. A transcranial Doppler has been developed to evaluate the middle cerebral artery and other intracranial vessels, using a low-frequency Doppler signal to penetrate the thin bone of the temporal and occipital regions.

Magnetic resonance (MR) imaging and MR angiography have been evaluated as a means of imaging the carotid arteries (Figure 5.1). These are highly sensitive imaging tools for the evaluation of patients with symptomatic cerebrovascular disease. MR imaging is more sensitive than computed

Table 5.1 Commonly used carotid duplex velocity and Doppler waveform criteria for determination of luminal stenosis of the internal carotid artery.

Stenosis (%)	Peak systolic velocity (cm/s)	End diastolic velocity (cm/s)	Spectral broadening
<30	<120	Any value	Minimal or absent
30–49	<120	Any value	Present
50–79	>120	<140	Present
80–99	>120	>140	Present

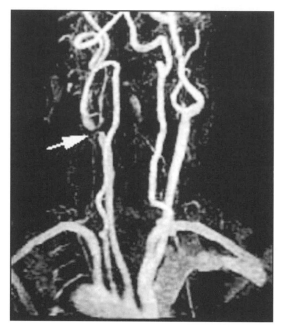

Figure 5.1 MR angiography of the bilateral carotid arteries and aortic arch. A high-grade stenosis is noted in the right carotid internal carotid artery (arrow).

tomography (CT) scanning for the detection of an acute stroke. MR imaging can detect a stroke immediately after the infarction occurs, whereas CT scanning cannot. MR angiography, which is evolving rapidly, permits evaluation of both the extracranial and intracranial cerebral circulations. The precision of MR angiography in determining the extent of stenosis, although improving rapidly, remains inferior to that achieved by conventional angiography. Nonetheless, MR angiography will likely play an increasingly important role in the diagnostic evaluation of patients with cerebrovascular disease.

Carotid angiography has been the traditional diagnostic tool for the evaluation of cerebrovascular disease. However, fewer hospitals now perform routine contrast angiography on all patients prior to surgery. This is partly because of the potential for angiographic-related complications as well as improved diagnostic accuracy of noninvasive imaging modalities. Angiography remains the only method that allows complete and detailed visualization of both the intracranial and extracranial arterial circulations. Complications associated with angiography include dye allergy, renal toxicity, particularly in patients with diabetes mellitus; chronic renal insufficiency; and neurologic complications, such as stroke, which range from 1–3%.[3]

Indications for intervention

Since operative intervention of carotid occlusive disease, or carotid endarterectomy, was first described in 1963 as a treatment strategy for stroke prevention,[4] this operation has been subjected to intense scrutiny to determine its clinical durability in various large-scale prospective randomized clinical trials. Presently, carotid endarterectomy is indicated for treatment of patients with hemispheric TIAs and stroke associated with carotid bifurcation occlusive disease. In addition, prophylactic carotid endarterectomy for asymptomatic patients with high-grade stenosis or complex ulcerated plaques is indicated. A brief overview of three important clinical trials, including the European Carotid Surgery Trial (ECST), the North American Symptomatic Carotid Endarterectomy Trial (NASCET), and the Asymptomatic Carotid Atherosclerosis Study (ACAS), will be discussed below.

Overview of ECST and NASCET

The benefit of carotid endarterectomy for patients with symptomatic cerebrovascular disease has recently been established by both the ECST and NASCET trials. These studies, randomized nearly 6000 patients in 200 hospitals around the world comparing "best medical therapy" against "best medical therapy" plus carotid endarterectomy. These studies documented a significant reduction in cerebrovascular events following the procedure compared with patients managed medically. Both trials showed that carotid endarterectomy conferred significant benefit in symptomatic patients with a 70–99% stenosis.[5–8] Although the NASCET trial observed a small but significant benefit in patients with 50–69% stenoses, the ECST trial found no evidence of benefit in patients with lesser degrees of the disease. The reason for these apparent discrepancies lies in the method for calculating degree of stenosis. ECST compared the residual luminal diameter against the diameter of the carotid artery at the level of the stenosis (usually the carotid bulb). NASCET compared the residual luminal diameter against the diameter of the internal carotid artery (ICA) at least 1 cm above the stenosis. As a consequence, ECST tends to systematically overestimate stenoses (as compared with NASCET), particularly in those with mild/moderate disease. In reality, a 60% NASCET stenosis is approximately equivalent to a 80% ECST.[7,8]

The ECST and NASCET trials have identified predictive factors that are associated with a significantly higher risk of late stroke in medically treated patients. These include; male sex, 90–94% stenosis, surface irregularity/ulceration, coexistent intracranial disease, no recruitment of intracranial collaterals, hemispheric symptoms, cerebral events within 2 months, multiple cerebral events, contralateral occlusion, multiple concurrent risk factors, and age >75 years.[5,7,8]

Overview of ACAS

The ACAS trial was a prospective study that randomized 1600 patients with asymptomatic stenosis of 60% or greater to either carotid endarterectomy and aspirin or aspirin alone.[9] This study was interrupted because of a significant benefit identified in patients undergoing carotid endarterectomy. At the time of interruption of the study, a relative reduction in stroke rate by 50% was observed by patients undergoing carotid endarterectomy. The benefit was much greater in men than women. This study used stroke as its primary endpoint. This group has since substantiated unequivocally the effectiveness of carotid endarterectomy in good-risk patients identified to have high-grade stenosis.

These prospective trials firmly established the role of carotid endarterectomy in the prevention of strokes in patients with high-grade carotid artery stenosis, regardless whether the lesion is symptomatic or asymptomatic. All the patients in these clinical trials were carefully selected, and the carotid endarterectomy was performed by surgeons with proven success and low complication rates. For patients with carotid occlusive disease to benefit from surgical intervention, the operation must be performed by experienced surgeons with proven low operative morbidity and mortality.

Carotid angioplasty and stenting

With the rapid advancement in endovascular therapy, carotid artery stenting has been shown to be safe and efficacious in the treatment of carotid occlusive disease in high-risk patients.[10–12] A recent consensus statement from the American Heart Association (AHA) highlighted that carotid stenting should only be offered to limited subgroups of patients, whereas the traditional carotid endarterectomy should remain the standard treatment in patients with carotid occlusive disease.[13] Similarly, a multidisplinary physician panel recently published a consensus statement advocating that carotid stenting should be reserved in specific subgroups of patients with carotid occlusive lesions. Briefly, they include various anatomical considerations, which include high carotid bifurcation (>C2 level), contralateral carotid occlusion, presence of tracheostomy, history of ipsilateral neck irradiation, prior radical neck dissection, or carotid endarterectomy. Moreover, the high-risk criteria include patients with one or more medical comorbidities, such as those with myocardial infarction or stroke in the previous 3 months. High-risk pulmonary dysfunction includes patients with steroid-dependent chronic obstructive pulmonary disease, or measured forced expiratory volume in 1 s less than 30% of predicted or less than 1 L/s. Lastly, high-risk cardiac dysfunction includes those with a left ventricular ejection fraction less than 30% (documented heart failure, stage 3 or 4 of the New York Heart Association classification).

The perceived advantages of carotid stenting over endarterectomy are largely related to its less invasiveness, since a percutaneous stenting procedure can potentially reduce patient anxiety that is commonly associated with a surgical procedure. However, one potential complication of carotid stenting that may have impeded the wide acceptance of this endovascular procedure is distal cerebral embolization. This phenomenon can occur as a result of catheter manipulation in a plaque-laden carotid bifurcation due to either balloon angioplasty or stent deployment.[14] Several clinical studies have implicated that distal embolization as a cause of perioperative stroke following carotid stenting.[15–17]

Techniques of carotid stenting

While carotid artery stenting can be performed successfully using a variety of catheter-based techniques, we describe herein a technical protocol routinely used in our clinical practice.

The patient is admitted on the day of the procedure and consented for arch aortic and carotid angiography with possible stent placement, in the event that a high-grade carotid stenosis is both present and anatomically suitable. The patient is given clopidogrel (Plavix, 75 mg/day) and aspirin (81 mg/day) beginning 3 days prior to the intervention. The carotid stenting procedure can be performed either in an angiosuite or an operating room using a mobile C-arm unit. Intravenous antibiotic (cephazollin, 1 gm) is given 30 min before the procedure. Neurological status of the patient is monitored after each step of the procedure. Throughout the intervention, continuous electrocardiogram with monitoring of the heart rate and blood pressure is done.

Local anesthesia with 1% lidocaine is used to anesthetize the groin region followed by percutaneous cannulation of the common femoral artery. Following the placement of a 6 Fr introducer sheath, an aortic arch angiogram in the left anterior oblique (LAO) projection using a pigtail catheter with power injection is performed. The diagnostic angiography consists of visualization of the origins of the brachiocephalic arteries from the aortic arch, both carotid bifurcations in several projections, both vertebral arteries, and intracranial study of both carotid arteries and dominant vertebral artery.

Selective cannulation of the carotid artery is performed using a 5 Fr diagnostic catheter (SIM2, JB2, H1, or vertebral catheter, Boston Scientific, Natick, MA) followed by advancement of a 0.035-in. Bentson guidewire into the proximal common carotid artery. Carotid angiogram is performed to assess the carotid anatomy. Once the decision to perform stenting is confirmed based on the carotid angiogram, intravenous (IV) bivalirudin bolus (0.75 mg/kg) followed by an infusion rate of 2.5 mg/kg/h is given, which is maintained throughout the procedure. With direct catheter selection of the common carotid artery, a 0.038 in. 260-cm long stiff glidewire is used to cannulate the ipsilateral external carotid artery. Next, the diagnostic catheter is withdrawn and a 7 Fr 90-cm shuttle sheath (Boston Scientific) is advanced into the common carotid artery over the stiff glidewire. Care must be taken not to advance the 90 cm shuttle sheath beyond the carotid bulb. The tracking of the guiding sheath over the guidewire in the common carotid artery is greatly facilitated by positioning the guidewire in the external carotid artery.

Selective digital carotid angiogram is performed via the sideport of the shuttle sheath to delineate the anatomy of the common, internal, and external carotid arteries. Biplanar intracranial injections are also performed to document cerebral vasculature. The Amplatz guidewire is next replaced with a 0.018-in. guidewire system with distal embolization device, which is used to cross the internal carotid lesion. Following the activation of the embolization device, a coaxial 4-mm by 4-cm angioplasty balloon is used to predilate the carotid lesion.

We prefer to use the monorail self-expanding stent (Wallstent by Boston Scientific, PRECISE nitinol stent by Cordis, or ACCULINK nitinol stent by Guidant) that is deployed across the internal carotid stenosis with proximal attachment in the distal common carotid artery. Poststenting balloon angioplasty may be performed using angioplasty balloon less than 5.5 mm in diameter depending on the appearance of the completion angiogram (Figure 5.2). Completion angiography includes biplanar carotid and cerebral views to document vascular anatomy and exclude cerebral thromboembolism.

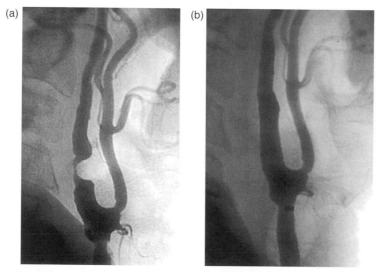

(a)　　　　(b)

Figure 5.2 Angiograms performing during an aortid artery stenting procedure. (a) Prestenting angiogram demonstrating a high-grade stenosis of the left internal carotid artery. (b) Completion angiogram demonstrating a satisfactory result following a Wallstent placement.

The poststenting balloon angiogram is perhaps the time when greatest amount of debris are embolizing to the cerebral circulation. To reduce this potential complication, several important technical principles must be kept in mind when performing poststenting balloon angioplasty: (1) use balloons that are no larger than 5.5 mm in diameter; (2) inflate the balloon to nominal, not beyond 4 atm pressures, and deflate slowly, and (3) accept a 10–15% residual stenosis, because this does not cause hemodynamic problems. In addition, the self-expanding stents have the tendency for progressive expansion, particularly if the stent is oversized appropriately.

The cerebral embolization protection device is deactivated, and the guidewire along with the shuttle sheath are next removed. The groin puncture site is closed with a 6 Fr femoral closure device (Perclose). The patient is to continue with oral clopidogrel for 1 month and aspirin therapy indefinitely.

Cerebral protection during carotid stenting

Despite reports of the relative safety of the carotid artery stenting procedure,[18–20] general concerns exist regarding the potential for neurological deficit as a result of embolic particles released from the carotid plaque during carotid balloon angioplasty and stenting procedure.[14,21] A study by Ohki and colleagues confirmed this phenomenon using an *ex vivo* model with human carotid plaques collected from carotid endarterectomy procedures.[14] The authors demonstrated that embolic particles were consistently produced from all plaques following stent placement.

In a transcranial Doppler study, which evaluated signals of cerebral embolization, Jordan and colleagues noted a mean of 7.4 emboli per stenosis with four neurological events among 40 patients undergoing carotid stenting procedure (10%).[17] In contrast, patients undergoing carotid endarterectomy had a mean of 8.8 emboli per stenosis with one neurological deficit among 75 patients (1.3%). The mean number of cerebral emboli was 56.8 in patients with neurologic deficit and 31.2 in those without ($p < 0.02$). The authors concluded that cerebral embolization was the predominant cause of acute neurological complications associated with carotid stenting.

The abundance of clinical evidence regarding the risk of neurological complication due to catheter-based carotid intervention has prompted many physicians to advocate routine use of distal protection devices to prevent cerebral embolization. Early studies have confirmed that significant amounts of embolic particles were routinely captured by the distal protection devices during carotid stenting.[22,23] In a carotid stenting study that utilized the PercuSurge GuardWire system (Medtronic, Minneapolis, MN) to prevent cerebral embolization, the number of embolic particles retrieved per patient ranged from 22 to 667 and a mean particle diameter was 203 ± 256 μm.[24]

Although no clinical study currently exists that proves embolization protection devices definitively reduces neurological sequelae due to carotid stenting, its benefit in improving clinical outcome in coronary intervention was recently

Table 5.2 Cerebral protection devices designed for carotid stenting.

Mechanisms of Cerebral Protection	Devices
Proximal balloon occlusion	Kachel balloon ArteriaA Parodi Antiembolization Catheter (ArteriA, San Francisco, CA)
Distal balloon occlusion	Henry-Amor balloon PercuSurg Guardwire (Medtronic, Sunnyvale, CA) Theron balloon
Distal carotid filter	ACCUNET (Guidant, Indianapolis, IN) Angioguard (Cordis, Warren, NJ) Bate floating filter (ArteriA, San Francisco, CA) Captura (Boston Scientific Corp., Natick, MA) Carotid Trap (Microvena, White Bear Lake, MN) E-Trap (Metamorphic Surgical Devices, Pittsburgh, PA) Filterwire (Embolic Protection Inc., San Carlos, CA) NeuroShield (MedNova, Inc., Galway, Ireland)

highlighted in the Saphenous Vein Graft Angioplasty Free of Emboli Randomized Trial (SAFER).[25] This was a prospective randomized study that evaluated 550 patients with stenotic saphenous vein graft following coronary artery bypass grafting (CABG) to either PercuSurge GuardWire-protected percutaneous transluminal coronary angioplasty (PTCA) or unprotected coronary intervention. The 30-day myocardial ischemic rate was 8.4% in the PercuSurge-protected group, in contrast to the 16.5% in the unprotected control group ($p < 0.01$). As the result of the clinical benefit demonstrated in the trial, the distal protection device is currently considered the standard of care in patients undergoing PTCA for high-grade coronary saphenous vein graft stenosis.

A variety of designs for cerebral protection devices currently exists in an effort to reduce distal embolization during carotid stenting procedures. Regardless of the device configuration, these devices can be grouped into three categories based on mechanisms by which the device prevents distal cerebral embolization, and they include (1) proximal balloon occlusion, (2) distal balloon occlusion, and (3) distal filter protection. Table 5.2 summarizes various cerebral protection devices based on these three protective mechanisms.

Proximal balloon occlusion devices

In devices that rely on the proximal occlusion principle, the common carotid flow is occluded using an occluding balloon attached to the guiding catheter that creates a reversal of flow in the internal carotid artery (Figure 5.3). Embolic particles released during carotid stenting are aspirated via the guiding catheter to prevent cerebral embolization. This proximal protection system provides cerebral protection before the passage of any type of device through

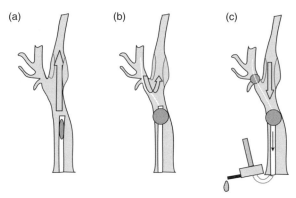

Figure 5.3 ArteriaA Parodi protection device is an example of a proximal balloon occlusion system that creates balloon occlusions in the external and common carotid arteries. This results in a reversal of flow in the internal carotid artery. Blood aspirated from the common carotid artery sheath is then filtered and returned to the circulation through a venous catheter.

the carotid stenosis, which potentially minimizes the likelihood of device-related cerebral embolization. These systems consist of a long introducer sheath with a balloon that is inflated in the common carotid artery. A second balloon, inflated in the external carotid artery, ensures the total blockade of the antegrade blood flow in the internal carotid artery. Proximal protection systems use the cerebral vascular connections of the circle of Willis. After occlusion of the common and external carotid artery, the collateral flow through the circle of Willis will create so-called backpressure, which will prevent antegrade flow in the internal carotid artery. After stent positioning, and before the deflation of the balloons in the common and external carotid artery, the blood present in the internal carotid artery – possibly containing dislodged debris – is aspirated and removed. The advantage of the proximal protection system is the fact that the entire procedure is carried out under protection and, if it is correctly applied, it should completely avoid any type of embolization. The disadvantages of the proximal protection system are that it is not tolerated by all patients, and a larger 10 Fr introducer sheath is typically required.

Distal balloon occlusion devices

In devices that use the distal balloon occlusion approach, an occlusion balloon attached to a guidewire is used to occlude the flow in the distal internal carotid artery (Figure 5.4). Embolic materials generated during carotid stenting are trapped by the distal balloon, which are removed by an aspiration catheter at the completion of the stenting procedure. This system consists of a 0.014-in. guide with a balloon on the distal portion that may be inflated and deflated through a very small channel contained in the guide itself (Percusurge/Guardwire, Medtronic Vascular, Santa Rosa, CA). The lesion is crossed with the guide, thereby positioning the balloon distally to the stenosis where it is inflated until the blood flow in the internal carotid artery is blocked.

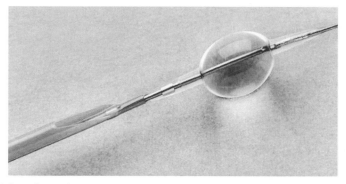

Figure 5.4 PercuSurge device is an example of the distal balloon occlusion device. The device captures potential embolic materials by the occluding balloon, which is placed distal to the carotid lesion.

Angioplasty and stenting are then performed. Once the procedure is completed, a catheter is advanced up to the distal balloon and the column of blood contained in the occluded internal carotid artery is aspirated. In this way, debris dislodged during the stent procedure is eliminated. The balloon is then deflated and the guide is removed. The advantages of distal occlusive balloons are their small diameter (less than 3 Fr crossing profile) and the good manoeuverability and flexibility of the system. Possible disadvantages are that the occlusion is not tolerated by 6–10% of patients and it is not possible to image the vessel with contrast medium during the inflation.[26]

Distal filter protection devices

In devices that incorporate a distal filter, cerebral protection is accomplished by trapping embolic particles in a temporary filter deployed during the carotid stenting procedure (Figure 5.5). Distal filter protection device consists of a metallic skeleton that is coated by a membrane of polyethylene or a net of nitinol wires that contain 80–200 mm diameter holes.[20] The filters are usually positioned at the distal portion of a 0.014-in. guide. During the procedure, the filters are enveloped into a delivery catheter in which they are advanced distally to the stenosis (Figure 5.6). After the lesion is crossed, the filter is opened by removing the delivery sheath. At the end of the stenting procedure, the filter is closed with use of a retrieval catheter, and the filter is removed from the carotid artery. In the presence of sharp stenoses from calcific or very fibrous plaques, passage of the closed filter may be impossible. Possible complications of the filter are vasospasm or no-flow due to occlusion of the pores by material embolized into the filter. Both complications, generally resolve after the removal of the filter device. A number of second- and third-generation protection filters exist. The technical characteristics of a good protection filter consist of a low profile (<3 Fr), an adequate torqueability to cross tortuous vessels, and when open, adequate apposition to the wall to ensure the best possible protection.

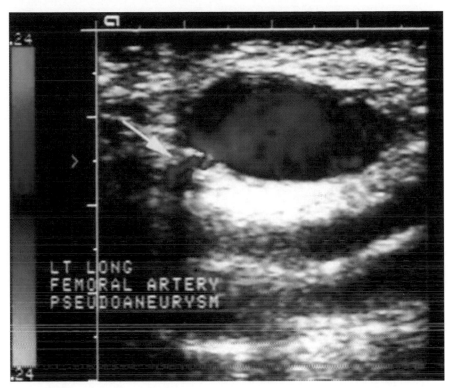

Plate 1 Duplex examination of pseudoaneurysm showing tract from the femoral artery into the pseudoaneurysm cavity.

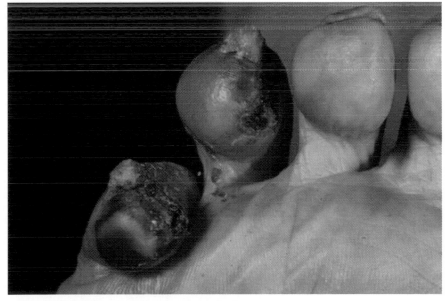

Plate 2 Toe ischemia as a result of distal embolization.

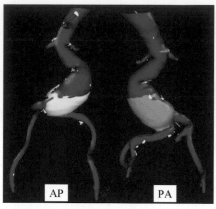

Plate 3 Compound angulation of the proximal aortic neck.

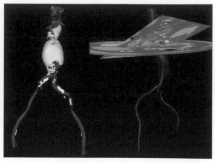

Plate 4 CT scan with 3-D reconstruction with center-line path and embedded orthogonal cut.

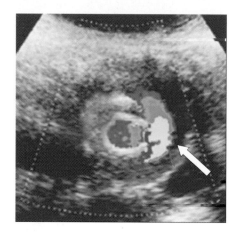

Plate 5 An abdominal duplex ultrasound demonstrates an endoleak as evidenced by the perigraft contrast flow (arrow).

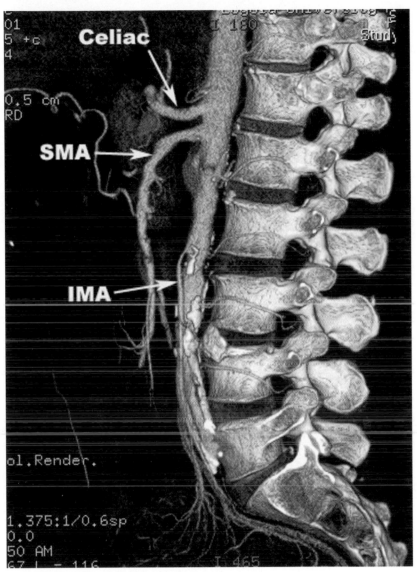

Plate 6 CT angiogram of the abdomen with 3-D reconstruction provides a clear view of the CA, SMA, and IMA.

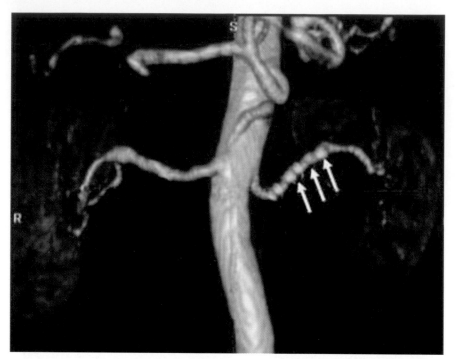

Plate 7 MRA of the abdominal aorta revealed the presence of a left renal artery fibromuscular dysplasia (arrows).

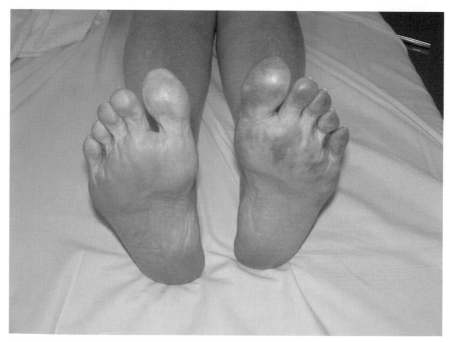

Plate 8 Stent-related restenosis can cause distal embolization resulting in the blue toe syndrome.

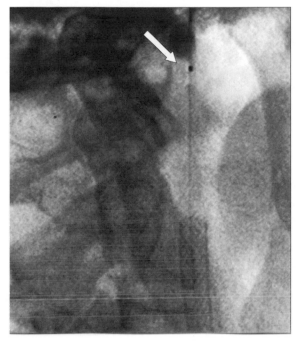

Figure 5.5 Intraoperative fluoroscopic view of the FilterWire distal protection device with a radio opaque marker (arrow) distal to the carotid stent.

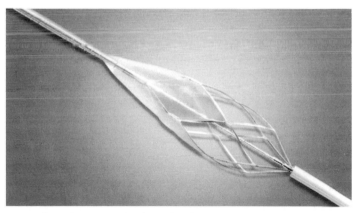

Figure 5.6 AngioGuard is an example of the distal filter protection device. It provides cerebral protection during carotid stenting by trapping embolic materials within the filter.

Results of clinical trials

Several recent studies have demonstrated a comparable clinical outcome of endovascular carotid intervention with carotid endarterectomy. Several important randomized prospective trials are summarized further.

Carotid and vertebral artery transluminal angioplasty study

As one of the early clinical investigations evaluating the efficacy of percutaneous carotid intervention, the Carotid and Vertebral Artery Transluminal Angioplasty Study (CAVATAS) evaluated patients with high-grade carotid stenosis undergoing intervention consisting of either carotid endarterectomy or balloon angioplasty.[27] The trial randomized 251 patients with high-grade carotid stenosis to balloon angioplasty and 253 cohort patients to endarterectomy.[27] The incidence of 30-day disabling stroke or death was similar between the endovascular and surgical groups, which were 6.4% and 5.9%, respectively. The overall stroke and death also remained similar between the two groups, which were 10.0% and 9.9%, respectively.[27] One significant finding from this study was a markedly reduced operative morbidity, such as cranial nerve palsy in the endovascular groups, which occurred in 8.7% in the endarterectomy groups while none in the endovascular group.

This prospective randomized study found that both treatment modalities had similar clinical outcomes after 3 years of follow-up even though the rate of severe restenosis is higher in the endovascular group (14% versus 4%) at 1-year follow-up. These findings were remarkable considering that no carotid distal embolization protection devices were available at the time of this clinical trial.

Stenting and angioplasty with protection in patients at high risk for endarterectomy trial

The Stenting and Angioplasty with Protection in Patients at High Risk for Endarterectomy (SAPPHIRE) trial is a prospective, randomized multicenter trial of carotid endarterectomy versus carotid artery stenting in high surgical risk patients.[28,29] The study, which employed the SMART nitinol stent and the AngioGuard emboli protection device (Johnson & Johnson, Cordis, Warren, NJ), enrolled 747 patients from 29 hospitals who were either asymptomatic with greater than 80% carotid stenosis or symptomatic with greater than 50% stenosis. Among the enrolled patients, 334 patients underwent randomization of 413, who were assigned to treatment. The study found that patients who were randomized to the carotid stenting with distal protection devices had a significantly lower rate of perioperative major events (death, stroke, or myocardial infarction) compared with patients randomized to endarterectomy (4.4% and 9.9% respectively). However, when comparing the rate of stroke alone, there is no significant difference between the two groups (3.1% and 3.3%, respectively), while patients who underwent carotid stent had significant decreased incidence of postoperative myocardial infarction comparing to endarterectomy (1.9% and 6.6%, respectively).[28,29] This trial confirms carotid stent with distal protection device is not inferior to the endarterectomy.

In parallel stenting and endarterectomy registries for 413 patients, who could not be randomized in the trial, 406 patients were enrolled in a stent registry and 7 patients in a surgical registry. The 30-day major adverse cardiac event rate was 7.8% in the stent group, in contrast to 14.3% in those who were enrolled in the endarterectomy registry. The study found a significantly improved short-term perioperative stroke and death rate in the stenting group when compared to the endarterectomy patients.[28,30] Researchers attributed this remarkable finding to the improved stent design as well as the use of routine cerebral protection devices.[28,30]

Carotid revascularization endarterectomy versus stent trial

Carotid Revascularization Endarterectomy versus Stent Trial (CREST) is jointly sponsored by Guidant Corporation (Indianapolis, IN) and the NIH.[31,32] The study will randomize symptomatic patients, who are at low surgical risk to either stenting or endarterectomy. The inclusion criteria are similar to the NASCET study. This study utilizes the ACCULINK nitinol stent (Guidant, Ternacula, CA) as well as the ACCUNET emboli prevention device (Guidant). The primary outcome events will include: (1) any stroke, myocardial infarction, or death during the 30-day perioperative or periprocedural period, or (2) ipsilateral stroke after 30 days. The trial is expected to enroll 2500 patients and be completed by 2007.

ACCULINK for revascularization for carotids in high risk patient registry (ARCHER) trial

This multicenter study conducted in both Europe and the United States involving 581 consecutive patients in three single arm trials is still ongoing. The results have been presented in the annual meetings of Society of Interventional Radiology and American College of Cardiology. This trial is sponsored by Guidant Corporation using ACCULINK stent and ACCUNET distal protection device in high-risk symptomatic patients with more than 50% stenosis or asymptomatic patients with over 80% stenosis. The ARCHeR 1 trial used just the stent, the ARCHeR 2 trial included the stent plus embolic protection, and the ARCHeR 3 trial used a newer version of the catheters for delivering the stent and embolic filter, which utilizes the rapid exchange system. The preliminary date showed that the 30-day adverse event rate counting all strokes, deaths, or heart attacks were 7.6, 8.6, and 8.3% for ARCHeR 1, 2, and 3 trials respectively. The incidence of major stroke or death in the first 30 days was remarkably low in all trials, and they were 3.8, 2.5, and 2.8%, for ARCHeR 1, 2, and 3 trials respectively.

Complications of carotid artery stenting

Although carotid percutaneous intervention is relatively safe, procedure-related complications that are specific to carotid angioplasty and stent have been reported particularly distal embolization, intraoperative hypotension and bradycardia, and restenosis.

The risk of cerebral embolization due to carotid intervention was underscored in CAVATAS trial, which compared the safety and efficacy of carotid endarterectomy with carotid balloon angioplasty, with and without stenting.[33] The study reported that a mean of 202±119 high-intensity embolization signals were produced during the carotid balloon angioplasty procedure, in contrast to a mean of 52 ± 64 high-intensity embolization signals produced during a carotid endarterectomy ($p < 0.05$).[33] The Leicester trial, which was another prospective randomized multicenter trial that compared the efficacy of carotid stenting versus endarterectomy, similarly reported that more cerebral embolization events occurred following carotid stenting than endarterectomy.[34] This trial was stopped because of the unacceptably high stroke death rate following carotid stenting (71%) compared with endarterectomy (0%) following the enrollment of only 17 patients. The neurological events due to stent-related cerebral embolization was illustrated by a recent study in which patients underwent diffusion-weighted MRI (DW-MRI) of the brain before and after carotid artery stenting.[35] Jaeger and colleagues analyzed the incidence of silent embolic cerebral infarctions in 67 patients with high-grade carotid stenosis with DW-MRI, and found new ipsilateral ischemic lesions that occurred after stent implantation in 29% of patients ($n = 20$).[35] This study further underscored the clinical presence of cerebral embolization due to carotid intervention.

Although bradycardia is frequently encountered during the carotid angioplasty and stent procedure, hemodynamic instability rarely develops. A retrospective single-center study analyzed 471 patients undergoing carotid stenting and found 7% patients developed severe hypotension and/or bradycardia despite routine premedication with atropine and adequate fluid balance.[36] The elderly patients and those with coronary diseases were at higher risk. Maintaining a good communication with the anesthesiologist and aggressive resuscitation are fundamental in reducing the risk of and preventing the complication of hemodynamic instability during the carotid procedure.

In-stent stenosis after carotid stenting has been demonstrated by several studies. Chakhtoura and associates reported 8% high-grade restentosis rate during their 18-month follow-up of 50 carotid stent procedures.[37] Similarly, Lal et al. performed 122 carotid stenting procedures and reported 5 year clinical significant in-stent stenosis of 6.4%.[38] Willfort-Ehringer and colleagues prospectively evaluated 125 carotid stent procedures using ultrasonography and demonstrated that the diameters of the self-expanding stents steadily increased over 2 years and the neointimal thickness increased up to 12 months, then stabilized thereafter.[39] They thus postulated that the neointimal proliferation prevails up to 12 month, which may give rise to rare stent recurrent stenosis. Stent expansion reduces this effect in the first year, and dominates in the second year. This might contribute to the good mid-term outcome of carotid stenting. As demonstrated by multiple studies, stent restenosis occurs not infrequently, and routine post-procedure evaluation is essential in identifying the hemodynamically significant stenosis and those patients that require reintervention.

References

1 Ingall T. Stroke – incidence, mortality, morbidity and risk. *J Insur Med* 2004; **36**:143–52.

2 O'Rourke F, Dean N, Akhtar N, Shuaib A. Current and future concepts in stroke prevention. *Cmaj* 2004; **170**:1123–33.

3 Willinsky RA, Taylor SM, TerBrugge K, Farb RI, Tomlinson G, Montanera W. Neurologic complications of cerebral angiography: prospective analysis of 2899 procedures and review of the literature. *Radiology* 2003; **227**:522–28.

4 Debakey ME, Crawford ES, Cooley DA, Morris GC, Jr., Garret HE, Fields WS. Cerebral Arterial Insufficiency: One to 11-Year Results Following Arterial Reconstructive Operation. *Ann Surg* 1965; **161**:921–45.

5 Coyne TJ, Wallace MC. Surgical referral for carotid artery stenosis – the influence of NASCET. North American Symptomatic Carotid Endarterectomy Trial. *Can J Neurol Sci* 1994; **21**:129–32.

6 Chang YJ, Golby AJ, Albers GW. Detection of carotid stenosis. From NASCET results to clinical practice. *Stroke* 1995; **26**:1325–28.

7 Naylor AR, Rothwell PM, Bell PR. Overview of the principal results and secondary analyses from the European and North American randomised trials of endarterectomy for symptomatic carotid stenosis. *Eur J Vasc Endovasc Surg* 2003; **26**:115–29.

8 Gasecki AP, Hachinski VC, Mendel T, Barnett HT. Endarterectomy for symptomatic carotid stenosis. Review of the European and North American Symptomatic Carotid Surgery Trials. *Nebr Med J* 1992; **77**:121–23.

9 Moore WS, Barnett HJ, Beebe HG, et al. Guidelines for carotid endarterectomy. A multidisciplinary consensus statement from the Ad Hoc Committee, American Heart Association. *Circulation* 1995; **91**:566–79.

10 Domenig C, Hamdan AD, Belfield AK, et al. Recurrent stenosis and contralateral occlusion: high-risk situations in carotid endarterectomy? *Ann Vasc Surg* 2003; **17**:622–28.

11 Hobson RW, 2nd, Lal BK, Chakhtoura E, et al. Carotid artery stenting: analysis of data for 105 patients at high risk. *J Vasc Surg* 2003; 37:1234–39.

12 Lin PH, Bush RL, Lubbe DF, et al. Carotid artery stenting with routine cerebral protection in high-risk patients. *Am J Surg* 2004; **188**:644–52.

13 Bettmann MA, Katzen BT, Whisnant J, et al. Carotid stenting and angioplasty: a statement for healthcare professionals from the Councils on Cardiovascular Radiology, Stroke, Cardio-Thoracic and Vascular Surgery, Epidemiology and Prevention, and Clinical Cardiology, American Heart Association. *Stroke* 1998; **29**:336–38.

14 Ohki T, Marin ML, Lyon RT, et al. Ex vivo human carotid artery bifurcation stenting: correlation of lesion characteristics with embolic potential. *J Vasc Surg* 1998; **27**: 463–71.

15 Gil-Peralta A, Gonzalez A, Gonzalez-Marcos JR, et al. Internal carotid artery stenting in patients with symptomatic atheromatous pseudoocclusion. *Cerebrovasc Dis* 2004; **17**: 105–12.

16 Mas JL, Chatellier G, Beyssen B. Carotid angioplasty and stenting with and without cerebral protection: clinical alert from the Endarterectomy Versus Angioplasty in Patients With Symptomatic Severe Carotid Stenosis (EVA-3S) trial. *Stroke* 2004; **35**: e18–20.

17 Jordan WD, Jr., Voellinger DC, Doblar DD, Plyushcheva NP, Fisher WS, McDowell HA. Microemboli detected by transcranial Doppler monitoring in patients during carotid angioplasty versus carotid endarterectomy. *Cardiovasc Surg* 1999; **7**:33–38.

18 Stankovic G, Liistro F, Moshiri S, *et al.* Carotid artery stenting in the first 100 consecutive patients: results and follow up. *Heart* 2002; **88**:381–86.

19 Ischinger TA. Carotid stenting: which stent for which lesion? *J Interv Cardiol* 2001; **14**:617–23.

20 Al-Mubarak N, Colombo A, Gaines PA, *et al.* Multicenter evaluation of carotid artery stenting with a filter protection system. *J Am Coll Cardiol* 2002; **39**:841–46.

21 DeMonte F, Peerless SJ, Rankin RN. Carotid transluminal angioplasty with evidence of distal embolization. Case report. *J Neurosurg* 1989; **70**:138–41.

22 Henry M, Amor M, Henry I, *et al.* Carotid stenting with cerebral protection: first clinical experience using the PercuSurge GuardWire system. *J Endovasc Surg* 1999; **6**: 321–31.

23 Criado FJ, Lingelbach JM, Ledesma DF, Lucas PR. Carotid artery stenting in a vascular surgery practice. *J Vasc Surg* 2002; **35**:430–34.

24 Whitlow PL, Lylyk P, Londero H, *et al.* Carotid artery stenting protected with an emboli containment system. *Stroke* 2002; **33**:1308–14.

25 Baim DS, Wahr D, George B, *et al.* Randomized trial of a distal embolic protection device during percutaneous intervention of saphenous vein aorto-coronary bypass grafts. *Circulation* 2002; **105**:1285–90.

26 Al-Mubarak N, Roubin GS, Vitek JJ, Iyer SS, New G, Leon MB. Effect of the distal-balloon protection system on microembolization during carotid stenting. *Circulation* 2001; **104**:1999–2002.

27 Endovascular versus surgical treatment in patients with carotid stenosis in the Carotid and Vertebral Artery Transluminal Angioplasty Study (CAVATAS): a randomised trial. *Lancet* 2001; **357**:1729–37.

28 Yadav JS. Carotid stenting in high-risk patients: design and rationale of the SAPPHIRE trial. *Cleve Clin J Med* 2004; **71** :S45–46.

29 Yadav JS, Wholey MH, Kuntz RE, *et al.* Protected carotid-artery stenting versus endarterectomy in high-risk patients. *N Engl J Med* 2004; **351**:1493–501.

30 Yadav JS. Study of Angioplasty with Protection in Patients at High Risk for Endarterectomy (SAPPHIRE) trial. Abstract presented at the American Heart Association meeting. Chicago, IL, 2002.

31 Hobson RW, 2nd. Update on the Carotid Revascularization Endarterectomy versus Stent Trial (CREST) protocol. *J Am Coll Surg* 2002; **194**:S9–14.

32 Hobson RW, 2nd, Howard VJ, Brott TG, Howard G, Roubin GS, Ferguson RD. Organizing the Carotid Revascularization Endarterectomy versus Stenting Trial (CREST): National Institutes of Health, Health Care Financing Administration, and industry funding. *Curr Control Trials Cardiovasc Med* 2001; **2**:160–64.

33 Crawley F, Stygall J, Lunn S, Harrison M, Brown MM, Newman S. Comparison of microembolism detected by transcranial Doppler and neuropsychological sequelae of carotid surgery and percutaneous transluminal angioplasty. *Stroke* 2000; **31**: 1329–34.

34 Naylor AR, Bolia A, Abbott RJ, *et al.* Randomized study of carotid angioplasty and stenting versus carotid endarterectomy: a stopped trial. *J Vasc Surg* 1998; **28**:326–34.

35 Jaeger HJ, Mathias KD, Hauth E, *et al.* Cerebral ischemia detected with diffusion-weighted MR imaging after stent implantation in the carotid artery. *AJNR Am J Neuroradiol* 2002; **23**:200–7.

36 Mlekusch W, Schillinger M, Sabeti S, *et al.* Hypotension and bradycardia after elective carotid stenting: frequency and risk factors. *J Endovasc Ther* 2003; **10**:851–59; discussion 860–61.

37 Chakhtoura EY, Hobson RW, 2nd, Goldstein J, *et al.* In-stent restenosis after carotid angioplasty-stenting: incidence and management. *J Vasc Surg* 2001; **33**:220–25; discussion 225–26.

38 Lal BK, Hobson RW, 2nd, Goldstein J, *et al.* In-stent recurrent stenosis after carotid artery stenting: life table analysis and clinical relevance. *J Vasc Surg* 2003; **38**:1162–68; discussion 1169.

39 Willfort-Ehringer A, Ahmadi R, Gruber D, *et al.* Arterial remodeling and hemodynamics in carotid stents: a prospective duplex ultrasound study over 2 years. *J Vasc Surg* 2004; **39**:728–34.

CHAPTER 6

Supra-aortic trunk and upper extremity arterial disease

Imran Mohiuddin, Eric J. Silberfein, Eric Peden

Arterial disease involving branches of the aortic arch and upper extremity vasculature have been described since the mid-nineteenth century.[1,2] The three branches of the aortic arch namely the innominate artery with its major branches, the right common carotid and the right subclavian, the left common carotid artery and the left subclavian artery are commonly referred to as the supra-aortic trunk. Aortic arch branch disease is defined as disease of these vessels resulting in flow-limiting stenosis or embolization of the brain or upper extremities. Although initial reports described inflammatory etiologies of the disease involving the supra-aortic trunk, more recently atherosclerosis has been defined as the most common cause of the disease in Western societies.[2] While the presence of the lesion alone represents an infrequent indication for operation, the incidence of this disease surpasses estimates with the majority of lesions being asymptomatic. The importance of the left internal mammary artery in coronary surgery has lent credence to attempts by some to prophylactically treat subclavian artery lesion.

Initial reports from the 1960s, described various types of open treatment for these lesions. Crawford was the first to report his 10 year experience with both extraanatomic and trans-sternal repair.[3] His preferred repair towards the end of his series was an extraanatomic approach because of decreased mortality. This extraanatomic approach soon became preferred owing to fewer complications. Many modern series have described excellent long-term patency rates combined with improved morbidity and mortality.[4,5]

With the evolution of vascular surgery to include endovascular procedures, physicians have debated regarding whether open or endovascular approach should be used as primary therapy. In 1981, the first report of retrograde balloon angioplasty of an innominate artery lesion was described.[6] Since then, many different endovascular treatments of the supra-aortic trunk have been reported.[7] While the long-term clinical data of endovascular interventions remains scarce, interventionalists should be familiar with the disease pattern and endovascular treatment modality of supra-aortic trunk and upper extremity arterial disease. In this chapter, the clinical features and endovascular therapy for disease involving the supra-aortic region is presented. Common problems and treatment complications of endovascular interventions are also discussed.

Etiology

The majority of arterial occlusive disease in the supra-aortic trunk and upper extremity tends to be atherosclerotic in nature. The pathophysiologic mechanisms of this disease involves the formation of atherosclerotic plaques with calcium deposition, thinning of the media, patchy destruction of muscle and elastic fibers, fragmentation of the internal elastic lamina, and thrombi composed of platelets and fibrin. Recent reports indicate an incidence of 70–100% of all trans-sternally treated occlusive lesions of the great vessels to be atherosclerotic in etiology.[5,8]

Atherosclerosis is also the most common cause of occlusive disease of the upper extremity arterial system. A report of 5000 patients from the joint study of extracranial arterial occlusion reported multiple vessel involvement including the upper extremity in nearly two-thirds of patients.[9] Due to the irregular nature of these plaques, embolic phenomenon can occur in as high as 30% of these patients.

Takayasu's arteritis is the next most common cause of arterial occlusive disease of the supra-aortic trunk in the United States, with the Mayo clinic series reporting a 22% incidence in patients requiring surgery.[10] Takayasu's arteritis results from an inflammatory reaction the exact etiology of which is unknown. Several hypothesis are present, the most common of which is an infectious agent. Most likely there is a multifactorial cause.[11] Initially, giant cells form within the media leading to destruction of its elastic fibers, which results in fibrosis. This fibrosis accounts for the long tapering stenotic lesions seen in this disease. Intimal damage can also lead to the development of atherosclerosis years after the inflammation has abated. Due to multiple vessel involvement low-flow states are often seen, which can result in global ischemic symptoms. Upper extremity claudication symptoms are also present in greater than half of the patients.[5] Embolic phenomenon is seen in less than one-third of patients.

Radiation-induced stenosis of the great vessels predisposes the arteries to atherosclerotic changes often in unusual locations. The duration of irradiation for the development is usually 10 years but variability has been reported. Both embolic and low-flow phenomenons have been reported. Other causative disorders include radiation arteritis secondary to Hodgkin's disease or malignancies of the neck, vasospastic disorders, thoracic outlet syndrome, trauma (gunshot or deceleration injuries), connective tissue disorders, and emboli. In this chapter, discussion is focused on the clinical features and endovascular treatment of diseases involving the supra-aortic branch and upper extremity arterial segment. Clinical data as well as treatment complications are also presented.

Clinical presentation

Atherosclerosis is the etiology present in the vast majority of patients with supra-aortic trunk and upper extremity arterial disease. The clinical presentation of these patients is well described. The typical patient is in their fifth or sixth decade of life. These patients generally have the same risk factors that are seen with coronary artery disease including age, smoking, hyperlipidemia, and genetic predisposition.[5] The presentation of these patients can be divided into two categories: embolic or stenotic.

Embolic phenomenon results in acute neurovascular symptoms in either the cerebral or upper extremity distribution. Typical neurologic symptoms include hemispheric events from the anterior circulation or ameurosis fugax similar to those seen in carotid bifurcation disease. Pure upper extremity emboli are also seen but are much less frequent. When they do occur, they are often distal presenting with cool and numb hand or fingers.

Flow-limiting stenotic lesions are typically seen in patients with upper extremity claudication and subclavian steal syndrome. Claudication is a loosely used term to describe exercise-induced ischemia, hand and arm cramping, and fatigue. Symptoms may progress along the spectrum of disease to rest pain and tissue loss, although this is much less common for upper extremity than in the lower extremity. Subclavian steal is a well-described clinical entity resulting from a proximal subclavian stenosis or occlusion. Although angiographically common, it is rarely symptomatic.[12] After upper extremity activity, blood flows retrograde down the vertebrobasilar system and "steals" blood from the posterior circulation. This results in dizziness, bilateral visual disturbances, and imbalance. More recently appreciated is the coronary-subclavian steal syndrome in patients with a diseased subclavian artery proximal to an internal mammary artery bypass to the coronary system. Arm exercise in that instance causes reversed flow in the mammary bypass to supply the arm and leads to coronary ischemia.

Patients with Takayasu's arteritis generally present before the age of 40. Early symptoms are often nonspecific including fevers and myalgia. Hypertension is frequent. As the disease progresses, flow-limiting fibrotic stenoses develop resulting in lightheadedness, photophobia, and visual changes. Subclavian steal and upper extremity claudication can also occur. Classically, there is absent pulses in one or both upper extremities.[11]

Patients with radiation-induced supra-aortic trunk and upper extremity disease often present at a younger age depending upon the time of their radiation exposure. They have angiographically atypical appearing lesions, which are diffuse rather than the focal lesions seen with typical atherosclerosis.[13] These patients can present with either embolic or flow-limiting symptoms.

Anatomical considerations

An endovascular approach to the treatment of supra-aortic trunk and upper extremity vascular disease requires an understanding of the vascular anatomy in this region. Figure 6.1 delineates the distribution of atherosclerotic occlusive disease involving the supra-aortic trunk in patients presenting with neurological symptoms. The natural curves combined with the tortuosity of

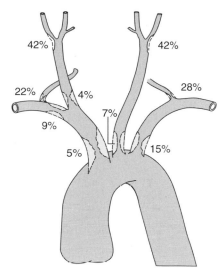

Figure 6.1 Anatomic distribution of atherosclerotic lesions causing neurological symptoms involving aortic arch branch vessels.

atherosclerosis mandate the use of a stiff wire and a long guiding sheath when doing interventions in this area. The innominate artery is the first major branch of the aortic arch. It usually ascends for a distance of 4-6 cm before bifurcating into the right subclavian and the right common carotid. This artery is often prone to being tortuous in elderly patients, which can at times preclude endovascular intervention. If the tortuousity involves the proximal subclavian artery, it can often mimic aneurysmal dilation on angiograms.

The right common carotid artery originates from the innominate while the left common carotid artery comes directly off the aorta. Despite their different origins, they have identical cervical courses. The carotid bifurcation is generally at C2/C3 near the superior horn of the thyroid cartilage.

The right subclavian artery originates from the innominate artery and then arches laterally and posteriorly behind the anterior scalene muscle. The left subclavian artery is usually the third branch of the aorta and initially ascends until the root of the neck where it arches laterally also traversing behind the anterior scalene muscle. There are two important branches of the subclavian: the vertebral and the internal mammary. It is important to realize that these two branches take off directly opposite from each other from the subclavian artery.

Frequently anatomic variants of the supra-aortic branches can be seen during either diagnostic or interventional procedures, which are demonstrated in Figure 6.2. The most common of these variants is the bovine arch. Other variants include aberrant left vertebral artery origin and an aberrant right subclavian artery originating from the proximal portion of the descending thoracic aorta. Physicians should be cognizant of these anatomic variants so that appropriate diagnostic catheters can be used for endovascular procedures.

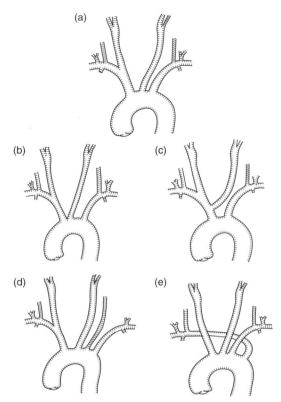

Figure 6.2 Commonly encountered normal and variant anatomical configurations of supra-aortic trunk. (a) Normal configuration. (b) Common origin of innominate and left common carotid artery. (c) Left common carotid artery arising from the innominate artery. (d) Aberrant left vertebral artery arising from the aortic arch proximal to the left subclavian artery. (e) Aberrant left subclavian artery arising from the descending thoracic aorta.

Diagnostic evaluation

Paramount to diagnosis is a good history and physical examination of the patient and should include an examination of the thoracic outlet and the entire upper extremity. In addition to a careful delineation of the patient's symptoms, a careful review of pertinent occupational, pharmacologic, and athletic risks should be elicited. The physical exam starts with a good pulse examination of the subclavian artery in the supraclavicular fossa, the axillary artery under the armpit, the brachial artery at the upper arm and elbow, and the radial and ulnar arteries at the wrist. A decreased or absent pulse in any site other than the supraclavicular fossa may indicate arterial occlusion. Both the infraclavicular and supraclavicular fossa should be palpated to help detect the presence of a subclavian aneurysm or cervical rib. Auscultation of the subclavian artery may detect the presence of a bruit to help establish the diagnosis of thoracic outlet compression to the artery. The blood pressure should be recorded in both arms. A systolic difference of greater than 20 mm Hg is likely to be significant and suggestive of proximal occlusive disease. Examination of the hand is not complete without an Allen test. Any part of the hand that does not blush is an indication of incomplete palmar arch.

Noninvasive testing is somewhat limited in the upper extremity due to the relative inaccessibility of the subclavian arteries to Doppler evaluation. However, the finding of a pressure difference between the arms and reversed flow in the ipsilateral vertebral artery by duplex scanning is highly suggestive of proximal subclavian stenosis. This reversed flow can be accentuated with hyperemia testing where a cuff is inflated in the arm and then released after a few minutes. If this phenomenon is not associated with symptoms, then further investigation may not be necessary. However, in a symptomatic patient or in a patient in whom an internal mammary artery (IMA) to left anterior descending artery (LAD) bypass has been performed, further investigation is necessary. MRA and CT angiography on modern machines can demonstrate lesions effectively, but dynamic information such as reversed flow in the ipsilateral vertebral artery leading to late filling of the distal subclavian artery or pressure gradients can only reliably be obtained with conventional angiography. Arteriography should be reserved for symptomatic patients or those in whom coronary-subclavian steal is suspected or might develop. In rare cases of aneurysms of the supra-aortic trunk, CT scanning or MRA of the chest can provide important information regarding the size of the aneurysm and its anatomic relationship to other mediastinal and neck structures. These scans should be obtained in addition to an arteriogram.

Although certainly not as common as carotid bifurcation disease, supra-aortic trunk disease does, at times, require intervention. The three patterns of presentation, namely ischemic symptoms, steal symptoms, or embolic phenomena are universally accepted as indications for intervention. In patients with symptoms suggestive of subclavian steal syndrome and concurrent carotid stenoses, the carotid stenosis is usually addressed first. If the carotid lesion is at the origin of the carotid required for carotid-subclavian bypass, then synchronous retrograde stenting of the common carotid artery origin prior to creating the bypass can be performed. Although endovascular therapy usually is aimed at the relief of symptoms, there a few situations in which intervention may be warranted in the asymptomatic patient. These include, the planned use of the ipsilateral IMA distal to a subclavian lesion, or the requirement for axillobifemoral grafting. Additional intervention may be required in patients who previously have undergone IMA grafting and develop coronary ischemia as a result of stenosis in the ipsilateral subclavian artery proximal to the origin of the IMA.

Endovascular treatment strategies

The different types of interventions can be divided based on the anatomic distribution: innominate, common carotid, and subclavian artery. For all of

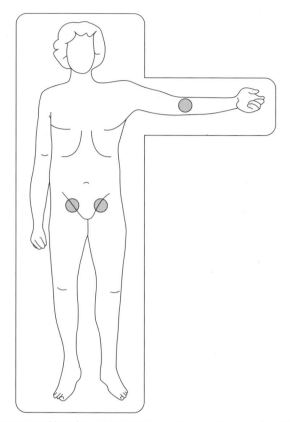

Figure 6.3 The proper position of a patient includes exposure and preparation of both groins and left upper extremity access sites.

these approaches, we usually start with a retrograde femoral technique and switch to other approaches only when needed. For this reason, it is imperative to prepare the patient for either approach (Figure 6.3). For all great vessel interventions, the preferred drug of choice in intraprocedural anticoagulation is bivalirudin, which is a direct thrombin inhibitor. This drug is usually given as a bolus then followed by a drip. This drug has a similar effect as heparin, yet it has a shorter half-life and can be simply turned off at the end of the case. Its use may be limited by high cost. In addition, after completion of stenting, patients are placed on clopidogrel for 1 month.

Innominate and common carotid artery interventions

Retrograde femoral artery approach for supra-aortic trunk interventions is preferred. If severe aortoiliac occlusive disease precludes a femoral approach, one can consider either a retrograde brachial artery access. Once the femoral artery is cannulated, a Bentson wire is placed followed by a 6-Fr introducer sheath placement. The guidewire is advanced until it bounces up off the ascending aorta. The Simmons-2 catheter is then reformed in the ascending aorta over the guidewire and used to select the common carotid or innominate artery. Alternatively, the Simmons-2 catheter can also be formed in the subclavian. Figure 6.4 illustrates two techniques on reforming this catheter. Once the vessel of interest is selectively cannulated, a guidewire exchange is performed in which a stiff angled Glidewire is used to cross the lesion and tip is placed either in the axillary or external carotid artery. Following the removal of the Simmons-2 catheter and introducer sheath, the placement of the Glidewire in the external carotid artery provides a sturdy tractability to allow a long guiding sheath to advance over the Glidewire. The guiding sheath is positioned just proximal to the lesion. For ostial lesions, the sheath may have to be positioned within the aortic arch. With tortuous vessels, it may be necessary to use an Amplatz wire to straighten out the curves. Alternatively, a second stiff wire may be placed adjacent to the Glidewire to function as a "buddy wire", which may facilitate in the tracking of the guiding sheath. There are various cerebral protection devices available in the market, which is discussed elsewhere in this book. Once the cerebral protection device is appropriately deployed, a balloon-expandable stent with diameter 8–10 mm is typically used for innominate or common carotid ostial lesion. Optimal treatment of ostial lesions requires the placement of the stent with 1–2 mm extending into the lumen of the aortic arch. If the innominate and left common carotid arteries share a common origin, or a bovine arch, care must be taken to avoid compression of either artery during stent deployment. This is best avoided by simultaneous placement of kissing stents in both arteries.

In the event that a retrograde brachial artery approach is performed for innominate artery intervention, the brachial artery access can be achieved by using a micropuncture kit and a 6-Fr introducer sheath. Systemic anticoagulant is administered and a Glidewire is carefully manipulated until it crosses the innominate artery lesion. The introducer sheath is exchanged for a guiding sheath, which is positioned just distal to the lesion. The stent is then deployed across the lesion as described previously. The disadvantage of this approach in innominate artery intervention is that there is no cerebral protection to prevent procedural-related embolization.

In common carotid ostial lesions that cannot be accessed from a retrograde femoral approach, one can consider a retrograde carotid artery cannulation via a cervical approach. Similarly, in patients with concomitant ipsilateral carotid bifurcation lesion and innominate or carotid ostial disease, a combined approach including carotid endarterectomy and retrograde innominate or carotid stenting can be performed. In the latter scenario, carotid endarterectomy should be performed first, either under local or general anesthesia. Just prior to the closure of the carotid arteriotomy, a 7-Fr introducer sheath is inserted in a retrograde fashion for stent placement. It is important to place a vascular clamp distal to the introducer sheath to minimize procedural-related embolization to the cerebral circulation. Once the retrograde stenting is completed, the sheath is removed followed by the closure of the arteriotomy

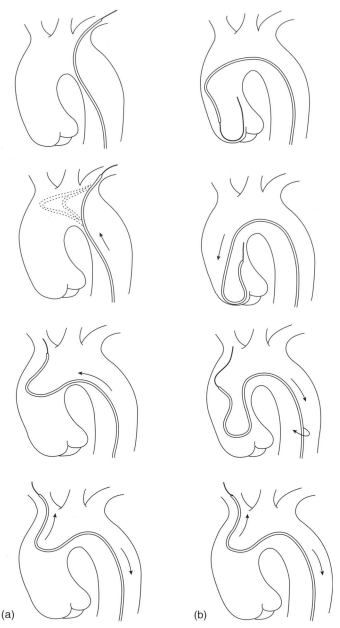

Figure 6.4 Reforming the Simmons catheter. (a) Reforming the Simmons using the subclavian artery. The left subclavian artery is selected. The catheter is then reformed by multiple, quick, and short advancements. Short, quick withdraws is used to select the artery of choice. (b) Reforming the Simmons using the ascending aorta. The guidewire is bounced superiorly off the aortic valve. The catheter is advanced until it forms over the wire. It is then rotated to attain the proper direction. By gently pull back the catheter, it will advance forward to cannulate the artery of choice.

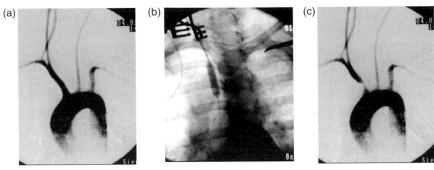

Figure 6.5 Placement of a proximal innominate artery stent via a retrograde right common carotid artery approach. (a) Initial angiogram, which shows the proximal innominate artery lesion. (b) A right common carotid artery cutdown was done, which provided an access for balloon angioplasty and stent placement. (c) Completion angiogram after deployment of balloon-expandable stent.

incision. In situations where carotid artery cutdown is performed solely for access purpose, an 18-gauge needle and a Bentson wires can be used to cross the proximal innominate or carotid artery lesion. A 6-Fr sheath is placed and through it the stent is deployed across the lesion. Figures 6.5 illustrates the placement of a proximal innominate artery stent via a right carotid cutdown approach. A 5-0 polypropylene suture can be placed around the introducer sheath in a figure-of-eight fashion to close the arteriotomy. Alternatively with diseased vessels or concomitant bifurcation disease, a carotid patch angioplasty is performed to widen the vessel lumen.

Subclavian artery interventions

Although these lesions can be approached either through a femoral or brachial access, our preference is to use the brachial artery. First, percutaneous access is obtained by using a micropuncture kit. An initial 5 or 6-Fr sheath allows placement of diagnostic catheters for angiography. If the lesion is located at the ostium of the subclavian artery and there is difficulty determining the anatomy, a separate puncture from the groin allows placement of a pigtail catheter in the aortic arch for simultaneous injections. Usually the lesion can be imaged from a catheter placed through the brachial puncture and if necessary, a pigtail can be advanced into the arch over a wire passed through the lesion.

Once the lesion is clearly identified, a guidewire is passed through the lesion into the aortic arch, preferably directed down the descending aorta. At this point, we generally give a small dose of heparin (2000–3000 units) and if tight, the lesion can be predilated with an undersized balloon to allow for easy passage of the stent. We prefer a balloon-expandable stent for accuracy of placement. If the lesion is involving the ostium, the stent should again be positioned to allow for 1–2 mm of overhang into the aortic arch. Careful inflation of the initial balloon and choice of size of the stent must be emphasized to minimize chances of rupture of the subclavian artery. Generally, a 6 or 7-Fr sheath is required, depending on the size of the device chosen. Although somewhat controversial, primary stenting of these lesions is our preference because of the calcified nature of the lesions and the predictable result achieved. Care must be taken to avoid stent covering of the vertebral and internal mammary arteries. Finally, a completion study is performed to confirm adequate result and lack of any complication.

Results from clinical series

The first case of innominate artery stenting was reported back in 1981.[6] Since then there have been multiple reports in the literature that have supported the use of endovascular therapy to treat great vessel disease. Early series reported patency rates of 96% at 36 months in patients treated with subclavian artery stents. Diethrich also reported on the successful use of Palmaz stents and Wallstents in the treatment of innominate artery lesions.[7,14] These early reports had stroke rates of less than 1%.[15] Higher complication rates were noted when common carotid intervention were performed in combination with endarterectomy.[16] Retrograde common carotid and innominate artery stent deployment was first described by Queral and Criado in their 4-year experience with 26 stent procedures.[17] They reported no strokes or deaths with distal cross-clamping. A comparison of stenting with traditional operative therapy for subclavian disease was reported by Hadjipetrou and associates.[18] In their series of 18 patients there were no strokes. This was compared with a 2–4% stroke rate in the literature for open repairs. They concluded that endovascular repair should be the first-line of therapy offered to patients. In a recent review of radiation-induced arterial lesions, there was a patency rate of 93% at 18 months in a series of 14 patients treated with common carotid artery stents. Diethrich and colleagues have also shown that angioplasty and stenting can be used successfully to treat patients with coronary-subclavian steal.[19] In their series of 14 patients, they had primary and assisted-primary patency rates of 86 and a 100% with a median follow-up of 29 months. In a recent study, Brountzos and colleagues reported their experience of primary stenting of subclavian and innominate artery in 48 symptomatic patients. The authors reported that common symptoms attributable to innominate and subclavian artery diseases include vertebrobasilar insufficiency (17%), upper limb ischemia (31%), angina (13%), and transient ischemia attack (18%).[20] Excellent technical and clinical success rates were achieved with primary stenting, which were 96% and 94%, respectively. Complications occurred in four patients (8%), which included puncture site hematoma, hand embolization, and transient cerebral ischemia. With a mean follow-up of 17 months, the authors reported cumulative primary patency rate was 91.7% and 77% at 12 and 24 months, respectively. In addition, cumulative secondary patency rate was 96.5% and 91.7% at 12 and 24 months, respectively.[20] Taken altogether, these clinical studies indicate that endovascular therapy is a safe and effective method to treat supra-aortic and upper extremity occlusive disease.

Common problems and complications

Inadvertent passage of a guidewire in the subintimal plane may lead to dissection and thrombotic occlusion. In addition, inflation of the balloon may cause plaque disruption and embolization. A complication that is rare but dreaded by interventionalists is vessel perforation. If unrecognized, this can potentially lead to death from exsanguinations. Complications that are seen most commonly with supra-aortic trunk interventions can be divided into three categories: embolic phenomenon, access site, and disruption.

Embolization is the most significant complication affecting supra-aortic trunk and upper extremity endovascular intervention. Although there is no data for supra-aortic trunk lesions, early data from the SAPPHIRE trial show that carotid stenting with cerebral protection has similar stroke rates to open surgery for the treatment of carotid bifurcation disease.[21] It is prudent to extrapolate this literature to supra-aortic trunk interventions and routinely use cerebral protection devices in order to limit embolization. If possible, avoid using the right retrograde brachial approach to treat innominate lesions as cerebral protection is difficult to obtain in this situation. While vertebrobasilar embolization is uncommon, there are patients who are posterior circulation dependant with antegrade flow through the vertebral artery. In this group of patients, embolization can be catastrophic and the use of cerebral protection while performing great vessel interventions is imperative. This underscores another reason to obtain carotid duplex prior to interventions of the great vessels in order to document the direction of flow in the vertebral arteries. The vertebral artery can also be occluded by the improper placements of stents across the ostia and by spreading of plaque during angioplasty. Embolization of plaque down the subclavian artery is the most common cause of acute upper extremity ischemia during endovascular procedures. Patients can present with sudden onset of cold, blue, ischemic lesions affecting one or more fingers, the "blue digit syndrome." These patients need to be recognized and treated rapidly with thrombolysis.[22]

The most frequently seen complications are related to the access site. They are similar to those seen with interventions in other areas and include bleeding, hematoma, and pseudoaneurysm. The majority of access site complications reported are from the cardiac catheterization literature where groin complication rates of 7% have been seen.[16,23] A significant degree of morbidity can also accompany brachial access.[16] The brachial artery is relatively small and can be collapsed and difficult to palpate because of proximal disease. Vasospasm is more common among arm vessels because they are small and prone to vasoconstriction. This type of access has also been associated with blue digit syndrome. Complications can be best avoided by adhering to the following principles: use of ultrasound to locate vessel, limiting the sheath size when possible, use of liberal doses of vasodilator through the sheath to minimize vasospasm, and adequate anticoagulation.

The subclavian artery is often described by experienced vascular surgeons as one of the most fragile arteries in the body. Vessel perforation in this area is certainly one of the most dreaded complications. Disruption can be caused by either balloon inflation or disruption. A recent report by Lin and associates discusses treatment options.[24] First, prompt recognition is essential as it prevents further blood loss. Exsanguination can be stopped by quickly passing a balloon over the guidewire and inflating over the disrupted artery. This underscores the reason to keep the guidewire in place until satisfactory completion of the

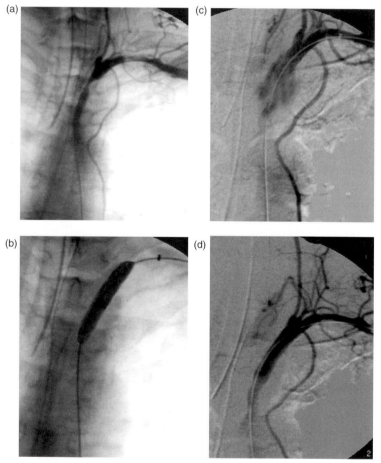

Figure 6.6 Subclavian artery disruption and subsequent treatment. (a) Left-sided subclavian artery stenosis proximal to the vertebral and internal mammary origins. (b) Dilation of the lesion. (c) Extravasation is noted. The balloon was advanced back across the lesion and inflated for 20 min. (d) Resolution of the extravasation. Should this approach fail, a covered stent/stent graft could be used to seal the leak if the anatomy is suitable, but emergency surgical consultation and repair must be considered.

procedure. The length of time to keep the balloon is unclear but at least 15 min is recommended. Doing so will often permanently seal the disruption. Figure 6.6 illustrates angioplasty, perforation, and subsequent sealing of a left subclavian artery. Alternatively a stent graft can be placed across the lesion. Although early reports have documented technical feasibility, long-term patency rates are unknown. By endovascular treatment of a disruption, one can also avoid the potential hazards of dissection in a acutely traumatized area.

References

1 Broadbent WH. Absence of pulsation in both radial arteries, vessels being full of blood. *Trans Med Soc Lond* 1875; **8**:165–68.

2 Takayasu M. Case of queer changes in central blood vessels of retina. *Acta Soc Ophthalmol Jpn* 1908; **12**:554.

3 Crawford ES, De Bakey ME, Morris GC, Jr., Howell JF. Surgical treatment of occlusion of the innominate, common carotid, and subclavian arteries: a 10 year experience. *Surgery* 1969; **65**:17–31.

4 Law MM, Colburn MD, Moore WS, Quinones-Baldrich WJ, Machleder HI, Gelabert HA. Carotid-subclavian bypass for brachiocephalic occlusive disease. Choice of conduit and long-term follow-up. *Stroke* 1995; **26**:1565–71.

5 Rhodes JM, Cherry KJ, Jr., Clark RC, *et al.* Aortic-origin reconstruction of the great vessels: risk factors of early and late complications. *J Vasc Surg* 2000; **31**:260–69.

6 Lowman BG, Queral LA, Holbrook WA, Estes JT, Bayly B. The treatment of innominate artery stenosis by intraoperative transluminal angioplasty. *Surgery* 1981; **89**: 565–68.

7 Diethrich EB. Endovascular management of brachiocephalic arterial occlusive disease. *Ann Vasc Surg* 2000; **14**:189–92.

8 Kieffer E, Sabatier J, Koskas F, Bahnini A. Atherosclerotic innominate artery occlusive disease: early and long-term results of surgical reconstruction. *J Vasc Surg* 1995; **21**:326–36; discussion 336–37.

9 Hass WK, Fields WS, North RR, Kircheff, II, Chase NE, Bauer RB. Joint study of extracranial arterial occlusion. II. Arteriography, techniques, sites, and complications. *JAMA* 1968; 203:961–68.

10 Cherry KJ, Jr., McCullough JL, Hallett JW, Jr., Pairolero PC, Gloviczki P. Technical principles of direct innominate artery revascularization: a comparison of endarterectomy and bypass grafts. *J Vasc Surg* 1989; **9**:718–23; discussion 723–24.

11 Johnston SL, Lock RJ, Gompels MM. Takayasu arteritis: a review. *J Clin Pathol* 2002; **55**:481–86.

12 Fields WS, Lemak NA. Joint Study of extracranial arterial occlusion. VII. Subclavian steal – a review of 168 cases. *JAMA* 1972; **222**:1139–43.

13 Mathes SJ, Alexander J. Radiation injury. *Surg Oncol Clin N Am* 1996; **5**:809–24.

14 Lobato AC, Quick RC, Phillips B, *et al.* Immediate endovascular repair for descending thoracic aortic transection secondary to blunt trauma. *J Endovasc Ther* 2000; **7**:16–20.

15 Diethrich EB, Cozacov JC. Subclavian stent implantation to alleviate coronary steal through a patent internal mammary artery graft. *J Endovasc Surg* 1995; **2**:77–80.

16 Sullivan TM, Gray BH, Bacharach JM, *et al.* Angioplasty and primary stenting of the subclavian, innominate, and common carotid arteries in 83 patients. *J Vasc Surg* 1998; **28**:1059–65.

17 Queral LA, Criado FJ. The treatment of focal aortic arch branch lesions with Palmaz stents. *J Vasc Surg* 1996; **23**:368–75.

18 Hadjipetrou P, Cox S, Piemonte T, Eisenhauer A. Percutaneous revascularization of atherosclerotic obstruction of aortic arch vessels. *J Am Coll Cardiol* 1999; **33**:1238–45.

19 Westerband A, Rodriguez JA, Ramaiah VG, Diethrich EB. Endovascular therapy in prevention and management of coronary-subclavian steal. *J Vasc Surg* 2003; **38**:699–703; discussion 704.

20 Brountzos EN, Petersen B, Binkert C, Panagiotou I, Kaufman JA. Primary stenting of subclavian and innominate artery occlusive disease: a single center's experience. *Cardiovasc Intervent Radiol* 2004; **27**:616–23.

21 Yadav JS, Wholey MH, Kuntz RE, *et al.* Protected carotid-artery stenting versus endarterectomy in high-risk patients. *N Engl J Med* 2004; **351**:1493–501.

22 Johnson SP, Durham JD, Subber SW, *et al.* Acute arterial occlusions of the small vessels of the hand and forearm: treatment with regional urokinase therapy. *J Vasc Interv Radiol* 1999; **10**:869–76.

23 Choussat R, Black A, Bossi I, Fajadet J, Marco J. Vascular complications and clinical outcome after coronary angioplasty with platelet IIb/IIIa receptor blockade. Comparison of transradial versus transfemoral arterial access. *Eur Heart J* 2000; **21**:662–67.

24 Lin PH, Bush RL, Weiss VJ, Dodson TF, Chaikof EL, Lumsden AB. Subclavian artery disruption resulting from endovascular intervention: treatment options. *J Vasc Surg* 2000; **32**:607–11.

CHAPTER 7

Thoracic aortic disease

Andy C. Chiou, Kristen L. Biggs, Peter H. Lin

Open surgical repair of thoracic aortic diseases such as enlarging aneurysms or symptomatic dissection has traditionally been regarded as the mainstay of therapy. Recent advances in aortic endovascular technology have led to the development of a less invasive and potentially safer therapeutic modality for aneurysmal disease of the descending thoracic aorta. Moreover, this technology may be appropriate for other diseases of the thoracic aorta, including traumatic disruptions and dissections. Contrary to endovascular repair of infrarenal aortic aneurysms, the evolution of thoracic stent grafts has progressed more slowly as there are only a limited number of devices currently undergoing clinical trials. Nonetheless, the enthusiasm for this technology persists as it may indeed hold the potential for the greatest patient benefit as conventional open surgical repair continues to offer serious morbidity and mortality rates.

Thoracic aorta disease is a broad term that encompasses several different disease entities. The types of disease that affect the thoracic aorta include: dissection, aneurysm, pseudoaneurysm, penetrating atherosclerotic ulcers, aortoesophageal and aortobronchial fistulas, and diseases of thoracic trauma, such as aortic transection. The most commonly encountered thoracic aorta diseases are dissections and aneurysms. The annual incidence of thoracic aortic aneurysms is six cases per 100,000 population.[1,2] True thoracic aortic aneurysms contain all three layers of the arterial wall, which can be classified as degenerative or secondary to infectious etiologies. Degenerative aneurysms can arise from atherosclerotic destruction of the medial arterial layer, or from intrinsic weakness associated with connective tissue disorders.

Thoracic aneurysms are fusiform in approximately 80% of cases and are saccular in 20%.[3,4] Fusiform aneurysms involve the descending thoracic aorta in 80% of cases and the ascending aorta or the arch in the remainder. In contrast, nearly 75% of all thoracic saccular aneurysms are found in the ascending aorta or the arch, with only 25% of cases being found in the descending aorta. Rupture of the thoracic aneurysm can result in mortality in 50–80% of these cases.[5] Nearly one-fourth of patients with thoracic aortic aneurysm have aneurysms elsewhere, typically affecting the abdominal aorta.[3]

In contrast to thoracic aneurysm, thoracic aortic dissection is mainly caused by high-pressure blood flow entering a tear in the intima and subsequently tracking within the arterial wall. It is the most common clinical catastrophe involving the aorta, which has an estimated incidence of 10 to 20 cases per million of population annually.[6] If a patient is untreated, this condition can result in a mortality rate of 90% after 3 months. Despite advances of surgical repair, operative mortality remained high until aggressive medical therapy became widely recognized as an effective treatment to patient stabilization in 1960s, which included intravenous beta-blocker and vasodilator therapy to control the underlying hypertension.[7] This permits stabilization of the dissection and is the mainstay of treatment for most patients who have dissections of the descending thoracic aorta. Operative or endovascular interventions are reserved in these patients when medical treatment fails or associated complications develop.

The development of catheter-based technology in vascular surgery has laid the foundation for advances in the treatment of thoracic aortic aneurysms. In contrast to the open thoracic aortic repair, the advantage of endovascular thoracic aortic repair is the avoidance of several important causes of morbidity associated with open surgery: surgical exposure of the aorta, aortic cross clamping, and opening and suturing of the diseased aorta. In this chapter, the clinical features and endovascular treatment options of descending thoracic aortic diseases, with particular emphasis on aortic aneurysms and dissection are discussed.

Etiology

Thoracic aortic aneurysm

Atherosclerotic medial degenerative disease accounts for more than 75% of thoracic aortic aneurysms.[3] Aortic dissection causes approximately 15% of all thoracic aortic aneurysms.[6] Marfans's and Ehlers–Danlos syndromes, mycotic aneurysm, and Takayasus's aortitis are less frequent culprits of remaining cases. Patients with nondissecting aneurysms (including degeneratives, Marfan's, or Ehlers–Danlos syndrome) and dissecting aneurysms have different associated risk factors that affect their clinical outcome. While both patient cohorts with thoracic aneurysms tend to have a high incidence of hypertension, patients with degenerative aneurysms typically have a higher incidence of coronary artery disease, renal insufficiency, cerebrovascular disease, and peripheral arterial occlusive disease than patients with dissecting aneurysm. The presence of these cardiovascular risk factors significantly influences the perioperative morbidity and long-term survival in this patient cohort.

Thoracic aortic dissection

Approximately 90% of patients with aortic dissection have either poorly controlled hypertension or a history of chronic hypertension. The condition occurs three to four times more frequently in hypertensive males and is most common in black patients. The patient is frequently a middle-aged black man with known hypertension who experiences sudden onset of excruciating, tearing back pain.[6] Hypertension causes excessive mechanical and metabolic strain on the media, which opposes arterial pressure within the aortic wall. Atherosclerosis is an associated risk factor in elderly patients with aortic dissection. These patients typically develop an aortic dissection secondary to an atherosclerotic penetrating ulcer, and they also frequently have underlying hypertension. The tear in the aorta commonly occurs in the descending thoracic aorta above the diaphragm. This aortic tear can result in a classic dissection, with multiple entry and a reentry tears.

Another important risk factor for aortic dissection is pregnancy, which is responsible for nearly half of aortic dissections in females below the age of 40 and usually occurs in the last trimester or during labor.[8] Aortic dissection in these patients can often result in dissection aneurysm. Rupture of a dissection aneurysm commonly occurs in these patients during the third trimester or the first stage of labor. Contributing factors of aortic dissection in pregnant patients include hypercirculation during the late gestational period, hypertension, and the loosened connective tissue owing to hormonal changes.[9] Many congenital disorders of elastic tissue may predispose the aorta to early dissection. These include Marfan, Turner, Noonan, and Ehlers–Danlos syndromes. A fundamental genetic derangement in the assembly and deposition of a newly discovered microfibrillar protein, fibrillin, occurs in Marfan's syndrome.[10] Lastly, blunt trauma occasionally causes aortic dissection, which may result in intimal rupture and dissecting hematoma. This condition is frequently observed following a sudden deceleration injury from an automobile accident, with resultant intimal tear of the descending thoracic aorta at the ligamentum arteriosum attachment. Dissection or aneurysm after an intimal tear caused by trauma may remain undetected for weeks or even years.

Clinical presentation

Most cases of thoracic aortic aneurysms are asymptomatic and are discovered incidentally on radiographic studies, appearing frequently as an unsuspected mass on a chest radiograph. When symptoms do occur, they are usually caused by compression of adjacent structures, dissection, or rupture. Rapid expansion can cause chest pain, hemoptysis, hematemesis, and hoarseness from compression of the laryngeal nerve, and stridor. Symptoms suggestive of thoracic aortic dissection vary depending on the location of the dissection. Involvement of the coronary arteries can be manifested as a myocardial infarction or pericardial tamponade, and valvular involvement may cause congestive heart failure. Patients often present with chest pain and commonly have a history of hypertension.

Diagnostic evaluation

If thoracic aorta disease is suspected, or if it has already been detected on other imaging studies, then further diagnostic evaluation is warranted. A contrast-enhanced computed tomography (CT) scan of the chest with three-dimensional reconstructions and thoracic aortography with a calibrated catheter are the two tests most commonly used to evaluate the extent of thoracic aortic disease. The main anatomic considerations that need to be evaluated for endoluminal stent-graft implantation are the presence of adequate proximal and distal aortic necks. The distance from the origin of the left subclavian artery to the proximal aspect of the aneurysm should be at least 2 cm. This distance allows adequate anchoring of the device and ensures that the stent graft does not inadvertently occlude the origin of the artery. If the aneurysm is adjacent to the left subclavian artery, a more favorable neck may be created by transposing the left subclavian artery onto the left common carotid artery or creating a left carotid-subclavian bypass grafting prior to endovascular repair. To avoid visceral vessel occlusion, the aneurysm should terminate between 2 and 3 cm proximal to the celiac artery. To minimize exclusion of intercostal arteries, the overall length of the stent graft should be kept to a minimum.

If a thoracic aortogram is performed, the pelvic vasculature is also studied to evaluate the diameter and tortuosity of the iliac and femoral arteries through which the stent graft will be accessed. Most thoracic aortic stent grafts require a sheath up to size 24-Fr in internal diameter. In the event that the iliac artery remains too narrow to accommodate the large introducer sheath, an adjunctive operative procedure may be required to create an iliac conduit through a retroperitoneal approach to permit stent-graft delivery.

For patients with intravenous contrast allergies or renal failure, magnetic resonance angiography (MRA) is an alternative for imaging the thoracic aorta. As this technology continues to improve, MRA may replace CT and contrast angiography as the gold standard in thoracic aortic diagnostic imaging. Transesophageal echocardiography (TEE) with color-flow mapping can also be used to evaluate thoracic disease or to assist in endovascular interventions. Many endovascular cases have been monitored intraoperatively with digital subtraction angiography and TEE.[11]

Indications for endovascular treatment

The specific applications of endoluminal repair using stent-graft devices in the thoracic aorta include a range of aneurysms, dissections, and traumatic lesions.

Thoracic aortic aneurysms

Clinical studies have shown various stent-graft devices are safe and effective in excluding descending thoracic aneurysm with successful mid-term follow-up results (Figure 7.1).[2,12–14] The devices used for thoracic aneurysms are usually much larger in diameter when compared to those used in infrarenal aortic aneurysm. Because of the large devices used in the thoracic aorta, this necessitates a self-expanding stent mechanism because balloons of this diameter are not readily available. However, balloon-expandable devices have also been successfully deployed to exclude aneurysms or dissections of the descending thoracic aorta.[15] Endovascular therapy is particularly applicable to localized or

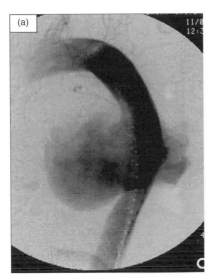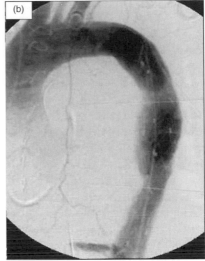

Figure 7.1 Endovascular repair of a descending thoracic aortic aneurysm: (a) Aortogram demonstrating a large symptomatic descending thoracic aneurysm. (b) Successful exclusion of the aneurysm was achieved with an endovascular stent graft.

saccular aneurysms of the descending thoracic aorta. It is similarly suited for focal anastomotic pseudoaneurysms involving the descending thoracic aorta.

Aortic dissection

Endoluminal stent-graft placement sometimes can be used in the management of type B aortic dissection. If possible, the stent graft should be positioned so that both the entry and exit points of the aortic tears are obliterated and any false aneurysm arising from the false lumen is depressurized. Because aortic dissection often involves a long segment of the thoracic aorta, it is often preferable to cover only the proximal aspect of the aortic dissection to reduce the likelihood of paraplegia due to intercostal artery exclusion.

Endovascular intervention in the treatment of descending thoracic aortic dissection, or type B dissection, is indicated in a limited number of situations, which are listed below:

1 Acute aortic rupture with associated back pain and hypotension. This condition requires urgent intervention and has a significant operative mortality.

2 An enlarging false-lumen aneurysm associated with a chronic aortic dissection. The patient may have a history of progressive widening of the mediastinum that is visible on follow-up chest radiographs, or an enlargement of the false lumen, which appears on sequential CT scans.

3 Branch artery involvement, involving the renal arteries, the mesenteric vessels, or the iliac arteries. Involvement of the renal arteries is suspected in cases with hypertension resistant to aggressive medical therapy or with deteriorating renal function. Mesenteric vessel involvement is suspected in patients who usually have postprandial abdominal pain. Iliac artery involvement is suspected in patients with changing femoral pulses. In the chronic setting, intermittent claudication is a sign of iliac artery involvement.

4 Progressive development of paraplegia. This occurs as a result of involvement of the spinal arteries that originate from the intercostal or lumbar arteries, which are affected by aortic dissection.

Aortic trauma, false aneurysms, and arteriovenous fistulas

The utility of endovascular stent grafts in traumatic aortic injury has great appeal because there is the potential to transform a challenging, hazardous open procedure involving thoracotomy into a simple, safe transluminal repair via a femoral artery access. Endografts can be used in the acute phase to achieve immediate hemostasis by excluding a vessel wall with active hemorrhage. Alternatively, it can be used in a late phase to manage thoracic false aneurysms or arteriovenous fistula. The technique may be particularly valuable when injuries occur to other vessels within the chest or the abdomen, including the subclavian artery or the visceral branches, and may be combined with interventional embolization techniques using coils, detachable balloons, or other occluding materials.[16–18] Successful repair of traumatic aortic rupture due to acute blunt trauma using aortic stent-graft implantation has also been reported (Figure 7.2).[5,17,19,20]

Devices for thoracic aortic aneurysm

Initially, experience with endovascular thoracic aneurysm repair was gained largely with home-made devices. Dake and associates reported the results of 13 patients implanted with a home-made device constructed of self-expanding stainless steel stents covered with Dacron grafts in 1994.[21] After a one-year

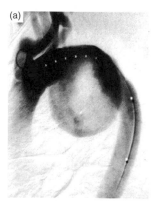
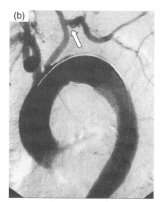
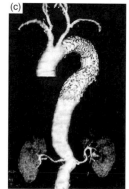

Figure 7.2 (a) Aortogram demonstrating a large traumatic aortic pseudoaneurysm in the descending thoracic aorta. (b) To increase the proximal endograft attachment, a left carotid-subclavian transposition was performed (arrow). The aneurysm was successfully excluded with an endograft. (c) Follow-up CT scan at 2 years demonstrated a successfully repaired thoracic aneurysm.

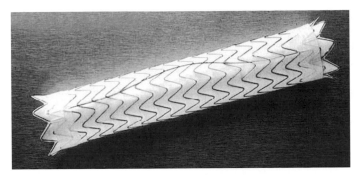

Figure 7.3 Gore TAG thoracic endoprosthesis.

follow-up period, only one patient required open conversion due to a progressively expanding aneurysm. Others have also proposed various custom-fabricated stent grafts, both with self-expanding and balloon-expandable stents.[18,22]

Existing devices for endoluminal thoracic aortic aneurysm treatment are currently in various phases of clinical investigation. Several commercial thoracic stent-graft devices undergoing clinical testing in the United States will be discussed. They include the Gore TAG device (WL Gore, Flagstaff, AZ), Zenith device (Cook, Bloomington, IN), and the Talent device (AVE/Medtronic Inc., Santa Rosa, CA).

The Gore TAG thoracic endoprosthesis (WL Gore) is constructed of radially reinforced ultrathin expanded polytetrafluoroethylene (ePTFE) graft material and in externally supported by nitinol wire (Figure 7.3). Stabilization bars are positioned 180° apart and span the length of the graft. Each device has an attached sleeve made of ePTFE that is sewn closed around the prosthesis and serves to constrain it during positioning. Grafts are available in diameters ranging between 26 and 40 mm, and lengths between 10 and 20 cm. Release of the graft begins in the mid-graft region to reduce distal displacement via a "wind-sock" effect. A three-lobed silicon balloon is used for modeling and for full expansion of the graft. The flexible catheter delivery system and the rapid deployment mechanism are great assets, particularly for deployment in curved segments of aorta within or close to the aortic arch. The delivery system and compatible introducer sheaths vary according to the diameter of the device and scale over a range of 20–24 Fr sheath.

The Zenith thoracic endovascular graft (Cook) uses a polyester weave and a covered stainless steel Z-stent construction. In this device, the proximal end is covered and has stainless steel hooks protruding through the graft fabric (Figure 7.4), which anchor the graft directly to the aortic wall. This also protects against distal stent-graft migration during high-velocity systolic blood flow. Full deployment of the top stent (with spikes) is released by pulling a trigger wire once optimal graft position is confirmed. The stents are modified Gianturco Z-stents, with small gaps left between each stent to allow some

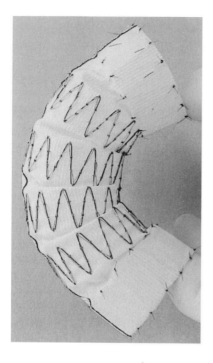

Figure 7.4 Zenith thoracic endovascular graft.

flexibility. Each end of the graft is held within a cap; inadvertent release during positioning within the aorta is prevented by a safety catch. The fall length of the graft material is stent supported to prevent graft torsion or compression. The stents are sutured onto the outside except at the points of proximal and distal attachment or seal. The stent grafts are available in a wide range of diameters and lengths. The delivery systems for Zenith device have profiles between 20 and 24-Fr. Device deployment is achieved by withdrawing an external sheath.

The talent thoracic stent-graft system (Medtronic) is composed of nitinol stent between layers of polyester graft. Individual stents are secured to the graft with suture (Figure 7.5). Between individual stents is the unsupported graft to allow for flexibility. The talent also has a longitudinal support bar. The proximal end of this stent graft is made in two configurations. It may be serrated (open web configuration) or may feature an open stent segment (bare wire configuration), which may be placed across the orifice of renal, mesenteric, left subclavian, or internal iliac arteries without occlusion of antegrade blood flow. Similar configuration is also available in the distal stent graft, which permits the uncovered device to anchor across the celiac artery. The delivery systems for Talent have profiles between 22 and 25 Fr. The system is available in diameters of 32–26 mm. A custom fabrication of a prosthesis based on an individual patient's anatomy is available from the manufacturer.

Anatomic characteristics must be considered when choosing particular devices. Increased flexibility and delivery systems of smaller profile facilitate

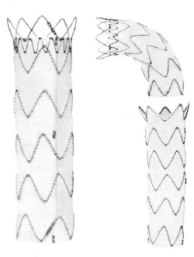

Figure 7.5 Talent thoracic stent-graft system.

deployment through severely angled aortic anatomy or iliac artery access vessels that are small, calcified, or tortuous. In patients with short proximal necks beyond the left subclavian artery, a device with an uncovered proximal stent may be beneficial. In terms of ease of use, the Gore TAG device has some advantages of enhanced flexibility. The maximum graft length available is of concern in the longer, more tortuous aneurysms in an effort to minimize the number of devices. The diameter of the device as well as the radial force of the underlying stent may on deployment provide a less-controlled release of the final device position.

Technique for endovascular repair of thoracic aneurysms

Following general preoperative medical assessment, including appropriate evaluation of the cardiopulmonary system, potential candidates for endovascular repair are evaluated by means of spiral CT scanning and aortography with calibrated catheter. Endovascular procedure is typically performed in a standard operating room with complete angiographic capabilities, with imaging done by either a portable digital radiographic C-arm unit or fixed angiographic system. Alternatively, the procedure may be performed in an OR-compatible interventional radiology laboratory. Either regional or general anesthesia can be used in this procedure. Ancillary procedures such as a carotid-to-subclavian bypass in order to lengthen the proximal landing site may be performed prior to endograft insertion. However, carotid-to-subclavian bypass is usually not necessary as occlusion of the left subclavian artery with a stent graft is well tolerated.[23] If ischemic symptoms of the arm are noted following endograft implantation, a bypass or transposition procedure may be performed electively in the postoperative period. Transesophageal echocardiography is used to help monitor accurate placement of the graft; it also provides real-time assessment of left ventricular function.

The patient is positioned on a radiolucent operating table in a supine position, and the chest is draped as for a standard left thoracotomy. This is done to facilitate a rapid conversion to an open chest procedure, if necessary. The patient's arms should be extended on arm tables to permit brachial artery access. The abdomen, pelvis, and groin of the patient are also draped for femoral, iliac, or retroperitoneal aortic access, depending on the preoperative pelvic arteriogram. A groin cutdown is performed to isolate the common femoral artery. Under direct visualization, a standard needle puncture is performed, and a 6-Fr angiographic sheath is introduced in the femoral artery. In the event that the femoral artery is severely diseased or inadequate for device insertion, the iliac artery can be exposed as an alternative site via a retroperitoneal incision. A 5-Fr pigtail catheter is introduced into the thoracic aorta to facilitate performance of an initial thoracic aortogram, which is obtained with the intensified image angled in a left anterior oblique position.

Brachial artery access is frequently helpful, which allows for periodic contrast agent injections through a catheter in the ascending aorta. It also permits passage of a stiff guidewire from the brachial artery to the femoral arteriotomy site, which may provide extra support for delivery system insertion in a patient with a tortuous iliac artery and aorta. If the procedure involves deliberate covering origin of the left subclavian artery, a right brachial artery access may be necessary. Intraoperative anticoagulation is established with intravenous heparin (100 U/kg). Activated clotting times are checked throughout the procedure to ensure that adequate systemic anticoagulation is maintained.

Following the identification of the proximal and the distal landing zones as demonstrated by the aortogram, a long 0.035 in. stiff guidewire is inserted via the angiographic catheter, which is then removed. The 6-Fr introducer sheath is withdrawn from the femoral artery. The artery is clamped, and the small arteriotomy incision is extended transversely to the diameter of the delivery system sheath.

The appropriate sheath size (20–24 Fr) for the chosen stent-graft system is inserted into the artery accessed and advanced to the desired proximal landing site depending on whether or not the origin of the left subclavian artery is to be deliberately covered. The actual delivery system is then introduced and the endovascular prosthesis deployed so as to have a 2 cm overlap with the nonaneurysmal aorta both proximally and distally. On occasion, a second or third prosthesis may be needed to gain additional length depending on the extent of disease in the descending aorta. Postdeployment balloon dilatation is performed to ensure not only full graft expansion including any overlap zones, but also complete contact with the aortic wall.

Once the stent-graft delivery system sheath is removed, a completion aortogram is obtained to ensure complete exclusion of the aortic aneurysm. The presence of any residual filling of the aneurysm, through either the superior or the inferior neck, is treated by placement of additional stent graft. If a perigraft endoleak persists, and is thought to be caused by poor apposition of the stent graft to the aortic wall, balloon dilatation of the stent graft can be considered. Following the removal of all sheaths and guidewires, the femoral artery is repaired with 6–0 Prolene sutures. The heparin may be reversed with intravenous protamine. The patient is extubated at the completion of the procedure. Chest X-ray is performed within the first 24 h following the procedure. A spiral CT scan is performed within 4 weeks of the procedure. Follow-up CT scans are done at 6 and 12 months and then at yearly intervals.

Adjunctive maneuvers in endovascular insertion of thoracic aortic stent grafts

Several adjunctive maneuvers may be performed to facilitate the endovascular insertion of thoracic stent grafts, and they include both technical and anesthetic maneuvers.

Placement of brachial-femoral guidewire

Insertion of a stiff guidewire from the brachial artery and exteriorized through the femoral artery may be helpful in selected cases when a tortuous aortic arch must be negotiated, especially with prostheses that have nonflexible deployment sheaths. A floppy guidewire is introduced initially through the right brachial access site and is negotiated through the arch and the descending aorta. A 5-Fr angiography catheter is passed over the floppy wire and is used to exchange a 260 cm stiff guidewire, which is pulled down from the aorta or the iliac artery and out of the femoral sheath using a snare catheter. Tension on both ends of the stiff wire may then be used to help the large access sheaths to traverse regions of angulation in the iliac vessels or within the aortic arch. The subclavian and the innominate arteries should be protected from direct trauma caused by the shearing of the stiff guidewire. This can be accomplished by placing an angiographic catheter over the guidewire within the aortic arch. Both the guidewire and angiographic catheter should remain together throughout the procedure.

Controlled hypotension to facilitate stent-graft deployment

Many early clinical studies have documented the propensity of stent-graft displacement or caudal movement during deployment, a phenomenon largely caused by the high blood flow in the descending aorta.[24–26] This scenario was particularly problematic if the stent graft is composed of a balloon-expandable stent attached to a graft material, particularly in many early clinical reports utilizing homemade devices. Many physicians have reported the benefit of controlled hypotension by lowering the mean arterial blood pressure to between 50–60 mm Hg by administration of intravenous sodium nitroprusside. This is performed just prior to the stent-graft deployment in an effort to reduce the risk of downstream migration caused by intraaortic blood flow during deployment. When the stent-graft position is appropriate and the blood pressure is optimal, the stent graft is deployed by rapidly withdrawing the sheath while the pusher mandrel is held firmly in position. Immediately after stent-graft deployment, the nitroprusside infusion is discontinued to normalize the blood pressure.

Adenosine-induced cardiac asystole during stent-graft deployment

The administration of intravenous adenosine to produce temporary cardiac asystole in order to enhance the precision of placement of thoracic endoluminal devices was first reported by Dorros and Cohn in 1996.[27] The effectiveness of this agent in transiently arresting cardiac flow during thoracic endovascular procedure has also been reported by others.[14,28,29] Administration of intravenous adenosine produced a predictable and reproducible period of asystole of 15–30 s before spontaneous return of sinus rhythm. Asystole allowed graft deployment without the risk of displacement by blood flow, particularly in the upper thoracic aorta. The bolus dose required to produce this effect ranged from 12 to 45 mg, and was reproducible in the same patient. No deleterious effects from transient cardiac asystole caused by adenosine infusion during endovascular thoracic aortic procedure have been reported in the literature. Most physicians agree that adenosine may be administered safely in selected cases, particularly those requiring precise deployment of the graft, high in the thoracic aorta.

Other technical maneuvers to facilitate stent-graft deployment

Various technical maneuvers have been described to facilitate the deployment of the devices with increased precision. These maneuvers include: (1) use of a flexible graft attachment system, which conforms more readily to angulated segments of the aortic neck; (2) use of a less flexible shaft on the deployment catheter, giving added support to the system; (3) endograft passage and deployment over a "super-stiff" guidewire; and (4) further support of the deployment catheter and endograft device by the use of a separate pusher catheter to prevent movement of the balloon when inflated. Efforts to decrease cardiac output during device deployment by means of the Valsalva maneuver have also been reported.[30]

Results from clincial series

Even though almost a decade has elapsed since Dake's reported his initial experience with thoracic aortic endografts,[21] the devices continue to be developed, redesigned, and undergo clinical investigations. However, several centers have reported their own experience with one or more devices, both commercially manufactured and "homemade", whether under the auspices of a clinical trial or for compassionate use in selected patients. Mitchell and colleagues reported one of the largest series regarding endovascular thoracic aortic aneurysm repair between 1992 and 1995 at Stanford University Medical Center.[26,31] Homemade devices were implanted for a variety of pathologic conditions of the thoracic aorta. The grafts were constructed of self-expanding, stainless steel Z-stents covered with Dacron. One early death (three total deaths) occurred secondary to graft failure and there were two cases of neurologic deficits. One late death occurred from aneurysm expansion with eventual rupture in a patient with a known endoleak. After a mean follow-up of 12.6 months, a second death had occurred that could possibly have resulted from aneurysm rupture as well. There was one open conversion. Overall, native aneurysm sac thrombosis was successful in 88% (39/44); this rate was achieved after additional interventions were performed (coil embolization in one patient and additional stent grafts in two patients). Problems encountered with this and other homemade devices were related to the bulky delivery system. Furthermore, the lack of columnar support resulted in the tendency of the grafts to "wind sock" with cardiac pulsations and thus, be misdeployed. Greenberg and colleagues similarly reported the results their early experience with homemade devices.[29] In this series, device design was altered over the course of the study period. Overall, in the 25 high-risk patients that were treated, the 30-day mortality rate was 12.5% of elective cases and 33% for urgent cases. The authors noted that four of five perioperative mortalities were directly associated with access failure, early delivery device failure, or other graft-related issues similar to those reported by Dake. Modifications were made to the delivery system and to the device (changing from a nonsupported body to a fully supported system with improved longitudinal strength). Patient selection criteria also evolved over the time span of this review. Later, patients who had extremely tortuous vessels or significant amounts of atheromatous debris seen within the aortic lumen were excluded after two patients succumbed from massive embolization early in the authors' experience.

Commercially manufactured devices continue to be implanted under FDA-approved trials or single-center Investigational Device Exemption, with several centers reporting initial experience with one or more stent-graft systems. In recent literature, Thompson and colleagues described the largest group of patients treated with a single device.[32] Forty-six patients underwent thoracic aortic endoluminal stent-graft implantation with the Gore TAG thoracic endoprosthesis for various aortic pathologies including two acute traumatic ruptures. Although these authors experienced a 100% technical success rate intraoperatively, one of the two perioperative deaths was device related. An iliac artery rupture during sheath perforation occurred while device deployment resulting in the patient's demise. No cases of paraplegia occurred and early endoleaks were treated with additional stent grafts. In the short-term follow-up of 8.5 months, patients in whom endografts were placed for thoracic aortic aneurysm experienced no increase in native sac diameter. Mean aneurysm shrinkage at 12 months was 0.85 cm.

Similarly, Cambria and associates recently reported their thoracic aorta stent-graft experience in 28 patients, 14 of whom received a custom-made device and 14 had the commercially available Excluder implanted.[33] Technical success was 96% as was complete exclusion of the thoracic lesion. There were no conversions and six endoleaks (21%) found on the discharge CT scan. Five of these sealed spontaneously and the sixth patient expired at 4 months postimplantation of unrelated causes. No cases of paraplegia occurred during the study timeframe, though, the authors did acknowledge in an addendum a single case of paraplegia had occurred in a patient with extensive thoracic disease, since the manuscript was submitted. Moreover, these authors noted that device deployment was both less complicated and more precise with the commercial device. Nonetheless, six patients sustained injuries to iliofemoral access arteries, with three patients needing direct surgical repair. These device-related complications occurred irrespective of the type of stent-graft construct placed.

A comparison of endovascular to open treatment of descending thoracic aortic aneurysms was reported by our group recently.[28] Successful deployment occurred in 95% patients implanted with either the Talent or Gore devices. When directly compared to a nonrandomized cohort of open controls, patients undergoing endoluminal repair had significantly shorter operating times, less intraoperative blood loss, and fewer intensive care unit and hospital days. Aneurysm shrinkage (6.8–4.9 cm) was observed at a follow-up of 12 months in the endograft group with no cases of endoleak. Two patients treated via endovascular means died during the follow-up time period, one from multisystem organ failure after successful endograft placement. The operative mortality rate in the open group was 10%, in contrast to zero in the endovascular group. Neither group had any cases of neurologic deficits.

Common problems and complications

Various complications that can result from thoracic stent placement have been reported in the literature. A brief discussion of some of these complications is provided.

Paraplegia

With the current knowledge of paraplegia following open thoracic aneurysm operation, it is well recognized that such a complication can be the result of interruption of the spinal blood flow due to either intercostal artery ligation or prolonged aortic cross-clamping. Multiple adjunctive measures have been performed and tested for spinal cord protection, however, the risk of postoperative paraplegia following an open operation continue to range from 6 to 21%. Clinical studies showed that endovascular repair similarly carry a risk of paraplegia due to occlusion of the intercostal arteries, but the incidence appears be less than 10%, and approximately 5% of affected patients experience a full recovery.[14,29,34] To date, the reported incidence of paraplegia appears to be significantly lower than with open surgical repair. In some cases, the onset of paraplegia has been delayed by 24 h or longer after the procedure. A recent study by Fattori and associates revealed no cases of paraplegia arose in their group of 70 patients, despite covering the entire descending thoracic aorta in 21 cases.[35]

Endoleak

Endoleak of a thoracic endovascular repair occurs when there is an incomplete seal of the endovascular devices at the proximal or the distal attachment site, which is termed a type I endoleak. A type II endoleak is characterized by a retrograde blood flow from intercostal arteries or other collateral vessels. In a recent series of patients treated with thoracic endovascular stent grafts involving between 50 to 70 patients, the endoleak rate has been reported as 7–10%.[36] The primary endoleak rate was somewhat higher in a study by Orend and associates at 20.3% (15 out of 74 patients).[19] The authors attribute this high rate to their initial endovascular stent placement criteria of 10 mm landing zones. After changing the landing zones to 20 mm, fewer endoleaks were encountered.

Device failure

Device failures, such as failure to properly deploy, stent fracture, or stent migration have also been described. Late changes in the graft structure, which can occur due to distortion, component breakage, or fabric tears, have been reported with devices used for repair of abdominal aneurysms. Further careful long-term follow-up of thoracic devices is required to ensure that mechanical device failure is not a limiting factor. Ellozy reported in a clinical study that 13% of patients developed stent fracture in their thoracic endografts at a mean of 20 months of follow-up.[37] Nine of these patients did not have an associated endoleak and were being followed with CT scans. When endoleak does occur with stent fracture, often operative repair is required to prevent further complications, such as aneurysm rupture.

Difficulty in delivering thoracic endografts

Because of the relative large profile of thoracic aortic endograft, a larger introducer sheath is typically required than the endovascular abdominal aortic aneurysm procedures. The sheath must often negotiate a tortuous route through the iliac system and the dilated, angulated aorta itself. Small arteries, atherosclerotic lesions, and angulation may prevent the sheath from reaching its deployment site or may result in kinking of the sheath, which prevents the graft from being released. In the event that ileofemoral artery is either tortuous or severely diseased, a retroperitoneal access through the common iliac artery may be achieved with an iliac conduit bypass graft to permit endograft delivery.

Conclusion

Of the various diseases that affect the thoracic aorta, aneurysms and dissections are the most frequently encountered. Thoracic aorta disease has been managed traditionally with surgical treatment, often involving thoracotomy, cross-clamping of the aorta, and substantial blood loss. Surgical repair has been associated with multiple serious complications, such as stroke, visceral ischemia, paraplegia, and cardiopulmonary compromise. Mortality rates have been uncomfortably high at 5–57%. Endovascular stent grafts offer a less invasive alternative to treatment of thoracic aorta disease. Morbidity and mortality rates for endovascular treatment of thoracic aorta disease rival and may surpass those for open surgical repair. These devices are still in investigational stages in the United States, but short-term data from international trials are extremely promising. For patients with prohibitive operative risks or contraindications to surgery, stent grafts may offer a treatment of choice where none existed previously. The introduction of endoluminally placed thoracic stent grafts into the vascular surgeon's repertoire may in fact revolutionize the treatment of thoracic aorta disease.

References

1 Elefteriades JA. Perspectives on diseases of the thoracic aorta. *Adv Cardiol* 2004; **41**: 75–86.

2 Ouriel K, Greenberg RK. Endovascular treatment of thoracic aortic aneurysms. *J Card Surg* 2003; **18**:455–63.

3 DeBakey ME, Noon GP. Aneurysms of the thoracic aorta. *Mod Concepts Cardiovasc Dis* 1975; **44**:53–58.

4 Bromley LL. Thoracic aneurysms. *Postgrad Med J* 1967; **43**:61–64.

5 Rittenhouse EA, Dillard DH, Winterscheid LC, Merendino KA. Traumatic rupture of the thoracic aorta: a review of the literature and a report of five cases with attention to special problems in early surgical management. *Ann Surg* 1969; **170**:87–100.

6 Prahlow JA, Barnard JJ, Milewicz DM. Thoracic aortic aneurysms and dissections. *J Forensic Sci* 1998; **43**:1244–49.

7 Dalen JE, Alpert JS, Cohn LH, Black H, Collins JJ. Dissection of the thoracic aorta. Medical or surgical therapy? *Am J Cardiol* 1974; **34**:803–8.

8 Immer FF, Bansi AG, Immer-Bansi AS, *et al.* Aortic dissection in pregnancy: analysis of risk factors and outcome. *Ann Thorac Surg* 2003; **76**:309–14.

9 Fabricius AM, Autschbach R, Doll N, Mohr W. Acute aortic dissection during pregnancy. *Thorac Cardiovasc Surg* 2001; **49**:56–57.

10 Robinson PN, Booms P. The molecular pathogenesis of the Marfan syndrome. *Cell Mol Life Sci* 2001; **58**:1698–707.

11 Criado E, Wall P, Lucas P, Gasparis A, Proffit T, Ricotta J. Transesophageal echo-guided endovascular exclusion of thoracic aortic mobile thrombi. *J Vasc Surg* 2004; **39**: 238–42.

12 Greenberg R, Harthun N. Endovascular repair of lesions of descending thoracic aorta: aneurysms and dissections. *Curr Opin Cardiol* 2001; **16**:225–30.

13 Criado FJ, Clark NS, McKendrick C, Longway J, Domer GS. Update on the Talent LPS AAA stent graft: results with "enhanced talent". *Semin Vasc Surg* 2003; **16**:158–65.

14 Criado FJ, Clark NS, Barnatan MF. Stent graft repair in the aortic arch and descending thoracic aorta: a 4-year experience. *J Vasc Surg* 2002; 36: 1121–28.

15 Parodi JC. Endovascular repair of aortic aneurysms, arteriovenous fistulas, and false aneurysms. *World J Surg* 1996; **20**:655–63.

16 Lin PH, Bush RL, Tong FC, Chaikof E, Martin LG, Lumsden AB. Intra-arterial thrombin injection of an ascending aortic pseudoaneurysm complicated by transient ischemic attack and rescued with systemic abciximab. *J Vasc Surg* 2001; **34**:939–42.

17 Kato N, Dake MD, Miller DC, *et al.* Traumatic thoracic aortic aneurysm: treatment with endovascular stent-grafts. *Radiology* 1997; **205**:657–62.

18 Dorros G, Avula S, Fox P, Rhomberg B, Werner P. Endovascular covered stent repair of an intercostal artery patch dehiscence from a descending thoracic aortic aneurysm graft. *J Endovasc Surg* 1996; **3**:299–305.

19 Orend KH, Scharrer-Pamler R, Kapfer X, Kotsis T, Gorich J, Sunder-Plassmann L. Endovascular treatment in diseases of the descending thoracic aorta: 6-year results of a single center. *J Vasc Surg* 2003; **37**:91–99.

20 Bell RE, Taylor PR, Aukett M, Sabharwal T, Reidy JF. Results of urgent and emergency thoracic procedures treated by endoluminal repair. *Eur J Vasc Endovasc Surg* 2003; **25**:527–31.

21 Dake MD, Miller DC, Semba CP, Mitchell RS, Walker PJ, Liddell RP. Transluminal placement of endovascular stent-grafts for the treatment of descending thoracic aortic aneurysms. *N Engl J Med* 1994; **331**:1729–34.

22 Chuter TA, Gordon RL, Reilly LM, Goodman JD, Messina LM. An endovascular system for thoracoabdominal aortic aneurysm repair. *J Endovasc Ther* 2001; **8**:25–33.

23 Hausegger KA, Oberwalder P, Tiesenhausen K, *et al.* Intentional left subclavian artery occlusion by thoracic aortic stent-grafts without surgical transposition. *J Endovasc Ther* 2001; **8**:472–76.

24 Kahn RA, Marin ML, Hollier L, Parsons R, Griepp R. Induction of ventricular fibrillation to facilitate endovascular stent graft repair of thoracic aortic aneurysms. *Anesthesiology* 1998; **88**:534–36.

25 Semba CP, Mitchell RS, Miller DC, *et al.* Thoracic aortic aneurysm repair with endovascular stent-grafts. *Vasc Med* 1997; **2**:98–103.

26 Mitchell RS, Miller DC, Dake MD. Stent-graft repair of thoracic aortic aneurysms. *Semin Vasc Surg* 1997; **10**:257–71.

27 Dorros G, Cohn JM. Adenosine-induced transient cardiac asystole enhances precise deployment of stent-grafts in the thoracic or abdominal aorta. *J Endovasc Surg* 1996; **3**:270–72.

28 Najibi S, Terramani TT, Weiss VJ, *et al.* Endoluminal versus open treatment of descending thoracic aortic aneurysms. *J Vasc Surg* 2002; **36**:732–37.

29 Greenberg R, Resch T, Nyman U, *et al.* Endovascular repair of descending thoracic aortic aneurysms: an early experience with intermediate-term follow-up. *J Vasc Surg* 2000; **31**:147–56.

30 Yano OJ, Faries PL, Morrissey N, Teodorescu V, Hollier LH, Marin ML. Ancillary techniques to facilitate endovascular repair of aortic aneurysms. *J Vasc Surg* 2001; **34**:69–75.

31 Mitchell RS, Miller DC, Dake MD, Semba CP, Moore KA, Sakai T. Thoracic aortic aneurysm repair with an endovascular stent graft: the "first generation". *Ann Thorac Surg* 1999; **67**:1971–74; discussion 1979–80.

32 Thompson CS, Gaxotte VD, Rodriguez JA, *et al.* Endoluminal stent grafting of the thoracic aorta: initial experience with the Gore Excluder. *J Vasc Surg* 2002; **35**:1163–70.

33 Cambria RP, Brewster DC, Lauterbach SR, *et al.* Evolving experience with thoracic aortic stent graft repair. *J Vasc Surg* 2002; **35**:1129–36.

34 Makaroun MS, Dillavou ED, Kee ST, *et al.* Endovascular treatment of thoracic aortic aneurysms: results of the phase II multicenter trial of the GORE TAG thoracic endoprosthesis. *J Vasc Surg* 2005; **41**:1–9.

35 Fattori R, Napoli G, Lovato L, *et al.* Descending thoracic aortic diseases: stent-graft repair. *Radiology* 2003; **229**:176–83.

36 Bell RE, Taylor PR, Aukett M, Sabharwal T, Reidy JF. Mid-term results for second-generation thoracic stent grafts. *Br J Surg* 2003; **90**:811–17.

37 Ellozy SH, Carroccio A, Minor M, *et al.* Challenges of endovascular tube graft repair of thoracic aortic aneurysm: midterm follow-up and lessons learned. *J Vasc Surg* 2003; **38**:676–83.

CHAPTER 8

Abdominal aortic aneurysm

W. Anthony Lee, Daniel J. Martin, Imran Mohiuddin

In spite of more than 45,000 patients undergoing elective repair of abdominal aortic aneurysm (AAA) each year in the United States, approximately 15,000 patients die annually as a result of ruptured aneurysm, making it the tenth leading cause of death in men in this country.[1] The incidence appears to be increasing and this is due in part to improvements in diagnostic imaging and more importantly a result of a growing elderly population. With early diagnosis and timely intervention, aneurysm rupture-related death is largely preventable. Conventional treatment of an AAA involves replacing the aneurysmal segment of the aorta with a prosthetic graft, with the operation performed through a large abdominal incision. Techniques for this open abdominal surgery have been refined, adapted, and extensively studied by vascular surgeons over the past four decades. Despite a well documented low perioperative mortality rate of 2–3% in large academic institutions, the thought of undergoing an open abdominal aortic operation often provokes a sense of anxiety in many patients due in part to the postoperative pain associated with the large abdominal incision as well as the long recovery time needed before the patient can return to normal physical activity.

The most common location of aortic aneurysms is the infrarenal aorta. Endovascular stent-graft placement represents a revolutionary and minimally invasive treatment for infrarenal AAAs that only requires 1–2 days of hospitalization, and the patient can return to normal physical activity within 1 week. The concept of utilizing an endoluminal device in the management of vascular disease was first proposed by Dotter and colleagues, who successfully treated a patient with iliac occlusion using transluminal angioplasty in 1964.[2] Nearly two decades later, Parodi and colleagues reported the first successful endovascular repair of AAA using a stent-graft device.[3] Since then, a variety of stent-graft technologies have been developed to treat AAA. The rapid innovation of this new treatment modality has undoubtedly captured the attention of patients with aortic aneurysms as well as physicians who practice endovascular therapy. Physicians in general should be knowledgeable regarding available treatment options of AAA in order to provide adequate evaluation and education to patients and their families. In this chapter treatment options for AAAs are outlined, including conventional repair and endovascular approach. Advantages and potential complications of these treatments are also addressed.

Etiology

The prevalence of AAA has been gradually increasing due to wider use of diagnostic imaging and population-based screening programs, and is currently estimated to be about 5–7% of the population who are 65 years or older. This translates to approximately 2.7 million Americans based on the 2000 US Census. It is now the tenth leading cause of death with 15,000 deaths annually. Risk factors for AAA include age (>65 years), male gender (4 : 1), family history (first degree relative), hypertension, smoking (>10 years), other aneurysms (thoracic aorta, femoral, and popliteal arteries), and Caucasian race.

The natural history of an AAA is to expand and rupture. AAA exhibits a "staccato" pattern of growth, where periods of relative quiescence may alternate with expansion. Therefore, while an individual pattern of growth cannot be predicted, average aggregate growth is approximately 3–4 mm/year. There is some evidence to suggest that larger aneurysms may expand faster than smaller aneurysms, but there is significant overlap between the ranges of growth rates at each strata of size.

Rupture risk appears to be directly related to aneurysm size as predicted by Laplace's Law. While more sophisticated methods of assessing rupture risk based on finite element analysis of wall stress is under active investigation, maximum transverse diameter remains the standard method of risk assessment for aneurysm rupture. In the past, AAA rupture risk has been overestimated. More recently, two landmark studies have served to better define the natural history of AAA.[4,5] Based on best available evidence, the annualized risk of rupture is given in Table 8.1. The rupture risk is quite low below 5.5 cm and begins to rise exponentially thereafter. This size can serve as an appropriate threshold for recommending elective repair provided one's surgical mortality is below 5%. For each size strata, however, women appear to be at a higher risk for rupture than men, and a lower threshold of 4.5–5.0 cm may be reasonable in good-risk patients. Although data is less compelling, a pattern of rapid expansion of >0.5 cm within 6-months can be considered a relative indication for elective repair. Aneurysms that fall below these indications may safely be followed with CT or ultrasound at 6-month intervals, with long-term outcomes equivalent to earlier surgical repair. Interestingly, in the ADAM study, 80% of all AAA who were followed in this manner eventually came to repair within 5 years.

Aneurysm diameter (cm)	Annualized Risk (%/year)
5–6	3–15
6–7	10–20
7–8	20–40
>8	30–50

Table 8.1 Risk of rupture of abdominal aortic aneurysm per year by diameter.

Unless symptomatic or ruptured, AAA repair is a prophylactic one. The rationale for recommending repair is predicated on the assumption that the risk of aneurysm rupture exceeds the combined risk of death from all other causes such as cardiopulmonary disease and cancer. On the other hand, our limitation in predicting timing and cause of death is underscored by the observation that over 25% of patients who were deemed unfit for surgical repair because of their comorbidities died from rupture of their aneurysms within 5 years.

Clinical symptoms

Most AAA are asymptomatic and they are usually found incidentally during workup for chronic back pain or kidney stones. Physical examination is neither sensitive nor specific except in thin patients. Large aneurysms may be missed in the obese, while normal aortic pulsations may be mistaken for an aneurysm in thin individuals. Rarely, patients present with back pain and/or abdominal pain with a tender pulsatile mass. These patients belong in the subset of "symptomatic" aneurysms. Patients with these symptoms must be treated for a rupture until proven otherwise. If the patient is hemodynamically stable and the aneurysm is intact on a CT scan, the patient is admitted for blood pressure control with intravenous antihypertensive agents and repaired usually within 12–24 h or at least during the same hospitalization. In contrast, patients who are hemodynamically unstable with a history of acute back pain and/or syncope, and a known unrepaired AAA or a pulsatile abdominal mass should be immediately taken to the operating room with a presumed diagnosis of a ruptured AAA.

Overall mortality of AAA rupture is 71–77%, which include all out-of-hospital and in-hospital deaths, as compared to 2–6% for elective open surgical repair.[6-8] Nearly half of all patients with ruptured AAA will die before reaching the hospital. For the remainder, surgical mortality is 45–50% and has not substantially changed in the last 30 years.

Relevant anatomy

An abdominal aortic aneurysm is defined as a pathologic focal dilation of the aorta that is greater than 30 mm or 1.5 times the adjacent diameter of the normal aorta. Male aortas tend to be larger than females and there is generalized growth of the aortic diameter with each decade of life. Almost 90% of AAA are infrarenal in location and have a fusiform morphology. There is a higher predilection for juxtarenal and suprarenal AAA in women as compared to men. Concomitant common iliac and/or hypogastric artery aneurysms can be found in 20–25% of patients. Although the etiology of most aortic aneurysms is atherosclerotic, clinically significant peripheral occlusive disease is unusual and present in less than 10% of all cases.

While extravascular anatomy is important for open surgical repair of AAA, intravascular anatomy and aortoiliac morphology are important for endovascular repair. Pertinent anatomic dimensions include the diameter of the proximal nondilated infrarenal aortic neck, which can range from 18 to 30 mm, common iliac artery, from 8 to 16 mm, and external iliac arteries, 6–10 mm. Morphologically, the aortic neck can manifest complex angulation above and below the renal arteries due to combination of elongation and anterolateral displacement by the posterior bulge of the aneurysmal aorta. (Plate 3, facing p. 80) Furthermore, the shape of the proximal neck is rarely tubular, but often is conical, reverse conical, or barrel shaped. Distally, the iliac arteries can have severe tortuosity with multiple compound turns. While not significant from hemodynamic standpoint, severe iliac calcifications combined with extreme tortuosity can pose a formidable challenge during endovascular repair.

Diagnostic evaluation

Preoperative evaluation should include routine history and physical examination with particular attention to (1) any symptoms referable to the aneurysm, which may impact the timing of repair, (2) history of pelvic surgery or radiation, in the event retroperitoneal exposure is required or interruption of hypogastric circulation is planned, (3) claudication suggestive of significant iliac occlusive disease, (4) lower extremity bypass or other femoral reconstructive procedures, and (5) chronic renal insufficiency or contrast allergy.

Cross-sectional imaging is required for definitive evaluation of AAA. While ultrasound is safe, widely available, relatively accurate and inexpensive, and therefore is the screening modality of choice, the CT scan remains the gold standard for determination of anatomic eligibility for endovascular repair. Size of the AAA may differ up to 1 cm between CT and ultrasound, and during longitudinal follow-up, comparisons should be made between identical modalities. With modern multirow detector scanners, a timed-bolus intravenous contrast enhanced, 2.5–3.0 mm slice spiral CT of the chest, abdomen, and pelvis can be performed in less than 30 s with a single breath hold. Extremely high-resolution images are obtained with submillimeter spatial resolution (Figure 8.1). Proper window level and width (brightness and contrast) is important for discrimination among aortic wall, calcific plaque, thrombus, and lumen. The only major drawback to CT is the risk of contrast nephropathy in diabetics and in patients with renal insufficiency.

The spiral technique further affords the ability for three-dimensional reconstruction. Three-dimensional reconstructions can yield important morphologic information that is critical to endovascular therapy. Using third-party software, these images can be viewed and manipulated on one's desktop PC and so-called "center-line" (transverse slices perpendicular to the central flow lumen of the aorta) diameter and length measurements obtained. (Plate 4, facing p. 80) Conventional angiography has a minimal role in the current management of AAA. Angiography is invasive with an increased risk of complications. Indications for angiography are isolated to concomitant iliac occlusive disease (present in less than 10% of patients with AAA) and unusual renovascular anatomy.

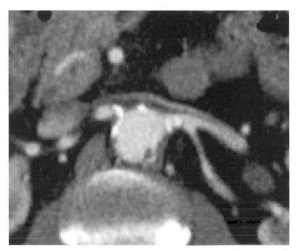

Figure 8.1 High-resolution contrast spiral CT angiogram.

Treatment

Over a decade has passed since the first report, by Parodi in 1991,[3] of human implantation of a home made stent graft for endovascular repair of an AAA. Although long-term data are scant and many issues regarding durability and efficacy remain controversial, multiple prospective clinical trials across different devices and, more recently, analysis of large Medicare administrative databases and meta-analyses of published literature, have consistently demonstrated significantly decreased operative time, blood loss, length of stay in hospital, and overall perioperative morbidity and mortality of endovascular repair as compared to open surgical repair. For patients who are at increased risk for surgery because of age or comorbidity, endovascular repair is a superior minimally invasive alternative. Several multicenter prospective randomized trials are currently underway both in the United States and Europe to compare the early and long-term differences between open and endovascular repair in good-risk patients.

The principle of endovascular repair of AAA involves a covered stent device (stent graft or endograft) that is fixed proximally and distally to nonaneurysmal aortoiliac segment and thereby endoluminally excluding the aneurysm from the aortic circulation. Unlike open surgical repair, the aneurysm sac is neither resected nor its branches, such as lumbar arteries or the inferior mesenteric artery, ligated. Currently, three devices are available for elective repair of intact infrarenal AAA: (1) Medtronic AneuRx (Santa Rosa, CA), (2) W.L. Gore Excluder (Flagstaff, AZ), and (3) Cook Zenith (Bloomington, IN). Despite some differences in physical appearance, mechanical properties, and materials, they are discussed collectively in this chapter. They are all modular devices consisting of a primary device or main body and one or two iliac limbs that insert into the main body to complete the repair. Depending on the device, there are varying degrees of flexibility in the choice of iliac limbs that can be matched to the main body, which can impact the customizability for a particular anatomy.

Anatomic eligibility for endovascular repair is mainly based on three areas: the proximal aortic neck, common iliac arteries, and the external iliac and common femoral arteries, which relate to the proximal and distal landing zones or fixation sites and the access vessels, respectively. The requirements for the proximal aortic neck are a diameter of 18–28 mm and a minimum length of 15 mm. Usually, multiple measurements of the diameter are taken along the length of the neck to assess its shape. All diameter measurements are mid-wall to mid-wall of the vessels. Secondary considerations include mural calcifications (<50% circumference), luminal thrombus (<50% circumference), and angulation (<45°). Presence of significant amount of any one of these secondary features in combination with a relatively short proximal neck may compromise successful short and long-term fixation of the stent graft and exclusion of the aneurysm. The usual distal landing zone is the common iliac artery. The external iliac artery may serve as an alternate site when the ipsilateral common iliac artery is aneurysmal or ectatic. The treatable diameters of common iliac arteries range from 8 to 20 mm and there should be at least 20 mm of apposable artery of uniform diameter to allow adequate fixation. And finally, at least one of the two common femoral and external iliac arteries must be at least 7 mm in diameter in order to safely introduce the main delivery sheath. Slightly smaller iliac diameters may be tolerated depending on the specific device and in the absence of severe tortuosity and calcific disease. Difficult access is one of the main causes of increased procedural times and intraoperative complications. Using these criteria, approximately 60% of all AAA are anatomic candidates for endovascular repair.

The next step in the preoperative planning is device selection. Typically, the proximal diameter of the main device is oversized by 10–20% of the nominal diameter of the aortic neck. Distally, the iliac limbs are oversized by 1–4 mm depending on the individual device's instructions for use. The biggest challenge to proper device selection remains determining the optimal length from the renal arteries to the hypogastric arteries. Despite availability of sophisticated three-dimensional reconstructions, the exact path that a device will take from the proximal aortic neck to the distal iliac arteries is difficult to predict. It is dependent on a host of factors related to the mechanical properties of the stent graft and the morphology of the aortoiliac flow lumen. "Plumb-line" measurements of axial CT images can be quite inaccurate, typically grossly underestimating the length, while center-line measurements usually overestimate the length. Angiographic measurements using a marker catheter are invasive, requires contrast and radiation exposure, and also inaccurate because it fails to take into account the stiffness of the stent graft. The consequences of not choosing the correct length of the device include inadvertent coverage of the hypogastric artery if too long and the need for additional devices if too short. In the former case, one incurs a 40% risk of ipsilateral hip and buttock claudication, whereas in the latter, one adds the cost of $2500 per extender to an already expensive procedure and introduces another component junction that can be a potential source of modular separation.

Procedural technique

Although endovascular AAA repair may be performed in any venue with appropriate digital fluoroscopic imaging capability, due to the need for absolute sterility and aseptic technique, it is most safely performed in a surgical suite. While a fixed floor or ceiling-mounted fluoroscopic equipment, as in a dedicated endovascular surgical suite, may provide some benefit in terms of image quality and duration of fluoroscopy without X-ray tube burn out, most endovascular AAA repairs can be safely performed with portable C-arm fluoroscopic equipment.

The patient is prepped and draped just as in open AAA repair. Patients with renal insufficiency should be started on perioperative oral N-acetylcysteine (Mucomyst) and sodium bicarbonate infusion to reduce the risk of contrast nephropathy.[9] A variety of anesthetic options may be used. Regional anesthesia may be appropriate for patients with pulmonary disease. There are reports of success with local anesthetics alone, as the incisions are typically smaller than a typical open inguinal hernia repair.[10,11]

Bilateral transverse oblique incisions are made just below the inguinal ligament to expose approximately 2–3 cm of common femoral arteries and obtain proximal control. Special attention is paid to avoid the groin crease to decrease the risk of wound complications. Some have advocated a completely percutaneous access using the "preclose" technique with the Perclose suture-mediated vascular closure device (Abbott Perclose, Redwood City, CA). Review of reported series on this technique suggest a technical success rate of 95% for medium size sheaths ranging from 12–16 Fr, and 75% success for 18–24 Fr sizes.

Transfemoral access is obtained using standard Seldinger technique. Initial soft-tipped starter guidewires are exchanged for stiff guidewires, which are advanced to the thoracic arch. Intravenous heparin at 80 IU/kg are administered and the ACT (activated clotting time) is maintained at 200–250 s. These guidewires provide the necessary support for the subsequent introduction of the large diameter delivery catheters and devices. In the absence of special anatomic considerations, the primary device is inserted through the right side and the contralateral iliac limb is inserted through the left side. After administration of heparin, the delivery catheter or the introducer sheath is advanced to the L1–L2 vertebral space, which typically marks the location of the renal arteries. An angiographic catheter is advanced from the contralateral femoral artery to the same level.

A road-mapping aortogram is obtained to localize the renal arteries. The primary device is rotated to the desired orientation and deployed just below the lowest renal artery. The angiographic catheter is replaced with a directional catheter and an angled guidewire and the opening for the contralateral limb on the main device is cannulated. Intrastent passage of the guidewire is confirmed and the angled guidewire is replaced with a stiff guidewire. The contralateral iliac limb is inserted into the docking opening of the primary device and deployed. For the Zenith device, there is a separate ipsilateral iliac limb that must be deployed to complete the repair. Depending on the accuracy of preoperative measurements, device selection, native anatomy, and technique, additional extenders may be required to achieve complete aneurysm exclusion and adequate fixation proximally and distally. Retrograde iliac angiograms are performed through the sheaths to locate the hypogastric arteries so as to prevent their inadvertent coverage. A completion angiogram is performed looking for patency of the renal and hypogastric arteries, the device limbs, proximal and distal fixation, and endoleak. Adjunctive interventions including additional devices, balloons, bare stents, etc. are performed as needed. The procedure is concluded with routine repairs of the femoral arteries and closure of the groin incisions. The patients are recovered in the recovery room for 2–4 h and admitted to the general care floor. Although in the past, patients were admitted to the Intensive Care Unit (ICU), this is rarely needed. Most patients can be started on a regular diet that evening and discharged the next morning.

Surveillance

Lifelong follow-up is essential to the long-term success after endovascular AAA repair. Indeed, one may go so far as to say that absence of appropriate follow-up is tantamount to not having had a repair at all. One postoperative surveillance algorithm is illustrated in Figure 8.2. A triple-phase (noncontrast, contrast, and delayed) spiral CT scan and a four-view (anteroposterior, lateral,

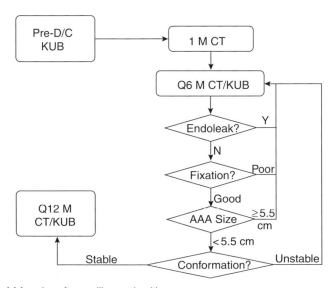

Figure 8.2 AAA endograft surveillance algorithm.

and two obliques) abdominal X-ray should be obtained within the first month. Subsequent imaging can be obtained at 6-month intervals in the first 1–2 years and yearly thereafter. After the first 6 months, patients who cannot travel easily may obtain their studies locally and submit them for review. The CT scan is for detection of endoleaks, subtle proximal migrations, and changes in the aneurysm size. The abdominal X-ray gives a "birds-eye" view of the overall morphology of the stent graft. Subtle changes in conformation of the iliac limbs relative to each other and/or the spine can provide early signs of impending component separation or loss of fixation. Further, stent fractures and/or suture breaks that can compromise long-term device integrity can sometimes only be detected on a plain film and not on a CT scan.

Results from clinical series

The primary success rate after endovascular repair of abdominal aortic aneurysm has been reported to be as high as 95%.[12-14] The less invasive nature of this procedure is appealing to many physicians and patients. In addition, virtually all reports indicate a decreased blood loss, transfusion requirements, length of ICU and hospital stay for endovascular repair of abdominal aortic aneurysms when compared to the standard surgical approach.[7,15,16] With the advent of bifurcated grafts and improved delivery systems in the future, the only real limitation will be cost. When evaluating the literature for results from clinical series, it is important to look at a comparison of endoluminal versus open repair, device specific outcome, and cost analysis studies.

Endovascular versus open repair

Early reports on results with endovascular repair were often flawed due to selection biases. This is because from its inception, endovascular repair has been used mostly in patients who are at higher risk for open repair. At the same time, only patients with favorable anatomy including less tortuosity and the presence of a suitable infrarenal neck were considered for endovascular repair. Randomization is also difficult because most patients who anatomically qualify for endovascular repair would withdraw from the study if randomized to open repair. Consequently, there are very few randomized-controlled trials that have compared outcomes in patients with similar risk factors and anatomy that are eligible for both types of repair. Two such European trials have recently published short-term outcome data that are unbiased in design.

The DREAM trial is a multicenter randomized trial that compared open versus endovascular repair among a group of 345 patients at 28 European centers utilizing multiple different devices including: Gore, AneuRx, and Zenith.[17] Patients were included only if they were considered to be candidates for both types of repairs. The operative mortality rate was 4.6% in the operative group versus 1.2% in the endoluminal group at 30 days. When looking at the combined rate of operative mortality and severe complications, there was an incidence of 9.8% in the open repair versus 4.7% in the endoluminal group. The difference here was largely due to the higher frequency of pulmonary complications seen in the open group. There was a higher incidence of graft-related complications in the endoluminal group. There was no difference in the nonvascular-local complication rate among the two groups. The EVAR-1 trial is also a multicenter randomized trial that compared open to endoluminal repair.[15] This study was conducted on 1082 patients at 34 centers in the United Kingdom utilizing all available devices. Short-term mortality at 30 days was 4.7% in the open and 1.7% in the endoluminal group. The in-hospital mortality rate was also increased in the open when compared to the endoluminal group (6.2–2.1%). As expected, the secondary-intervention rate was higher in the endoluminal group (9.8–5.8%). Complication rates were not reported with the EVAR-1 trial. There are criticisms that can be applied to both of these trials. Patients had to be eligible for either type of repair in order to be included in the study. Consequently, these findings cannot be generalized for patients who are too sick to undergo open surgery or in those patients whose anatomy precludes them from undergoing endovascular repair. At the time of writing this chapter, there were other randomized trials that were ongoing including the Open versus Endovascular Repair (OVER) trial in the United States and the Anevrisme de l'aorte abdominale: Chirugie versus Endoprothese (ACE) trial in France that may yield further information.[18]

Device specific outcome

Device specific outcomes have been evaluated by several leading researchers and are summarized in Table 8.2. Matsumura and associates compared endoluminal to open repair using the Excluder device.[16] In their review, they demonstrated a 30-day mortality rate of 1% along with an endoleak rate of 17 and 20% at 1- and 2-year intervals.[16] The limb narrowing, limb migration, and trunk migration were all 1% at 2 years. There were no deployment failures or early conversions. There was an annual 7% reintervention rate. Aneurysm growth was demonstrated in 14% of patients at 2 years. The Zenith device by Cook has been studied by Greenberg and associates.[14] In their review, they compared standard surgical repair to endoluminal repair in low-risk patients as well as endoluminal repair in high-risk patients. They reported a 30-day

Table 8.2 30-day mortality, 1-year aneurysm growth, migration, endoleak, and freedom from rupture rates for the Gore, Zenith, AneuRx, and Talent LPS devices.

	30-day mortality (%)	Aneurysm growth (%)	Freedom from rupture (%)	Migration (%)	Endoleak (%)
Gore[16]	1	14	Not reported	1	17
Zenith[14]	3.5	Not reported	98.9–100	5.3	7.4
AneuRx[13]*	2.8	11.5	98.4	9.5	13.9
Talent LPS[19]	0.8	0–3	100	2–3	10

* 4-year data for AneuRx device.

mortality rate of 3.5%, which was equal to the open group. The rate of endoleak was 7.4 and 5.4% at 1 and 2-year intervals. There was a 5.3% migration of 5 mm at 1 year. Freedom from rupture was 100% in the low-risk and 98.9% in the high-risk endoluminal group at 2 years. Experience with the AneuRx device has been reported by Zarins and associates.[13] In their 4-year review, they found a 30-day mortality rate of 2.8%. Endoleak rate at 4-years was 13.9%, aneurysm enlargement was 11.5%, stent-graft migration was 9.5%. Freedom from rupture was noted to be 98.4% at 4 years. Criado and associates have reported on their 1-year experience with the Talent LPS device by Medtronic.[12,19] They report a 30-day mortality rate of 0.8%. Endoleak rate was 10%. Three deployment failures were noted and freedom from rupture was 100%. Aneurysm growth and migration rates were divided into three different neck-size groups. Patients with a wide neck (>26 mm) had a 3% growth and migration rate. Narrow-neck patients (<26 mm) had a 1% growth rate and a 2% migration neck. Interestingly, short-neck patients (<15 mm) had no aneurysm growths and a 2% migration rate.

Cost analysis

The current climate of cost containment and limited reimbursement for heathcare services mandates a critical analysis of the economic impact of any new medical technology on the market. The in hospital costs for both endovascular and open repair include graft cost, OR fees, radiology, pharmacy, ancillary care, ICU charges, and floor charges. Despite the improved morbidity and mortality rates, several early studies have reported no cost benefit with the application of endovascular repair.[20 22] The limiting factor appears to be the cost of the device. Despite commercialization of endovascular repair, the device costs are still in the range of $5000–6000 with no signs of abating. A recent report by Angle and associates further corroborates previous studies.[23] In their review, despite a decreased hospital and ICU stays and utilization of pharmacy and respiratory services, cost of endovascular repair was 1.74 times greater than the standard surgical approach. In addition, these cost analysis studies are centered on in-hospital costs and do not even begin to address secondary costs such as postoperative surveillance that is required with endovascular repair.

Common problems and complications

Problems and complications with endovascular AAA repair are myriad and can occur both during implantation and its subsequent follow-up. Some of the more common ones are reviewed here.

Difficult access

Access is the first step of any interventional procedure. The relatively large diameters of the delivery catheters of current devices, which range from 20 to 24 Fr require a minimum of 6.5–7.0 mm diameter common femoral and external iliac arteries. This is particularly problematic for women, whose arteries tend to be smaller than men's, and in patients with concomitant iliac occlusive disease, which may not be hemodynamically significant but may narrow the lumen sufficiently enough to prevent safe passage of the large sheaths. Difficult access to the aorta is one of the most common sources of life-threatening intraoperative complications and can add 1–2 h to the length of the procedure.

Overzealous insertion of the sheaths and delivery catheters can lead to catastrophic iliac artery rupture, typically with complete avulsion of the external iliac artery from the common iliac artery, as the latter is tethered down to the posterior pelvis by the hypogastric artery. This is manifested by a sudden "give" felt by the operator and rapid onset of hypotension. The diagnosis is usually obvious and expeditious proximal surgical or endovascular balloon control must be obtained to prevent exsanguinating hemorrhage.

Disease isolated to the femoral arteries can be overcome by extending the groin incision and exposing the less-diseased distal external iliac artery under the inguinal ligament. In cases of more diffuse iliofemoral disease, adjunctive techniques include balloon angioplasty, serial dilation, and a retroperitoneal iliac conduit. For this last technique, through a retroperitoneal exposure an 8- or 10-mm prosthetic conduit is anastomosed to the distal common iliac artery in an end-to-side manner. Although direct iliac puncture has been described, this is actually a very awkward method of arterial access given the stiffness of the delivery catheter and angle of insertion, and is prone to excessive bleeding during the procedure. The distal end of the conduit is exteriorized, occluded, and the conduit pressurized and directly punctured like an artery. After the procedure, the iliac conduit may be transected and oversewn near its base or converted into an iliofemoral bypass depending on the strength of the external iliac or femoral arterial pulse. The dictum that "if you think of an iliac conduit, you should do it" should be generally followed.

In 10% of cases, the femoral artery requires a more complicated repair beyond simple arteriotomy closure.[24] Usually this is from a posterior plaque fracture during the insertion of the delivery catheter. Local femoral endarterectomy, tacking down the edge of the distal plaque, and closure with a prosthetic patch angioplasty is typically required to prevent acute postoperative femoral thrombosis and limb ischemia.

Difficult contralateral limb opening cannulation

While direct cannulation of the contralateral limb opening can be easily accomplished in majority of cases, in the balance of the remaining cases, due to operator skill, aortoiliac morphology, position of the stent graft, and other unpredictable factors, cannulation may be extremely difficult. After difficult access, cannulation of the contralateral limb opening is the second rate-limiting step during endovascular AAA repair. One technique that can facilitate this step has been "cross-limb" deployment of the primary body (Figure 8.3). The trajectory of the iliac arteries as it joins the aorta is such that the catheter and the guidewire tend to point to the opposite wall and slightly anteriorly. Orienting the contralateral opening ipsilateral to the side of insertion places the

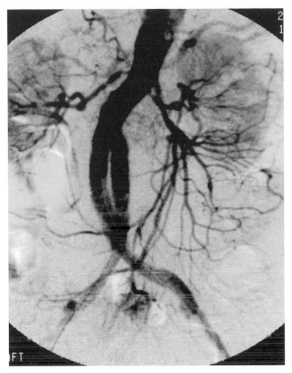

Figure 8.3 Cross-limb deployment of a bifurcated stent graft.

opening in close proximity to the cannulating wire. Other technical adjuncts include frequent changes of the C-arm angle to gain a different perspective as one reconstructs the 3-D spatial relationship between the guidewire and the opening from the 2-D fluoroscopic images.

When attempts at direct cannulation fail, two options include snaring an ipsilateral guidewire directed over the flow divider of the primary device and an aortouni-iliac (AUI) conversion. The former approach (and its variant from the left brachial artery) is almost always successful and the need for AUI conversion occurs in less than 1% of cases.

Common iliac artery aneurysm

Concomitant common iliac and hypogastric artery aneurysms may be present in up to 20% of all AAA. While uncomplicated ectasias may be treated with larger diameter cuffed iliac limbs or "bell-bottom" technique of using aortic cuffs in the iliac position, frank iliac aneurysms greater than 20–22 mm in diameters are best completely excluded. In these situations, the external iliac artery provides the alternative fixation site for the iliac limb. The backbleeding from the excluded hypogastric artery may be treated either by revascularization or simple occlusion. In the former case, the hypogastric artery is disconnected from the common iliac artery aneurysm and is bypassed or transposed

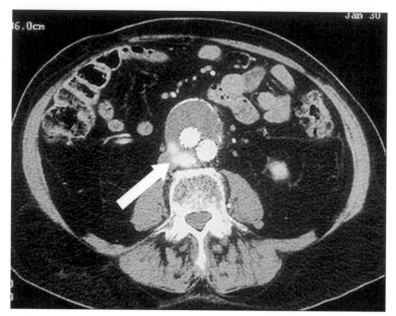

Figure 8.4 An endoleak is detected in the CT scan as evidenced by the perigraft contrast flow (arrow).

to the external iliac artery. In the latter instance, the hypogastric artery is coil embolized before the actual endovascular repair.

Endoleak

An endoleak is an extravasation of contrast outside the stent graft and within the aneurysm sac. It can be present in up to 20–30% of all endovascular AAA repairs in the early postoperative period.[25,26] In general, over half of these endoleaks will resolve spontaneously during the first 6 months resulting in a 10% incidence of chronic endoleaks in all cases beyond the first year of follow-up. Endoleaks can be detected using conventional angiography, contrast CT, MRA (magnetic resonance angiography), and color-flow duplex ultrasound (Figure 8.4 & Plate 5, facing p. 80). Although there is no recognized gold standard, in practice, angiography is considered the least sensitive but most specific for characterizing the source of the endoleak, while the CT scan is the most sensitive but least specific. Widespread availability and reliability that is relatively independent of the technique have made the CT scan the de facto standard imaging modality for postoperative surveillance. Conversely, routine use of duplex ultrasound and MRA has been limited by the lack of proper equipment and local expertise. On the other hand, investigational techniques such as time-resolved MRA may provide greater sensitivity and specificity than either angiography or CT in the future.

Four types of endoleaks have been described. Type I endoleak refers to fixation-related leaks that occur at the proximal or distal attachment sites. These represent less than 5% of all endoleaks and are seen as an early blush of contrast into the aneurysm sac from the proximal or distal ends of the device during completion angiography.[25-27] Although seen as marker of poor patient selection or inadequate repair, over 80% of these leaks spontaneously seal in the first 6 months. Persistent type I endoleaks, on the other hand, require prompt treatment. Type II endoleak refers to retrograde flow originating from a lumbar, inferior mesenteric, accessory renal, or hypogastric artery. They are the most common type of endoleak accounting for 20–30% of all cases and about half resolve spontaneously. On angiography, they are seen as a late filling of the aneurysm sac from a branch vessel(s). Type II endoleaks carry a relatively benign natural history and do not merit intervention unless associated with aneurysm growth. Type III endoleaks refer to failure of device integrity or component separation from modular systems. If detected intraoperative or in the early perioperative period, it is usually from inadequate overlap between two stent grafts, while in the late period, it may be from a fabric tear or junctional separation from conformational changes of the aneurysm. Regardless of the etiology or timing, these should be promptly repaired. And lastly, type IV endoleak refers to the diffuse, early blush seen during completion angiography due to graft porosity and/or suture holes of some Dacron-based devices. It does not have any clinical significance and usually cannot be seen after 48 h and heparin reversal. Endoleaks that have initially been considered type IV but persist become type III endoleaks by definition, as it indicates a more significant material defect than simple porosity or a suture hole.

Endotension

In approximately 5% of cases after an apparently successful endovascular repair, the aneurysm continues to grow without any demonstrable endoleak.[28] This phenomenon has been described as endotension. Although it was initially thought that an endoleak was really present but simply not detected, cases have been reported where the aneurysm has been surgically opened and the contents were completely devoid of any blood and no extravasation could be found. The mechanism of continued pressurization of the aneurysm sac following successful exclusion from the arterial circulation remains unsolved at this time. One putative mechanism has been linked to a transudative process related to certain expanded polytetrafluoroethylene (ePTFE) graft materials.[29] More importantly, however, the natural history of these enlarging aneurysms without endoleaks is unknown, but to date there has been no evidence to suggest that they carry an increased risk of rupture. Conservatively speaking, until further long-term data becomes available, if the patient is a suitable surgical risk, elective open conversion should be considered.

Secondary interventions

There is approximately 10–15% per year risk of secondary interventions following endovascular AAA repair.[30,31] These procedures are critical in the long-term success of the primary procedure in prevention of aneurysm rupture and aneurysm-related death. These secondary procedures, in order of frequency, include proximal or distal extender placement for migrations, highly selective or translumbar embolization for type II endoleaks, direct surgical or laparoscopic branch vessel ligations, bridging cuffs for component separations, and late open surgical conversions.

Rupture

Multiple large series have reported that an annual rupture rate of approximately 1–1.5% per year after endovascular repair.[32,33] The EUROSTAR registry reports a rupture rate of 2.3% over 15.4 months in patients with an endoleak, compared with 0.3% in those without endoleak.[33] Various causes of late ruptures have been reported in the literature, although presence of a persistent endoleak with aneurysm enlargement remains a common culprit for this complication. It has been shown that even successfully excluded aneurysm can lead to the development of attachment-site leaks and device failure, caused in part by aneurysm remodeling resulting in stent migration or kinking.[34,35]

Treatment of rupture may be open conversion or endovascular stent-graft placement. May and associates reported a mortality rate of 43% in those patients who underwent open conversion.[36] Emergent endovascular repair should be considered in these patients since it is potentially much faster and likely to cause physiologic stress than open conversion. Several reports have shown that endovascular repair can be performed successfully in patients previously treated with endoluminal prostheses.[37,38]

Conclusion

The management of AAA has been revolutionized by developments in endovascular technology. This minimally invasive treatment represents an exciting alternative to the conventional open repair. Short-term clinical reports have shown that endovascular stent grafting is technically feasible and efficacious. Moreover, the procedure is associated with less operative blood loss, shorter hospital stay, decreased morbidity, and reduced convalescence period compared to the conventional operation.

While our understanding of endovascular technology continues to evolve, this new treatment clearly provides the greatest benefit to high-risk patients who otherwise would not tolerate an open repair. Minimizing the risk of endoleaks will be critical to the long-term success of this procedure. Judicious application of this new technology and long-term patient surveillance are essential to ensuring positive outcomes with endovascular repair of AAA.

References

1 Cruz CP, Drouilhet JC, Southern FN, Eidt JF, Barnes RW, Moursi MM. Abdominal aortic aneurysm repair. *Vasc Surg* 2001; **35**:335–44.

2 Dotter CT, Judkins MP. Transluminal treatment of arteriosclerotic obstruction. Description of a new technic and a preliminary report of its application. *Circulation* 1964; **30**:654–70.

3 Parodi JC, Palmaz JC, Barone HD. Transfemoral intraluminal graft implantation for abdominal aortic aneurysms. *Ann Vasc Surg* 1991; **5**:491–99.

4 Lederle FA, Johnson GR, Wilson SE, *et al.* The aneurysm detection and management study screening program: validation cohort and final results. Aneurysm Detection and Management Veterans Affairs Cooperative Study Investigators. *Arch Intern Med* 2000; **160**:1425–30.

5 The U.K. Small Aneurysm Trial: design, methods and progress. The UK Small Aneurysm Trial participants. *Eur J Vasc Endovasc Surg* 1995; **9**:42–48.

6 Ouriel K, Greenberg RK, Clair DG. Endovascular treatment of aortic aneurysms. *Curr Probl Surg* 2002; **39**:242–345.

7 Makaroun MS, Chaikof E, Naslund T, Matsumura JS. Efficacy of a bifurcated endograft versus open repair of abdominal aortic aneurysms: a reappraisal. *J Vasc Surg* 2002; **35**:203–10.

8 Chaikof EL, Lin PH, Brinkman WT, *et al.* Endovascular repair of abdominal aortic aneurysms: risk stratified outcomes. *Ann Surg* 2002; **235**:833–41.

9 Bush RL, Lin PH, Bianco CC, *et al.* Endovascular aortic aneurysm repair in patients with renal dysfunction or severe contrast allergy: utility of imaging modalities without iodinated contrast. *Ann Vasc Surg* 2002; **16**:537–44.

10 Lippmann M, Lingam K, Rubin S, Julka I, White R. Anesthesia for endovascular repair of abdominal and thoracic aortic aneurysms: a review article. *J Cardiovasc Surg (Torino)* 2003; **44**:443–51.

11 Bush RL, Lin PH, Lumsden AB. Endovascular management of abdominal aortic aneurysms. *J Cardiovasc Surg (Torino)* 2003; **44**:527–34.

12 Criado FJ, Wilson EP, Fairman RM, Abul-Khoudoud O, Wellons E. Update on the Talent aortic stent graft: a preliminary report from United States phase I and II trials. *J Vasc Surg* 2001; **33**:S146–49.

13 Zarins CK. The US AneuRx Clinical Trial: 6-year clinical update 2002. *J Vasc Surg* 2003; **37**:904–8.

14 Greenberg RK, Chuter TA, Sternbergh WC, 3rd, Fearnot NE. Zenith AAA endovascular graft: intermediate-term results of the US multicenter trial. *J Vasc Surg* 2004; **39**: 1209–18.

15 Greenhalgh RM, Brown LC, Kwong GP, Powell JT, Thompson SG. Comparison of endovascular aneurysm repair with open repair in patients with abdominal aortic aneurysm (EVAR trial 1), 30-day operative mortality results: randomised controlled trial. *Lancet* 2004; **364**:843–48.

16 Matsumura JS, Brewster DC, Makaroun MS, Naftel DC. A multicenter controlled clinical trial of open versus endovascular treatment of abdominal aortic aneurysm. *J Vasc Surg* 2003; **37**:262–71.

17 Prinssen M, Verhoeven EL, Buth J, *et al.* A randomized trial comparing conventional and endovascular repair of abdominal aortic aneurysms. *N Engl J Med* 2004; **351**:1607–18.

18 Lederle FA. Abdominal aortic aneurysm – open versus endovascular repair. *N Engl J Med* 2004; **351**:1677–79.

19 Criado FJ, Fairman RM, Becker GJ. Talent LPS AAA stent graft: results of a pivotal clinical trial. *J Vasc Surg* 2003; **37**:709–15.

20 Bertges DJ, Zwolak RM, Deaton DH, *et al.* Current hospital costs and medicare reimbursement for endovascular abdominal aortic aneurysm repair. *J Vasc Surg* 2003; **37**:272–79.

21 Seiwert AJ, Wolfe J, Whalen RC, Pigott JP, Kritpracha B, Beebe HG. Cost comparison of aortic aneurysm endograft exclusion versus open surgical repair. *Am J Surg* 1999; **178**: 117–20.

22 Quinones-Baldrich WJ. Achieving cost-effective endoluminal aneurysm repair. *Semin Vasc Surg* 1999; **12**:220–25.

23 Angle N, Dorafshar AH, Moore WS, *et al.* Open versus endovascular repair of abdominal aortic aneurysms: what does each really cost? *Ann Vasc Surg* 2004; **18**:612–18.

24 Liewald F, Scharrer-Pamler R, Gorich J, *et al.* Intraoperative, perioperative and late complications with endovascular therapy of aortic aneurysm. *Eur J Vasc Endovasc Surg* 2001; **22**:251–56.

25 Buth J, Harris PL, Van Marrewijk C, Fransen G. Endoleaks during follow-up after endovascular repair of abdominal aortic aneurysm. Are they all dangerous? *J Cardiovasc Surg (Torino)* 2003; **44**:559–66.

26 Baum RA, Stavropoulos SW, Fairman RM, Carpenter JP. Endoleaks after endovascular repair of abdominal aortic aneurysms. *J Vasc Interv Radiol* 2003; **14**:1111–17.

27 Buth J, Harris PL, van Marrewijk C, Fransen G. The significance and management of different types of endoleaks. *Semin Vasc Surg* 2003; **16**:95–102.

28 Dubenec SR, White GH, Pasenau J, Tzilalis V, Choy E, Erdelez L. Endotension. A review of current views on pathophysiology and treatment. *J Cardiovasc Surg (Torino)* 2003; **44**:553–57.

29 Lin PH, Bush RL, Katzman JB, *et al.* Delayed aortic aneurysm enlargement due to endotension after endovascular abdominal aortic aneurysm repair. *J Vasc Surg* 2003; **38**:840–42.

30 Verhoeven EL, Tielliu IF, Prins TR, *et al.* Frequency and outcome of re-interventions after endovascular repair for abdominal aortic aneurysm: a prospective cohort study. *Eur J Vasc Endovasc Surg* 2004; **28**:357–64.

31 Flora HS, Chaloner EJ, Sweeney A, Brookes J, Raphael MJ, Adiseshiah M. Secondary intervention following endovascular repair of abdominal aortic aneurysm: a single centre experience. *Eur J Vasc Endovasc Surg* 2003; **26**:287–92.

32 Zarins CK, White RA, Hodgson KJ, Schwarten D, Fogarty TJ. Endoleak as a predictor of outcome after endovascular aneurysm repair: AneuRx multicenter clinical trial. *J Vasc Surg* 2000; **32**:90–107.

33 Harris PL, Vallabhaneni SR, Desgranges P, Becquemin JP, van Marrewijk C, Laheij RJ. Incidence and risk factors of late rupture, conversion, and death after endovascular repair of infrarenal aortic aneurysms: the EUROSTAR experience. European Collaborators on Stent/graft techniques for aortic aneurysm repair. *J Vasc Surg* 2000; **32**:739–49.

34 Krohg-Sorensen K, Brekke M, Drolsum A, Kvernebo K. Periprosthetic leak and rupture after endovascular repair of abdominal aortic aneurysm: the significance of device design for long-term results. *J Vasc Surg* 1999; **29**:1152–58.

35 Politz JK, Newman VS, Stewart MT. Late abdominal aortic aneurysm rupture after AneuRx repair: a report of three cases. *J Vasc Surg* 2000; **31**:599–606.

36 May J, White GH, Yu W, *et al.* Conversion from endoluminal to open repair of abdominal aortic aneurysms: a hazardous procedure. *Eur J Vasc Endovasc Surg* 1997; **14**:4–11.

37 Ramaiah VG, Thompson CS, Rodriguez-Lopez JA, DiMugno L, Olsen D, Diethrich EB. Endovascular repair of AAA rupture 20 months after endoluminal stent-grafting. *J Endovasc Ther* 2001; **8**:125–30.

38 Teufelsbauer H, Prusa AM, Prager M, *et al.* Endovascular treatment of a multimorbid patient with late AAA rupture after stent-graft placement: 1-year follow-up. *J Endovasc Ther* 2002; **9**:896–900.

CHAPTER 9

Mesenteric artery occlusive disease

Panagiotis Kougias, Mitchell Cox, Peter H. Lin

Vascular occlusive disease of the mesenteric vessels is a relatively uncommon but potentially devastating condition that generally presents in patients over 60 years of age, is three times more frequent in women, and has been recognized as an entity since 1936.[1] The incidence of such a disease is low and represents 2% of the revascularization operations for atheromatous lesions. The most common cause of mesenteric ischemia is atherosclerotic vascular disease. Autopsy studies have demonstrated splanchnic atherosclerosis in 35–70% of cases.[2] Other etiologies exist and include fibromuscular dysplasia, nodose panarteritis, arteritis, and celiac artery compression from a median arcuate ligament, but they are unusual and have an incidence of $\frac{1}{9}$ compared to that of atherosclerosis.

Chronic mesenteric ischemia is related to a lack of blood supply in the splanchnic region and is caused by disease in one or more visceral arteries: the celiac trunk, the superior mesenteric artery (SMA), and the inferior mesenteric artery (IMA). Mesenteric ischemia is thought to occur when two of the three visceral vessels are affected with severe stenosis or occlusion; however in as many as 9% of cases a single vessel is only involved (SMA in 5% and celiac trunk in 4% of cases).[3,4] This disease process may evolve in a chronic fashion, as in the case of progressive luminal obliteration due to atherosclerosis. On the other hand, mesenteric ischemia can occur suddenly, as in the case of thromboembolism. Despite recent progress in perioperative management and better understanding in pathophysiology, mesenteric ischemia is considered as one of the most catastrophic vascular disorders with mortality rates ranging from 50–75%. Delay in diagnosis and treatment are the main contributing factors in its high mortality. It is estimated that mesenteric ischemia accounts for 1 in every 1000 hospital admissions in this country. The prevalence is rising due in part to the increased awareness of this disease, the advanced age of the population, and the significant comorbidity of these elderly patients. Early recognition and prompt treatment before the onset of irreversible intestinal ischemia are essential to improve the outcome.

Anatomy and pathophysiology

Mesenteric arterial circulation is remarkable for its rich collateral network. Three main mesenteric arteries provide the arterial perfusion to the gastrointestinal system: the celiac artery (CA), the SMA, and the IMA. In general, CA provides arterial circulation to the foregut (distal esophagus to duodenum), hepatobiliary system, and spleen; the SMA supplies the midgut (jejunum to mid-colon); and the IMA supplies the hindgut (mid-colon to rectum). The CA and SMA arise from the ventral surface of the infradiaphragmatic suprarenal abdominal aorta, while the IMA originates from the left lateral portion of the infrarenal aorta. These anatomic origins in relation to the aorta are important when a mesenteric angiogram is performed to determine the luminal patency. In order to fully visualize the origins of the CA and SMA, it is necessary to perform both an anterioposterior and a lateral projection of the aorta since most arterial occlusive lesions occurs in the proximal segments of these mesenteric trunks.

Because of the abundant collateral flow between these mesenteric arteries, progressive diminution of flow in one or even two of the main mesenteric trunks is usually tolerated, provided that uninvolved mesenteric branches can enlarge over time to provide sufficient compensatory collateral flow. In contrast, acute occlusion of a main mesenteric trunk may result in profound ischemia due to lack of sufficient collateral flow. Collateral network between the CA and the SMA exist primarily through the superior and inferior pancreaticoduodenal arteries. The IMA may provide collateral arterial flow to the SMA through the marginal artery of Drummond, the arc of Riolan, and other unnamed retroperitoneal collateral vessels termed meandering mesenteric arteries (Figure 9.1). Lastly, collateral visceral vessels may provide important arterial flow to the IMA and the hindgut through the hypogastric arteries and the hemorrhoidal arterial network.

Regulation of mesenteric blood flow is largely modulated by both hormonal and neural stimuli, which characteristically regulate systemic blood flow. In addition, the mesenteric circulation responds to the gastrointestinal contents. Hormonal regulation is mediated by splanchnic vasodilators, such as nitric oxide, glucagon, and vasoactive intestinal peptide. Certain intrinsic vasoconstrictors, such as vasopressin, can diminish the mesenteric blood flow. On the other hand, neural regulation is provided by the extensive visceral autonomic innervation.

Clinical manifestation of mesenteric ischemia is predominantly postprandial abdominal pain, which signifies that the increased oxygen demand of digestion is not met by the gastrointestinal collateral circulation. The postprandial pain frequently occurs in the mid-abdomen, suggesting that the diversion of blood flow from the SMA to supply the stomach impairs perfusion to the small bowel. This leads to transient anaerobic metabolism and acidosis. Persistent or profound mesenteric ischemia will lead to mucosal compromise with release of intracellular contents and by-products of anaerobic metabolism to the splanchnic and systemic circulation. Injured bowel mucosa allows unimpeded influx of toxic substances from the bowel lumen with systemic consequences. If full-thickness necrosis occurs in the bowel wall, intestinal perforation ensues, which will lead to peritonitis. Concomitant atherosclerotic disease in cardiac

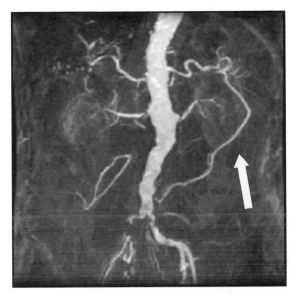

Figure 9.1 An aortogram showing a prominent collateral vessel, which is the arc of Riolan in a patient with an IMA occlusion. This vessel network provides collateral flow between the SMA and IMA.

or systemic circulation frequently compounds the diagnostic and therapeutic complexity of mesenteric ischemia.

Types of mesenteric artery occlusive disease

There are four major types of visceral ischemia involving the mesenteric arteries, which include: (1) acute embolic mesenteric ischemia; (2) acute thrombotic mesenteric ischemia; (3) chronic mesenteric ischemia; and (4) nonocclusive mesenteric ischemia. Despite the variability of these syndromes, a common anatomic pathology is involved in these processes. The SMA is the most commonly involved vessel in acute mesenteric ischemia. Acute thrombotic mesenteric ischemia frequently occurs in patients with underlying mesenteric atherosclerosis, which usually involves the origin of the mesenteric arteries while sparing the collateral branches. The development of collateral vessels is more likely when the occlusive process is a gradual rather than a sudden ischemic event. In acute embolic mesenteric ischemia, the emboli typically originate from a cardiac source and frequently occur in patients with atrial fibrillation or following myocardial infarction (Figures 9.2 & 9.3). Nonocclusive mesenteric ischemia is characterized by a low flow state in otherwise normal mesenteric arteries. In contrast, chronic mesenteric ischemia is a functional consequence of a long-standing atherosclerotic process, which typically involves at least two of the three main mesenteric vessels: the CA, SMA, and the IMA.

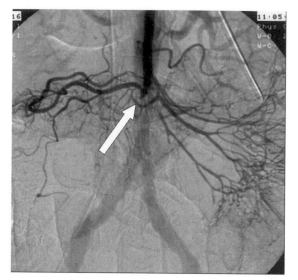

Figure 9.2 An anteroposterior view of a selective SMA angiogram showed an abrupted cutoff of the middle colic artery, which was caused by an emboli due to atrial fibrillation.

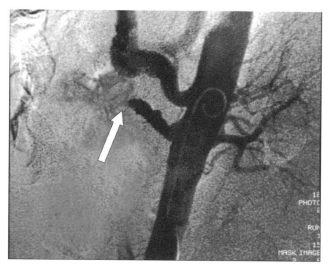

Figure 9.3 A lateral mesenteric angiogram showing an abrupted cutoff of the proximal SMA, which is consistent with SMA embolism.

Several less common syndromes of visceral ischemia involving the mesenteric arteries can also cause serious debilitation. Chronic mesenteric ischemic symptoms can occur due to extrinsic compression of the CA by the diaphragm, which is termed "the median arcuate ligament syndrome." Acute visceral ischemia may occur following an aortic operation, due to ligation of the IMA in the absence of adequate collateral vessels. Furthermore, acute visceral ischemia may develop in aortic dissection that involves the mesenteric arteries, or after coarctation repair. Finally, other unusual causes of ischemia include mesenteric arteritis, radiation arteritis, and cholesterol emboli.

Clinical presentation

Abdominal pain, out of proportion to physical findings, is the classic presentation in patients with acute mesenteric ischemia and occurs frequently following an embolic or thrombotic ischemic event of the SMA. Clinical manifestations may include sudden onset of abdominal cramps in patients with underlying cardiac or atherosclerotic diseases. The abdominal pain is often associated with bloody diarrhea, as a result of mucosal sloughing secondary to ischemia. Fever, diarrhea, nausea, vomiting, and abdominal distention are some common but nonspecific manifestations. Diffuse abdominal tenderness, rebound, and rigidity are ominous signs and usually herald bowel infarction.

Symptoms of thrombotic mesenteric ischemia may initially be more insidious than those of embolic mesenteric ischemia. Approximately 70% of patients with chronic mesenteric ischemia have a history of abdominal angina. In these patients, the chronicity of mesenteric atherosclerosis is important as it permits collateral vessel formation. The precipitating factor leading to chronic mesenteric occlusion is often due to an unrelated illness, which results in dehydration, such as diarrhea or vomiting that may further confuse the actual diagnosis. If the diagnosis is not recognized promptly, symptoms may worsen, which can lead to progressive abdominal distention, oliguria, increasing fluid requirements, and severe metabolic acidosis.

Abdominal pain is only present in approximately 70% of patients with nonocclusive mesenteric ischemia. When present, the pain is usually severe but may vary in location, character, and intensity. In the absence of abdominal pain, progressive abdominal distention with acidosis may be an early sign of ischemia and impending bowel infarction. The diagnosis of nonocclusive mesenteric ischemia should be considered in elderly patients with sudden abdominal pain, who have any of the following risk factors: congestive heart failure, acute myocardial infarction with cardiogenic shock, hypovolemic or hemorrhagic shock, sepsis, pancreatitis, and administration of digitalis or vasoconstrictor agents such as epinephrine.

Diagnostic studies

Various clinical possibilities should be considered in a patient with an acute onset of severe abdominal pain. Perforated gastroduodenal ulcer, intestinal obstruction, pancreatitis, cholecystitis, and nephrolithiasis occur more commonly than acute mesenteric ischemia. Laboratory evaluation is neither sensitive nor specific in distinguishing these various diagnoses. In the setting of mesenteric ischemia, complete blood count (CBC) may reveal hemoconcentration and leukocytosis. Metabolic acidosis develops as a result of anaerobic metabolism. Elevated serum amylase and lactate levels are nonspecific findings. Hyperkalemia and azotemia may occur in the late stages of mesenteric ischemia.

Plain abdominal radiographs may provide helpful information to exclude other causes of abdominal pain such as intestinal obstruction, perforation, or volvulus, which may exhibit symptoms mimicking intestinal ischemia. Pneumoperitoneum, pneumatosis intestinalis, and gas in the portal vein may indicate infarcted bowel. In contrast, radiographic appearance of an adynamic ileus with a gasless abdomen is the most common finding in patients with acute mesenteric ischemia.

Upper endoscopy, colonoscopy, or barium radiography does not provide any useful information when evaluating acute mesenteric ischemia. Moreover, barium enema is contraindicated if the diagnosis of mesenteric ischemia is being considered. The intraluminal barium can obscure accurate visualization of mesenteric circulation during angiography. In addition, intraperitoneal leakage of barium can occur in the setting of intestinal perforation, which can lead to added therapeutic challenges during mesenteric revascularization.

Diagnosis of chronic mesenteric ischemia can be more challenging. Usually, prior to the evaluation by a vascular service, the patients have undergone an extensive workup for the symptoms of chronic abdominal pain, weight loss, and anorexia. Rarely, the vascular surgeon is the first to encounter a patient with the above symptoms. In this situation, it is advisable to keep in mind that mesenteric ischemia is a rare entity, and that a full diagnostic workup that should include CT scan of the abdomen and evaluation by a gastroenterologist should be performed. Mesenteric occlusive disease may coexist with malignancy and symptoms of mesenteric vessel stenosis may be the result of extrinsic compression by a tumor.

Duplex ultrasonography is a valuable noninvasive means of assessing the patency of the mesenteric vessels. Moneta and associates, evaluated the use of duplex ultrasound in the diagnosis of mesenteric occlusive disease in a blinded prospective study.[5,6] A peak systolic velocity in the SMA >275 cm/s demonstrated a sensitivity of 92%, specificity of 96%, and an overall accuracy of 96% for detecting >70% stenosis. The same authors found sensitivity and specificity of 87 and 82%, respectively with an accuracy of 82% in predicting >70% celiac trunk stenosis. Duplex has been successfully used for follow-up after open surgical reconstruction or endovascular treatment of the mesenteric vessels to assess recurrence of the disease. Finally, spiral-computed tomography with 3-D reconstruction as well as magnetic resonance angiogram (MRA) has been promising in providing clear radiographic assessment of the mesenteric vessels (Figure 9.4; Plate 6, facing p. 80).

The definitive diagnosis of mesenteric vascular disease is made by biplanar mesenteric arteriography, which should be performed promptly in any patient with suspected mesenteric occlusion. It typically shows occlusion or near-occlusion of the CA and SMA at or near their origins from the aorta. In most cases, the IMA has been previously occluded secondary to diffuse infrarenal

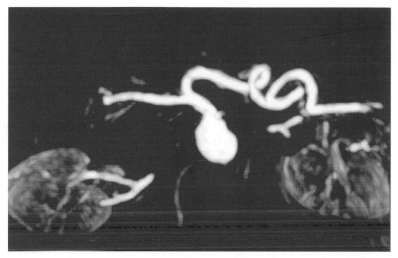

Figure 9.4 A sagital view of a MRA provides a clear view of the luminal patency of the SMA.

aortic atherosclerosis. The differentiation of the four different types of mesenteric arterial occlusion may be suggested with biplanar mesenteric arteriogram. Mesenteric emboli typically lodge at the orifice of the middle colic artery, which creates a "miniscus sign" with an abrupt cutoff of a normal proximal SMA several centimeters from its origin on the aorta.

Mesenteric thrombosis, in contrast, occurs at the most proximal SMA, which tapers off at 1–2 cm from its origin. In the case of chronic mesenteric occlusion, the appearance of collateral circulation is usually present. Nonocclusive mesenteric ischemia produces an arteriographic image of segmental mesenteric vasospasm with a relatively normal appearing main SMA trunk. Mesenteric arteriography can also play a therapeutic role. Once the diagnosis of nonocclusive mesenteric ischemia is made on the arteriogram, an infusion catheter can be placed at the SMA orifice and vasodilating agents, such as papaverine, can be administered intraarterially. The papaverine infusion may be continued postoperatively to treat persistent vasospasm, a common occurrence following mesenteric reperfusion. Transcatheter thrombolytic therapy has little role in the management of thrombotic mesenteric occlusion. Although thrombolytic agents may transiently recannulate the occluded vessels, the underlying occlusive lesions require definitive treatment. Furthermore, thrombolytic therapy typically requires a prolonged period of time to restore perfusion and the intestinal viability may be difficult to assess.

A word of caution would be appropriate here regarding patients with typical history of chronic intestinal angina, who present with an acute abdomen and classical findings of peritoneal irritation. Arteriography is the gold standard for the diagnosis of mesenteric occlusive disease, however, it can be a time consuming diagnostic modality. In this group of patients, immediate exploration for assessment of intestinal viability is the best choice.

Endovascular treatment strategies

Indications for intervention and patient selection

Classic symptoms of chronic mesenteric occlusive disease include "food fear," postprandial abdominal pain, and weight loss. The goals of revascularization in patients with symptomatic chronic mesenteric ischemia are to relieve symptoms, improve nutritional status, and prevent intestinal infarction. Endovascular treatment of mesenteric artery stenosis or short segment occlusion by balloon dilatation or stent placement represents a less invasive therapeutic alternative, particularly in patients whose medical comorbidities place them at a high operative risk category. Endovascular therapy is also suited in patients with recurrent disease or anastomotic stenosis following previous open mesenteric revascularization. Prophylactic mesenteric revascularization is rarely performed in the asymptomatic patient undergoing an aortic procedure for other indications.[7] However, the natural history of untreated chronic mesenteric ischemia may justify revascularization in some minimally symptomatic or asymptomatic patients if the operative risks are acceptable, since the first clinical presentation may be acute intestinal ischemia in as many as 50% of the patients, with a mortality rate that ranges from 15 to 70%.[8] This is particularly true when the SMA is involved. Mesenteric angioplasty and stenting is particularly suitable for this patient subgroup, given its low morbidity and mortality. Because of the limited experience with stent use in mesenteric vessels, appropriate indications for primary stent placement have not been clearly defined. Guidelines generally include calcified ostial stenoses, high-grade eccentric stenoses, chronic occlusions, and significant residual stenosis >30%, or the presence of dissection after angioplasty. Restenosis after PTA is also an indication for stent placement.[3,8–11]

Technique

To perform endovascular mesenteric revascularization, intraluminal access is performed via a femoral or brachial artery approach. Once an introducer sheath is placed in the femoral artery, an anterioposterior and lateral aortogram just below the level of the diaphragm is obtained with a pigtail catheter to identify the origin of the CA and SMA. Initial catheterization of the mesenteric artery can be performed using a variety of selective angled catheters, which include the RDC, Cobra-2, Simmons I (Boston Scientific/Meditech, Natick, MA), or SOS Omni catheter (Angiodynamics, Queensbury, NY). Once the mesenteric artery is cannulated, systemic heparin (5000 IU) is administered intravenously. A selective mesenteric angiogram is then performed to identify the diseased segment, which is followed by the placement of a 0.035 in. or less traumatic 0.014–0.018 in. guidewire to cross the stenotic lesion. Once the guidewire is placed across the stenosis, the catheter is carefully advanced over the guidewire across the lesion. In the event that the mesenteric artery is severely angulated as it arises from the aorta, a second stiffer guidewire (Amplatz or Rosen Guidewire, Boston Scientific) may be exchanged through the catheter to facilitate the placement of a 6-Fr guiding sheath (Pinnacle, Boston Scientific).

With the image intensifier angled in a lateral position to fully visualize the proximal mesenteric segment, a balloon angioplasty is advanced over the guidewire through the guiding sheath and positioned across the stenosis. The balloon diameter should be chosen based on the vessel size of the adjacent normal mesenteric vessel. Once balloon angioplasty is completed, a postangioplasty angiogram is necessary to document the procedural result. Radiographic evidence of either residual stenosis or mesenteric artery dissection constitutes suboptimal angioplasty results, which warrants mesenteric stent placement. Moreover, atherosclerotic involvement of the proximal mesenteric artery or vessel orifice should be treated with a balloon-expandable stent placement. These stents can be placed over a low profile 0.014 in. or 0.018 in. guidewire system. It is preferable to deliver the balloon-mounted stent through a guiding sheath, which is positioned just proximal to the mesenteric orifice while the balloon-mounted stent is advanced across the stenosis. The stent is next deployed by expanding the angioplasty balloon to its designated inflation pressure. The balloon is then deflated and carefully withdrawn through the guiding sheath.

Completion angiogram is performed by hand injecting a small volume of contrast through the guiding sheath. It is critical to maintain the guidewire access until satisfactory completion angiogram is obtained. If the completion angiogram reveals suboptimal radiographic results, such as residual stenosis or dissection, additional catheter-based intervention can be performed through the same guidewire. These interventions may include repeat balloon angioplasty for residual stenosis or additional stent placement for mesenteric artery dissection. During the procedure, intraarterial infusion of papaverine or nitroglycerine can be used to decrease vasospasm. Administration of antiplatelet agents is also recommended, for at least 6 months or even indefinitely if other risk factors of cardiovascular disease are present.[4,9,12]

Thrombolytic therapy for acute mesenteric ischemia
Catheter-directed thrombolytic therapy is a potentially useful treatment modality for acute mesenteric ischemia, which can be initiated with intraarterial delivery of thrombolytic agent into the mesenteric thrombus at the time of diagnostic angiography. Various thrombolytic medications, including urokinase (Abbokinase, Abbott Laboratory, North Chicago, IL) or recombinant tissue plasminogen activator (Activase, Genentech, South San Francisco, CA) has been reported to be successful in a small series of case reports. Catheter-directed thrombolytic therapy has a higher probability of restoring mesenteric blood flow success, when performed within 12 h of symptom onset. Successful resolution of a mesenteric thrombus will facilitate the identification of the underlying mesenteric occlusive disease process. As a result, subsequent operative mesenteric revascularization or mesenteric balloon angioplasty and stenting may be performed electively to correct the mesenteric stenosis. There

are two main drawbacks with regards to thrombolytic therapy in mesenteric ischemia. Percutaneous catheter-directed thrombolysis does not allow the possibility to inspect the potentially ischemic intestine, following restoration of the mesenteric flow. Additionally, a prolonged period of time may be necessary in order to achieve successful catheter-directed thrombolysis, due in part to serial angiographic surveillance to document thrombus resolution. An incomplete or unsuccessful thrombolysis may lead to delayed operative revascularization, which may further necessitate bowel resection for irreversible intestinal necrosis. Therefore, catheter-directed thrombolytic therapy for acute mesenteric ischemia should only be considered in selected patients under a closely scrutinized clinical protocol.

Treatment of nonocclusive mesenteric ischemia

The treatment of nonocclusive mesenteric ischemia is primarily pharmacologic with selective mesenteric arterial catheterization followed by infusion of vasodilatory agents, such as tolazoline or papaverine. Once the diagnosis is made on the mesenteric arteriography (Figure 9.5), intraarterial papaverine is given at a dose of 30–60 mg/h. This must be coupled with the cessation of other vasoconstricting agents. Concomitant intravenous heparin should be administered to prevent thrombosis in the cannulated vessels. Treatment strategy thereafter is dependent on the patient's clinical response to the vasodilator therapy.

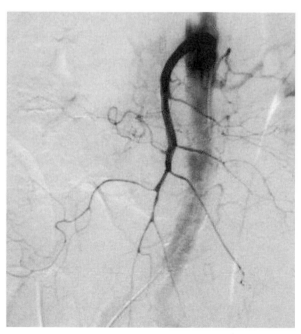

Figure 9.5 Mesenteric arteriogram showing nonocclusive mesenteric ischemia as evidenced by diffuse spasm of intestinal arcades, with poor filling of intramural vessels.

If abdominal symptoms improve, mesenteric arteriography should be repeated to document the resolution of vasospasm. The patient's hemodynamic status must be carefully monitored during papaverine infusion, as significant hypotension can develop in the event that the infusion catheter migrates into the aorta, which can lead to systemic circulation of papaverine. Surgical exploration is indicated if the patient develops signs of continued bowel ischemia or infarction as evidenced by rebound tenderness or involuntary guarding. In these circumstances, papaverine infusion should be continued intraoperatively and postoperatively. The operating room should be kept as warm as possible, and warm irrigation fluid and laparotomy pads should be used to prevent further intestinal vasoconstriction during exploration.

Treatment of celiac artery compression syndrome

Abdominal pain due to narrowing of the origin of the CA may occur as a result of extrinsic compression or impingement by the median arcuate ligament (Figure 9.6). This condition is known as celiac artery compression syndrome or

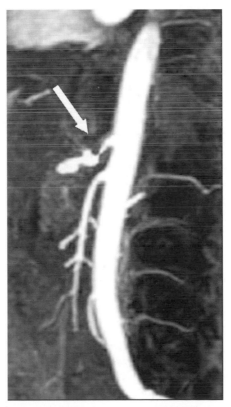

Figure 9.6 A lateral projection of the MRA of the aorta showing a chronic compression of the CA by the median arcuate ligament.

median arcuate ligament syndrome. The CA compression syndrome has been implicated in some variants of chronic mesenteric ischemia. Most patients are young females between 20 and 40 years of age. Abdominal symptom is nonspecific but the pain is localized in the upper abdomen, which may be precipitated by meals. The treatment goal is to release the ligamentous structure that compresses the proximal CA and correct any persistent stricture by bypass grafting. In a number of reports on endovascular management of chronic mesenteric ischemia, the presence of CA compression syndrome has been identified as a major factor of technical failure and recurrence. Therefore, angioplasty and stenting should not be undertaken if extrinsic compression of the CA by the median arcuate ligament is suspected, based on preoperative imaging studies, instead open surgical treatment should be performed.[13–15]

Results from clinical series

The first successful percutaneous angioplasty of the SMA was reported in 1980.[16] Since 1995, 11 series and multiple scattered case reports have reported results from endovascular management of mesenteric occlusive disease. In a recent literature review AbuRahma et al.[17] showed that endovascular intervention had overall technical success rate of 91%, early and late pain relief 84 and 71%, respectively, and 30-day morbidity and mortality rates of 16.4 and 4.3%, respectively. The average patency was 63% during an average 26-month follow-up. In our review of the literature from series since 1995, restenosis was developed in 22% of patients during 24.5 months of average follow-up. The long-term clinical relief without reintervention was 82%. Among the patients that had a technical failure, 15 were ultimately diagnosed with median arcuate ligament syndrome and underwent successful surgical treatment, an observation that emphasizes the need for careful patient selection. Interestingly, the addition of selective stenting after PTA that was started in 1998, while it slightly increases the technical success rate is not correlated with any substantial overall clinical benefit or improved long-term patency rates. In contrast to the endovascular treatment, open surgical techniques have achieved an immediate clinical success that approaches 100%, surgical mortality rate from 0 to 17%, and an operative morbidity rate that ranges from 19 to 54% in a number of different series.[18–29] AbuRahma and colleagues reported their experience of endovascular interventions of 22 patients with symptomatic mesenteric ischemia due to either SMA or CA stenosis.[30] They noted an excellent initial technical and clinical success rates, which were 96% (23/24) and 95% (21/22), respectively, with no perioperative mortality or major morbidity. During a mean follow-up of 26 months (range 1–54), the primary late clinical success rate was 61% and freedom from recurrent stenosis was 30%. The freedom from recurrent stenosis at 1, 2, 3, and 4 years were 65, 47, 39, and 13%, respectively. The authors concluded that mesenteric stenting, which provides excellent early results, is associated with a relatively high incidence of late restenosis.[30]

Several studies have attempted to compare the endovascular to standard open surgical approach.[18,19] The results of the open surgery appear to be more durable, but tend to be associated with higher morbidity and mortality rates and an overall longer hospital stay. In one study that compared the clinical outcome of open revascularization with percutaneous stenting for patients with chronic mesenteric ischemia, 28 patients underwent endovascular treatment and 85 patients underwent open mesenteric bypass grafting.[7] While both patient cohorts had similar baseline comorbidities and symptom durations, there was no difference in early in-hospital complication or mortality rate. Moreover, both groups had similar 3-year cumulative recurrent stenosis and mortality rate. However, patients treated with mesenteric stenting had a significantly higher incidence of recurrent symptoms. The authors concluded that operative mesenteric revascularization should be offered to patients with low surgical risks.[7]

Based on the above results, one could argue that mesenteric angioplasty and stenting demonstrate an inferior technical and clinical success rate. Long-term patency rates appear to be superior with the open technique. There is a general consensus, however, that the endovascular approach is associated with lower morbidity and mortality rates and is therefore more suitable for high-risk patients. Lack of standardization in these series makes comparison or pooling of results difficult, however, general comments can be made. Practices representing standard-of-care for stent placement today, such as perioperative heparinization and short-term antiplatelet therapy were not routinely used in the series under review. Their broad application could substantially improve the outcome after angioplasty and stenting. Stent characteristics might have also been of importance, since the first stents used had diminished radial force, favoring recoil of densely calcified lesions. Routine use of postoperative surveillance using arterial duplex was not consistently reported. Early diagnosis of restenosis and prompt reintervention can also improve long-term patency. Drug-eluting stents that have revolutionized the management of coronary syndromes are expected to soon be used in the peripheral arterial circulation but they were absent during the early experience of mesenteric stenting.

Complications are not common and rarely become life threatening. These include access site thrombosis, hematomas, and infection. Dissection can occur during PTA and is easily managed with placement of a stent. Balloon-mounted stents are preferred over the self-expanding ones because of the higher radial force and the more precise placement. Distal embolization has also been reported but it never resulted in acute intestinal ischemia, likely due to the rich network of collaterals already developed.[17]

Conclusion

Mesenteric ischemia is a rare but life-threatening condition. Open surgical reconstruction was traditionally considered the treatment of choice. Endovascular strategies have recently emerged and offer a viable alternative, associated with decreased morbidity and mortality. It is anticipated that by improving technical skills, advances in technology and refinement of stent characteristics, as well as introduction of drug-eluting stents will broaden the indications for stent placement, improve the overall efficacy and patency rates, and finally redefine the role of the endovascular approach.

References

1 Dunphy J. Abdominal pain of vascular origin. *Am J Med Sci* 1936; **192**:109–12.
2 Zelenock GB, Graham LM, Whitehouse WM, Jr., *et al.* Splanchnic arteriosclerotic disease and intestinal angina. *Arch Surg* 1980; **115**:497–501.
3 Maspes F, Mazzetti di Pietralata G, Gandini R, *et al.* Percutaneous transluminal angioplasty in the treatment of chronic mesenteric ischemia: results and 3 years of follow-up in 23 patients. *Abdom Imaging* 1998; **23**:358–63.
4 Allen RC, Martin GH, Rees CR, *et al.* Mesenteric angioplasty in the treatment of chronic intestinal ischemia. *J Vasc Surg* 1996; **24**:415–21; discussion 421–23.
5 Moneta GL, Yeager RA, Dalman R, Antonovic R, Hall LD, Porter JM. Duplex ultrasound criteria for diagnosis of splanchnic artery stenosis or occlusion. *J Vasc Surg* 1991; **14**:511–18; discussion 518–20.
6 Moneta GL, Lee RW, Yeager RA, Taylor LM, Jr., Porter JM. Mesenteric duplex scanning: a blinded prospective study. *J Vasc Surg* 1993; **17**:79–84; discussion 85–86.
7 Kasirajan K, O'Hara PJ, Gray BH, *et al.* Chronic mesenteric ischemia: open surgery versus percutaneous angioplasty and stenting. *J Vasc Surg* 2001; **33**:63–71.
8 Rose SC, Quigley TM, Raker EJ. Revascularization for chronic mesenteric ischemia: comparison of operative arterial bypass grafting and percutaneous transluminal angioplasty. *J Vasc Interv Radiol* 1995; **6**:339–49.
9 Nyman U, Ivancev K, Lindh M, Uher P. Endovascular treatment of chronic mesenteric ischemia: report of five cases. *Cardiovasc Intervent Radiol* 1998; **21**:305–13.
10 Matsumoto AH, Angle JF, Spinosa DJ, *et al.* Percutaneous transluminal angioplasty and stenting in the treatment of chronic mesenteric ischemia: results and longterm followup. *J Am Coll Surg* 2002; **194**:S22–31.
11 Pietura R, Szymanska A, El Furah M, Drelich-Zbroja A, Szczerbo-Trojanowska M. Chronic mesenteric ischemia: diagnosis and treatment with balloon angioplasty and stenting. *Med Sci Monit* 2002; **8**:PR8–12.
12 Hallisey MJ, Deschaine J, Illescas FF, *et al.* Angioplasty for the treatment of visceral ischemia. *J Vasc Interv Radiol* 1995; **6**:785–91.
13 Park WM, Gloviczki P, Cherry KJ, Jr., *et al.* Contemporary management of acute mesenteric ischemia: factors associated with survival. *J Vasc Surg* 2002; **35**:445–52.
14 Park WM, Cherry KJ, Jr., Chua HK, *et al.* Current results of open revascularization for chronic mesenteric ischemia: a standard for comparison. *J Vasc Surg* 2002; **35**:853–59.
15 Sheeran SR, Murphy TP, Khwaja A, Sussman SK, Hallisey MJ. Stent placement for treatment of mesenteric artery stenoses or occlusions. *J Vasc Interv Radiol* 1999; **10**:861–67.
16 Furrer J, Gruntzig A, Kugelmeier J, Goebel N. Treatment of abdominal angina with percutaneous dilatation of an arteria mesenterica superior stenosis. Preliminary communication. *Cardiovasc Intervent Radiol* 1980; **3**:43–44.
17 AbuRahma AF, Stone PA, Bates MC, Welch CA. Angioplasty/stenting of the superior mesenteric artery and celiac trunk: early and late outcomes. *J Endovasc Ther* 2003; **10**:1046–53.

18 Rose SC, Quigley TM, Raker EJ. Revascularization for chronic mesenteric ischemia: comparison of operative arterial bypass grafting and percutaneous transluminal angioplasty. *J Vasc Interv Radiol* 1995; **6**:339–49.

19 Kasirajan K, O'Hara PJ, Gray BH, *et al*. Chronic mesenteric ischemia: open surgery versus percutaneous angioplasty and stenting. *J Vasc Surg* 2001; **33**:63–71.

20 Derrow AE, Seeger JM, Dame DA, *et al*. The outcome in the United States after thoracoabdominal aortic aneurysm repair, renal artery bypass, and mesenteric revascularization. *J Vasc Surg* 2001; **34**:54–61.

21 Mateo RB, O'Hara PJ, Hertzer NR, Mascha EJ, Beven EG, Krajewski LP. Elective surgical treatment of symptomatic chronic mesenteric occlusive disease: early results and late outcomes. *J Vasc Surg* 1999; **29**:821–31; discussion 832.

22 Moneta GL, Lee RW, Yeager RA, Taylor LM, Jr., Porter JM. Mesenteric duplex scanning: a blinded prospective study. *J Vasc Surg* 1993; **17**:79–84; discussion 85–86.

23 Foley MI, Moneta GL, Abou-Zamzam AM, Jr., *et al*. Revascularization of the superior mesenteric artery alone for treatment of intestinal ischemia. *J Vasc Surg* 2000; **32**:37–47.

24 Zelenock GB, Graham LM, Whitehouse WM, Jr., *et al*. Splanchnic arteriosclerotic disease and intestinal angina. *Arch Surg* 1980; **115**:497–501.

25 Johnston KW, Lindsay TF, Walker PM, Kalman PG. Mesenteric arterial bypass grafts: early and late results and suggested surgical approach for chronic and acute mesenteric ischemia. *Surgery* 1995; **118**:1–7.

26 McAfee MK, Cherry KJ, Jr., Naessens JM, *et al*. Influence of complete revascularization on chronic mesenteric ischemia. *Am J Surg* 1992; **164**:220–24.

27 Cunningham CG, Reilly LM, Stoney R. Chronic visceral ischemia. *Surg Clin North Am* 1992; **72**:231–44.

28 Rheudasil JM, Stewart MT, Schellack JV, Smith RB, 3rd, Salam AA, Perdue GD. Surgical treatment of chronic mesenteric arterial insufficiency. *J Vasc Surg* 1988; **8**:495–500.

29 McMillan WD, McCarthy WJ, Bresticker MR, *et al*. Mesenteric artery bypass: objective patency determination. *J Vasc Surg* 1995; **21**:729–40; discussion 740–41.

30 AbuRahma AF, Stone PA, Bates MC, Welch CA. Angioplasty/stenting of the superior mesenteric artery and celiac trunk: early and late outcomes. *J Endovasc Ther* 2003; **10**:1046–53.

CHAPTER 10

Renal artery occlusive disease

Peter H. Lin, Rakesh Safaya, W. Todd Bohannon

Obstructive lesions of the renal artery can produce hypertension resulting in a condition known as renovascular hypertension, which is the most common form of hypertension amenable to therapeutic intervention. Renovascular hypertension is believed to affect 5–10% of all hypertensive patients in the United States.[1] Patients with renovascular hypertension are at an increased risk for irreversible renal dysfunction, if inadequate pharmacologic therapies are used to control the blood pressure. The majority of patients with renal artery obstructive disease have vascular lesions of either atherosclerotic disease or fibrodysplasia involving the renal arteries. The proximal portion of the renal artery represents the most common location for the development of atherosclerotic disease. It is well established that renal artery intervention, either by surgical or endovascular revascularization, provides an effective treatment for controlling renovascular hypertension as well as preserving renal function. The decision for intervention must encompass the full spectrum of clinical, anatomic, and physiologic considerations of the patient to yield the optimal benefit-risk balance.

Pathology of renal artery stenosis

Approximately 80% of all renal artery occlusive lesions are caused by atherosclerosis, which typically occur near the renal artery ostia and are usually less than 1 cm in length (Figure 10.1).[2] Atherosclerotic lesion involving the renal artery origin accounts for more than 95% of reported cases of renovascular hypertension.[3] Patients with this disease commonly present during the sixth decade of life. Men are affected twice as frequently as women. Moreover, they typically have other atherosclerotic disease varieties involving the coronary, mesenteric, cerebrovascular, and peripheral arterial circulation. Atherosclerotic occlusive lesions involving the proximal renal artery typically occur as a spillover of diffuse aortic atherosclerosis, which are bilateral in more than two-thirds of patients. When a unilateral lesion is present, the disease process affects the right and left renal artery with similar frequency. Medial and intimal accumulations of fibrous plaque and cholesterol-laden foam cells are typical of the diseased renal artery wall. In more advanced disease, characteristics of complicated atherosclerotic plaques such as hemorrhage, necrosis, calcification, and luminal thrombus are commonly present in the renal artery wall.[4]

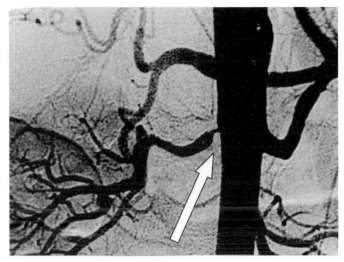

Figure 10.1 Occlusive disease of the renal artery typically involves the renal ostium (arrow), as a result of the aortic disease progression.

The second most common cause of renal artery stenosis is fibromuscular dysplasia, which accounts for 20% of cases.[5] Fibromuscular dysplasia of the renal artery represents a heterogeneous group of lesions that produces specific pathologic lesions in various regions of the vessel wall including the intima, media, or adventitia. The most common variety consists of medial fibroplasia, in which thickened fibromuscular ridges alternate with attenuated media producing the classic angiographic "string of beads" appearance (Figure 10.2).[6] The cause of medial fibroplasia remains unclear but appears to be associated with modification of the arterial smooth muscle cells in response to estrogenic stimuli during the reproductive years, unusual traction forces on affected vessels, and mural ischemia from impairment of vasa vasorum blood flow.[5] Fibromuscular hyperplasia usually affects the distal two-thirds of the main renal artery, and the right renal artery is affected more frequently than the left. The entity occurs most commonly in young, often multiparous women. Other, less common causes of renal artery stenosis include renal artery aneurysm (compressing the adjacent normal renal artery), arteriovenous malformations, neurofibromatosis, renal artery dissections, renal artery trauma, Takayasu's arteritis, and renal arteriovenous fistula.

Clinical features

Renovascular hypertension is the most common sequelae of renal artery occlusive disease. Although the prevalence of renovascular hypertension is less than 5% in the general hypertensive population, this is one of the few treatable forms of hypertension. The prevalence of renovascular hypertension among patients

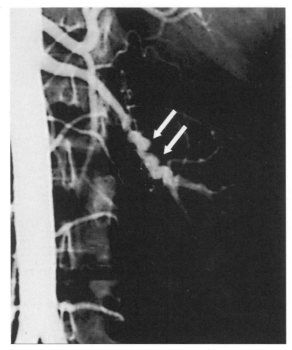

Figure 10.2 Abdominal aortogram revealed a left renal artery fibromuscular dysplasia with the typical "string of beads" appearance (arrows).

with diastolic blood pressures greater than 100 mm Hg is about 2%. It is even more frequent in patients who have severe diastolic hypertension, which can affect as many as 30% in those with a diastolic pressure over 125 mm Hg.[1,2]

Clinical features suggestive of renovascular hypertension include (1) systolic and diastolic upper abdominal bruits, (2) diastolic hypertension of greater than 115 mm Hg, (3) rapid onset of hypertension after the age of 50 years, (4) a sudden worsening of mild to moderate essential hypertension, or (5) development of hypertension during childhood. Physical examination can provide an important diagnostic feature in detecting renovascular hypertension, particularly with the presence of an abdominal bruit located in the epigastrium or in either of the upper abdominal quadrant. This finding is present in more than 75% of patients with renovascular hypertension, in contrast to less than 5% of those with essential hypertension.[7] Hypertensive patients who are resistant to pharmacologic therapy is also more likely to be associated with renovascular hypertension. In addition, those who develop renal function deterioration while receiving multiple antihypertensive drugs, particularly ACE inhibitors, may have underlying occlusive lesion involving the renal artery.

All patients with significant hypertension, especially elevated diastolic blood pressure, must be considered as suspect for renovascular disease. Young adults with hypertension, have a great deal to gain by avoiding lifelong treatment if renovascular hypertension is diagnosed and corrected. Appropriate diagnostic studies and intervention must be timely instituted to detect the possibility of renovascular hypertension in patients with primary hypertension, who present for clinical evaluation.

Diagnostic evaluation

The diagnostic requisites for renovascular hypertension include, both hypertension and renal artery stenosis. Nearly all diagnostic studies for renovascular hypertension evaluate either the anatomic stenosis or renal parenchymal dysfunction attributed to the stenosis. The benefits and limitations of these tests are important in the proper selection of patients for renal artery intervention.

Conventional renal artery angiography is critical to the evaluation of patients with possible renovascular hypertension. Intraarterial digital subtraction angiography is a useful modification of conventional studies in assessing the presence of renal artery occlusive disease. This technique allows use of smaller quantities of contrast agents compared with conventional arteriography, and it reduces the possibility of contrast-induced nephrotoxicity, which is of particular importance in patients with compromised renal function. A flush aortogram is performed first, so that any accessory renal arteries can be detected and the origins of all the renal arteries are adequately displayed. The presence of collateral vessels circumventing a renal artery stenosis strongly supports the hemodynamic importance of the stenosis. A pressure gradient of 10 mm Hg or greater is necessary for collateral vessel development, which is also associated with activation of the renin-angiotensin cascade.

Selective catheterization of the renal vein via a femoral vein approach for assessing renin activity is a more invasive test of detecting the functional status of renal artery disease. If unilateral disease is present, the affected kidney should secrete high levels of renin while the contralateral kidney should have low renin production. A ratio between the two kidneys, or the renal vein renin ratio (RVRR), of greater than 1.5 is indicative of functionally important renovascular hypertension, and it also predicts a favorable response from renovascular revascularization. Since this study assesses the ratio between the two kidneys, it is not useful in patients with bilateral disease since both kidneys may secrete abnormally elevated renin levels.

The renal:systemic renin index (RSRI) is calculated by subtracting systemic renin activity from individual renal vein renin activity and dividing the remainder by systemic renin activity. This value represents the degree of renin that an individual kidney secretes. In normal individuals without renovascular hypertension, the renal vein renin activity from each kidney is typically 24% or 0.24 higher than the systemic level. As the result, the total of both kidneys' renin activity is usually 48% or 0.48 greater than the systemic activity. This value of 0.48 reflects a steady state of renal renin activity.

The RSRI of the affected kidney in patients with renovascular hypertension is greater than 0.24. In the case of unilateral renal artery stenosis with normal contralateral kidney, the increase in ipsilateral renin release is normally balanced by suppression of the contralateral kidney renin production, which results in a drop in its RSRI to less than 0.24. Bilateral renal artery disease may negate the contralateral compensatory response, and the autonomous release of renin from both diseased kidneys may result in the sum of the individual RSRIs to be considerably greater than 0.48. The prognostic value of ischemic kidney renin hypersecretion (RSRI more than 0.48) and contralateral kidney renin suppression (RSRI between 0.0 and 0.24) as a means of discriminating between expected cured and favorable surgical response has been firmly studied. However, the prognostic accuracy of RSRI remains limited, in that approximately 10% of patients with favorable surgical response following renovascular revascularization do not exhibit contralateral renin suppression. The clinical usefulness of RSRI must be applied with caution in the management of patients with renovascular hypertension.

Magnetic resonance angiography, particularly with gadolinium contrast enhancement, has become a useful diagnostic tool for renal artery occlusive disease because of its ability to provide high-resolution images (Figures 10.3 & 10.4; Plate 7, facing p. 80). The minimally invasive nature of magnetic resonance angiography plus the low risk of nephrotoxicity of gadolinium contrast makes it an appealing diagnostic modality. With continuous refinement in imaging software, it will likely become a widely accepted imaging modality in patients suspected of renovascular hypertension.

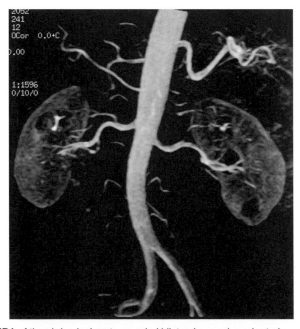

Figure 10.3 MRA of the abdominal aorta revealed bilateral normal renal arteries.

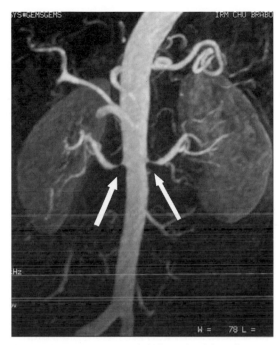

Figure 10.4 MRA of the abdominal aorta revealed bilateral ostial renal artery stenosis.

Abdominal renal artery ultrasonography is a noninvasive test of assessing renal artery stenosis, both by visualization of the vessel and by measurement of the effect of stenosis on blood flow velocity and waveforms. The presence of a severe renal artery stenosis correlates with peak systolic velocities of greater than 180 cm/s and the ratio of these velocities to those in the aorta is greater than 3.5. However, many renal artery ultrasounds are difficult to perform or interpret due to obesity or increased bowel gas pattern. In addition, renal ultrasonography does not differentiate among renal artery stenoses exceeding 60% cross-sectional stenosis. Because this test is highly dependent on the operator's expertise, its role as an effective screening test remains limited.

Treatment indications for renal artery disease

The therapeutic goal in patients with renovascular disease is two-fold. The first is to cure or improve high blood pressure thereby preventing the long-term deleterious systemic sequelae of hypertension on target organ systems, such as the cerebral, coronary, pulmonary, and peripheral circulations. The second goal is to preserve and possibly improve the renal function.

Prior to 1990, the most common treatment modality in patients with renal artery occlusive disease was surgical revascularization, with either renal artery bypass grafting or renal artery endarterectomy. The advancement of endovascular therapy in the past decade has led to various minimally invasive treatment strategies such as renal artery balloon angioplasty or stenting to control hypertension or to preserve renal function. The indications for endovascular treatment for renal artery occlusive disease includes, at least a 70% stenosis of one or both renal arteries and at least one of the following clinical criteria:

- inability to adequately control hypertension despite appropriate antihypertensive regimen;
- chronic renal insufficiency related to bilateral renal artery occlusive disease or stenosis to a solitary functioning kidney;
- dialysis-dependent renal failure in a patient with renal artery stenosis but without another definite cause of end-stage renal disease;
- recurrent congestive heart failure or flash pulmonary edema not attributable to active coronary ischemia.

Endovasuclar treatment modalities

Endovascular treatment of renal artery occlusive disease was first introduced by Grüntzig in 1978, who successfully dilated a renal artery stenosis using a balloon catheter technique.[8] This technique requires passage of a guidewire under fluoroscopic control typically from a femoral artery approach to, across the stenosis in the renal artery. A balloon-dilating catheter is passed over the guidewire and positioned within the area of stenosis and inflated to produce a controlled disruption of the arterial wall. Alternatively, a balloon-mounted expandable stent can be used to primarily dilate the renal artery stenosis. Completion angiography is usually performed to assess the immediate results. The technical aspect of an endovascular renal artery revascularization is discussed below.

Renal artery access and guiding sheath placement

Access to the renal artery for endovascular intervention is typically performed via a femoral artery approach, although a brachial artery approach can be considered in the event of severe aortoiliac occlusive disease, aortoiliac aneurysm, or severe caudal renal artery angulation. Once an introducer sheath is placed in the femoral artery, an anteriopposterior (AP) aortogram is obtained with a pigtail catheter placed in the suprarenal aorta to best visualize the left renal artery. In contrast, an aortogram with a 15–30° left anterior oblique (LAO) angulation is best to visualize the right renal artery. In patients with renal dysfunction, a selective renal catheterization can be performed without the initial aortogram. However, a diseased accessory or duplicating renal artery may be left undetected. Alternative noniodinated contrast agents, such as carbon dioxide and gadolinium, should be used in endovascular renal intervention in patients with renal dysfunction or allergic reactions.

Initial catheterization of the renal artery can be performed using a variety of selective angled catheters, which include the RDC, RC-2, Cobra-2,

Simmons I, or SOS Omni catheter (Boston Scientific/Medi-Tech, Natick, MA; Cook, Bloomington, IN; Medtronic, Santa Rosa, CA, Cordis, Warren, NJ; or Angiodynamics, Queensbury, NY). Once the renal artery is cannulated, systemic heparin (5000 IU) is administered intravenously. A selective renal angiogram is then performed utilizing a hand-injection technique with isoosmolar contrast (Visipaque 270, Nycomed Amersham, Princeton, NJ). Once the diseased renal artery is identified, a 0.035 in. or smaller profile 0.018–0.014 in. coronary guidewire is used to cross the stenotic lesion. Once the guidewire traverses across the renal artery stenosis, the catheter is carefully advanced over the guidewire across the lesion. A vasodilator (e.g. glycerol trinitrite 150 μg) is administered in the renal artery through the catheter to minimize the possibility of renal artery spasm. In the event that the renal artery is severely angulated as it arises from the aorta, a second stiffer guidewire (Amplatz or Rosen Guidewire, Boston Scientific) may be exchanged through the catheter to facilitate the placement of a 45-cm 6-Fr renal guiding sheath (Pinnacle, Boston Scientific). It is important to maintain the distal wire position without movement in the tertiary renal branches during guiding sheath placement to reduce the possibility of parenchymal perforation. Once the guiding sheath along its tapered obturator is advanced into the renal artery over the guidewire, the obturator is removed so that the guiding sheath is positioned just proximal to the renal ostium. Selective renal angiogram is performed to ensure the proper positioning of the guiding sheath.

Renal artery balloon angioplasty
With the image intensifier angled to maximize the visualization of the proximal renal artery, a balloon angioplasty is advanced over the guidewire through the guiding sheath and positioned across the renal artery stenosis. The balloon diameter should be chosen based on the vessel size of the adjacent normal renal artery segment. Various compliant angioplasty balloon catheters (CrossSail, Guidant, St. Paul, MN; or Gazelle, Boston Scientific) can be used for renal artery dilatation. We recommend choosing an angioplasty balloon less than 4 mm in diameter for the initial renal artery dilatation. The luminal diameter of the renal artery can be further assessed by measuring the known diameter of a fully inflated angioplasty balloon and comparing it to the renal artery dimension. Such a comparison may provide a reference guide to determine the necessity of renal artery dilatation with a larger diameter angioplasty balloon.

Renal artery stent placement
Once balloon angioplasty of the renal artery is completed, a postangioplasty angiogram is performed to document the procedural result. Radiographic evidence of either residual stenosis or renal artery dissection constitutes suboptimal angioplasty results, which warrants an immediate renal artery stent placement. Moreover, atherosclerotic involvement of the renal artery usually involves the vessel orifice, which typically requires a balloon-expandable stent placement. Various types of balloon-expandable stents can be considered

in this scenario (Express SD, Boston Scientific; Racer, Medtronic; or Palmaz Genesis, Cordis Endovascular). These stents can be placed over a low profile 0.014 or 0.018 in. guidewire system. It is preferable to deliver the balloon-mounted stent through a guiding sheath via a groin approach. The guiding sheath is positioned just proximal to the renal orifice while the balloon-mounted stent is advanced across the renal artery stenosis. A small amount of contrast material can be given through the guiding sheath to ensure an appropriate stent position. Next, the stent is deployed by expanding the angioplasty balloon to its designated inflation pressure, which is typically less than 8 atm. The balloon is then deflated and carefully withdrawn through the guiding sheath.

Completion angiogram is performed by hand injecting a small volume of contrast though the guiding sheath. It is critical to maintain the guidewire access until satisfactory completion angiogram is obtained. If the completion angiogram reveals suboptimal radiographic results, such as residual stenosis or dissection, additional catheter-based intervention can be performed through the same guidewire. These interventions may include repeat balloon angioplasty for residual stenosis or additional stent placement for renal artery dissection.

Completion angiogram

Prior to removal of the guidewire and sheath, a completion angiogram is performed (Figure 10.5). A small volume of contrast via hand injection through the sheath may be warranted, if contrast limitations are necessary, but these images have less detail when compared to a flush aortogram. If a flush aortogram is indicated, it is preferred to use a tandem wire technique in order to maintain wire access across the recently stented lesion. The sheath is withdrawn into the infrarenal aorta while maintaining guidewire position across the stented segment of renal artery and a second wire is advanced into the

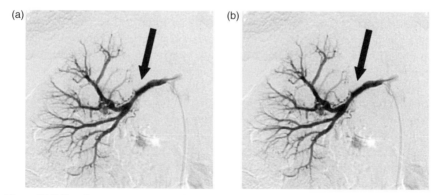

(a) (b)

Figure 10.5 Renal artery stenting: (a) focal lesion in the renal artery (arrow) and (b) poststenting angiogram reveals a satisfactory result following a renal artery stenting placement (arrow).

supra-diaphragmatic aorta. Over this second wire and through the guide sheath a 4 Fr pigtail catheter is placed in the suprarenal position. A power injection is performed and the flush aortogram reviewed for assessment of the stenting procedure. If secondary intervention is indicated, the original 0.014 in. wire that remains in its original position is used to recross the lesion safely.

Technical tips

1 The renal arteries often originate either anteriorly or posteriorly, and the initial diagnostic evaluation of the renal artery origins may be improved with oblique image intensifier views.

2 Catheter selection for initial access to the renal artery will depend on the patient's anatomy. Most visceral branches can be easily accessed with a selective catheter, such as the Simmons 1 Glidecath (Boston Scientific/Medi-Tech, Natick, MA, USA).

3 Arterial perforation or parenchymal injury is possible with injudicious guidewire advancement. One should be very conscious of the tip of the wire, which should maintain a fixed position throughout the procedure.

4 The saved image of the fully expanded initial angioplasty balloon will help estimate the native artery diameter and the optimal stent size. When using a compliant balloon, inflation pressure corresponds with variable balloon diameter.

5 Care must be taken to not over dilate and risk rupture of the renal artery.

6 Stents placed for ostial lesions should extend into the aorta approximately 2 mm.

7 Always the package insert for balloon and stent system for sheath and guidewire compatibility, balloon compliance, nominal, deployment and rated burst pressures should be read.

Results from clinical series

Percutaneous transluminal balloon angioplasty

Fibromuscular dysplasia of the renal artery is the most common treatment indication for percutaneous transluminal balloon angioplasty. Patients with symptomatic fibromuscular dysplasia such as hypertension or renal insufficiency, usually respond well to renal artery balloon angioplasty alone.[9,10] In contrast, balloon angioplasty generally is not an effective treatment for patients with renal artery stenosis or proximal occlusive disease of the renal artery, due to the high incidence of restenosis with balloon angioplasty alone.[7,11] In the latter group of patients, the preferred endovascular treatment is a renal artery stent placement.

The long-term benefit of renal artery balloon angioplasty in patients with fibromuscular dysplasia was reported by Surowiec and colleagues.[9] They followed 14 patients who underwent 19 interventions on 18 renal artery segments. The technical success rate of balloon angioplasty for fibromuscular dysplasia was 95%. Primary patency rates were 81, 69, 69, and 69% at 2, 4, 6, and 8 years, respectively. Assisted primary patency rates were all 87% at 2, 4, 6, and 8 years, respectively. The restenosis rate was 25% at 8 years. Clinical benefit, as defined by either improved or cured hypertension, was found in 79% of patients over-all, with two-thirds of patients having maintained this benefit at 8 years. The authors concluded that balloon angioplasty is highly effective in symptomatic fibromuscular dysplasia with excellent durable functional benefits.[9]

The utility of balloon angioplasty in renal artery stenosis has also been stud-ied clinically. Jaarsveld and associates performed a prospective study in which patients with renal artery stenosis were randomized to either drug therapy or balloon angioplasty treatment.[12] A total of 106 patients with 50% diameter stenosis or greater plus hypertension or renal insufficiency were random-ized in the study. Routine follow-ups were performed at 3 and 12 months. The authors reported that the baseline blood pressure was 179/104 mm Hg and 180/103 mm Hg in the angioplasty and drug-therapy groups respect-ively. At 3 months, there was no difference in the degree to which blood pressure was controlled between the two groups. However, the degree and dose of antihypertensive medications was slightly lowered in the balloon angioplasty group. In the drug-therapy group, 22 patients crossed over the balloon angioplasty group at 3 months because of persistent hypertension despite treatment with three or more drugs or because of a deterioration in renal function. At 12 months, there were no significant differences between the angioplasty and drug-therapy groups in systolic and diastolic blood pres-sures, daily drug doses, or renal function. The authors concluded that in the treatment of patients with hypertension and renal artery stenosis, percu-taneous transluminal balloon angioplasty alone offer minimal advantage over antihypertensive-drug therapy.

Renal artery stenting

Endovascular stent placement is the treatment of choice for patients with symp-tomatic or high-grade renal artery occlusive disease. This is due in part to the high incidence of restenosis with balloon angioplasty alone, particularly in the setting of ostial stenosis. Renal artery stenting is also indicated for renal artery dissection caused by balloon angioplasty or other catheter-based interven-tions. Numerous studies have clearly demonstrated the clinical efficacy of renal artery stenting when compared to balloon angioplasty alone in patients with high-grade renal artery stenosis. Currently, there are two balloon-expandable stents that have received the Food and Drug Administration approval for renal artery implantation. These are the (1) Bridge extra support balloon-expandable stent (Medtronic) and (2) Palmaz balloon-expandable stent (Cordis Endovascular).

White and colleagues conducted a study to evaluate the role of renal artery stenting in patients with poorly controlled hypertension and renal artery lesions that did not respond well to balloon angioplasty alone.[13] Balloon-expandable stents were placed in 100 consecutive patients with 133 renal artery stenoses. Of these, 67 of the patients had a unilateral renal artery stenosis treated and 33 had bilateral renal artery stenoses treated with stents placed in both renal arteries. The technical success of the procedure was 99%. The mean blood pressure values were $173 \pm 25/88 \pm 17$ mm Hg prior to stent implantation and $146 \pm 20/77 \pm 12$ mm Hg, 6 months after renal artery stenting ($p < 0.01$). Angiographic follow-up with 67 patients (mean 8.7 ± 5 months) demonstrated restenosis, as defined by 50% or greater luminal narrowing, occurred in 15 patients (19%). The study concluded that renal artery stenting is a highly effective treatment for renovascular hypertension, with a low angiographic restenosis rate. In another similar study, Blum and colleagues prospectively performed renal artery stenting in 68 patients (74 lesions) with ostial renal artery stenosis and suboptimal balloon angioplasty.[14] Patients were followed for a mean of 27 months with measurements of blood pressure and serum creatinine, duplex sonography, and intraarterial angiography. Patency rate at 5 year was 84.5% (mean follow-up was 27 months). Restenosis occurred in 8 of 74 arteries (11%), but after reintervention the secondary 5-year patency rate was 92.4%. Blood pressure was cured or improved in 78% of patients. The authors concluded that primary stent placement is an effective treatment for renal artery stenosis involving the ostium.

The clinical utility of renal artery stenting in renal function preservation was analyzed by several studies, which measured serial serum creatinine levels to determine the response of renal function following endovascular intervention.[15,16] In a study reported by Harden and colleagues, who performed 33 renal artery stenting in 32 patients with renal insufficiency, they noted that renal function improved or stabilized in 22 patients (69%).[16] In a similar study, Watson and associates evaluated the effect of renal artery stenting on renal function by comparing the slopes of the regression lines derived from the reciprocal of serum creatinine versus time.[15] With a total of 61 renal stenting performed in 33 patients, the authors found that after stent placement, the slopes of the reciprocal of the serum creatinine (1/Scr) were positive in 18 patients and less negative in 7 patients. The study concludes that in patients with chronic renal insufficiency due to obstructive renal artery stenosis, renal artery stenting is effective in improving or stabilizing renal function.

The clinical outcome of several large clinical studies of renal artery stenting in the treatment of renovascular hypertension or chronic renal insufficiency is shown in Table 10.1. These studies uniformly demonstrated an excellent technical success rate with low incidence of restenosis or procedural-related complications.[13,14,17–22] A similar analysis was reported by Leertouwer and colleagues, who performed a meta-analysis of 14 studies encompassing 678 patients with renal arterial stent placement in comparison with renal balloon angioplasty for renal arterial stenosis.[23] The study found that renal arterial stent placement proved highly successful, with an initial adequate performance in 98%. The overall cure rate for hypertension was 20%, whereas hypertension was improved in 49%. Renal function improved in 30% and stabilized in 38% of the patients. The restenosis rate at follow-up of 6–29 months was 17%. Renal stenting resulted in a higher technical success rate and a lower restenosis rate when compared to balloon angioplasty alone.

Recent endovascular advances have led to the development and refinement of embolization protection devices for endovascular intervention. The intent of the distal protection device is to capture any atherosclerotic debris caused by balloon angioplasty or stent placement without embolizing the renal parenchyma. Henry and associates performed distally protected renal stenting in 28 patients with 32 high-grade renal artery lesions.[24] All interventions were performed with the PercuSurge Guardwire device (Medtronic), which consisted of a temporary occlusion balloon that was inflated to provide parenchymal protection. Technical success with distal protection devices and renal stenting was 100%. Visible debris was aspirated from all patients. Blood pressure or renal function improvement was noted in three-fourths of patients at 6-months follow-up. This study suggested a possible utility of embolization protection device in renal artery intervention. Further clinical investigations are underway to validate the benefit of distally protected renal artery stenting.

Common problems and complications

While endovascular therapy of renal artery occlusive disease is considerably less invasive than conventional renal artery bypass operation, complications relating to this treatment modality can occur. In a study in which Guzman and colleagues compared the complications following renal artery angioplasty and surgical revascularization, the authors noted that major complication rate following endovascular and surgical treatment were 17 and 31 %, respectively. In contrast, significantly greater minor complications were associated with the endovascular cohort, which was 48%, in contrast to 7% in the surgical group.[25] In a prospective randomized study that compared the clinical outcome of renal artery balloon angioplasty versus stenting for renal ostial atherosclerotic lesion, comparable complications rates were found in the two groups, which were 39 and 43%, respectively. However, the incidence of restenosis rate at 6 months was significantly higher in the balloon angioplasty cohort than the stenting group, which was 48% in contrast to 14% at 6 months. This study underscores the clinical superiority of renal stenting compared to renal balloon angioplasty alone in patients with ostial stenosis.[26]

Deterioration in renal function, albeit transient, is a common complication following endovascular renal artery intervention. It is in part caused by the effects of iodinated contrast and transient renal dysfunction can occur within 48 h following the interventions. In most cases, supportive care with adequate fluid hydration is sufficient to reverse the renal dysfunction. However, transient hemodialysis may become necessary in approximately 1% of patients. Another procedural-related complications is renal artery atheroembolization, which can occur due to catheter-associated manipulations, including catheter manipulation in the aorta, crossing the stenosis, or balloon inflation and stent placement. The onset is more insidious, which can

Table 10.1 Clinical outcome of renal artery stent placement in the treatment of renovascular hypertension and renal insufficiency.

Author	Year	Patient No.	Technical Success	Follow-up (months)	Renal insufficiency (%)		Renovascular hypertension (%)		Complications (%)	Restenosis (%)
					Stable	Improved	Cured	Improved		
Iannone[20]	1996	63	99	10	45	36	4	35	13	14
Harden[16]	1997	32	100	6	34	34	N/A	N/A	3	13
Blum[14]	1997	68	100	27	N/A	N/A	16	62	0	11
White[13]	1997	100	99	6	N/A	20	N/A	N/A	2	19
Shannon[22]	1998	21	100	9	29	43	N/A	N/A	9	0
Rundback[21]	1998	45	94	17	N/A	N/A	N/A	N/A	9	25
Dorros[18]	1998	163	100	48	N/A	N/A	3	51	11	N/A
Henry[19]	1999	210	99	25	N/A	29	19	61	3	9
Bush[17]	2001	73	89	20	21	38	13	61	12	16

occur several days following interventions, and its clinical manifestations may include livedo reticularis or skin rash in the flank region. The diagnosis may be further supported with an elevated ESR level and eosinophilia. In an efforts to reduce the clinical complication of renal artery atheroembolism, physicians have to utilize distal protection device during renal artery intervention.[24] Preliminary studies have demonstrated clinical efficacy of distally protected renal artery stenting in minimizing procedural-related renal dysfunction. Further studies are undoubtedly warranted to validate its clinical efficacy.

Conclusion

Percutaneous transluminal balloon angioplasty is an effective treatment for renal artery fibromuscular dysplasia. In contrast, renal artery stenting is a proven treatment modality for renovascular hypertension and ischemic nephropathy caused by ostial renal artery stenoses. Endovascular interventions of renal artery occlusive disease provide excellent technical success and durable functional benefits. Devices used in endovascular renal artery intervention, such as guidewire, guiding sheaths, angioplasty balloons, and stents, are constantly undergoing further refinement to create lower profiles and ease of use. Future endovascular intervention of the renal artery may involve distal protection devices to reduce distal embolization. These technological improvements will likely confer even greater technical and clinical success in the management of renal artery occlusive disease.

References

1 Zoccali C, Mallamaci F, Finocchiaro P. Atherosclerotic renal artery stenosis: epidemiology, cardiovascular outcomes, and clinical prediction rules. *J Am Soc Nephrol* 2002; **13**:S179–83.

2 Klassen PS, Svetkey LP. Diagnosis and management of renovascular hypertension. *Cardiol Rev* 2000; **8**:17–29.

3 Gill KS, Fowler RC. Atherosclerotic renal arterial stenosis: clinical outcomes of stent placement for hypertension and renal failure. *Radiology* 2003; **226**:821–26.

4 Chade AR, Rodriguez-Porcel M, Grande JP, *et al*. Distinct renal injury in early atherosclerosis and renovascular disease. *Circulation* 2002; **106**:1165–71.

5 Vuong PN, Desoutter P, Mickley V, *et al*. Fibromuscular dysplasia of the renal artery responsible for renovascular hypertension: a histological presentation based on a series of 102 patients. *Vasa* 2004; **33**:13–18.

6 Mounier-Vehier C, Lions C, Jaboureck O, *et al*. Parenchymal consequences of fibromuscular dysplasia renal artery stenosis. *Am J Kidney Dis* 2002; **40**:1138–45.

7 Krijnen P, van Jaarsveld BC, Steyerberg EW, Man in 't Veld AJ, Schalekamp MA, Habbema JD. A clinical prediction rule for renal artery stenosis. *Ann Intern Med* 1998; **129**:705–11.

8 Grüntzig A. Percutaneous transluminal angioplasty. *AJR Am J Roentgenol* 1981; **136**:216–17.

9 Surowiec SM, Sivamurthy N, Rhodes JM, *et al*. Percutaneous therapy for renal artery fibromuscular dysplasia. *Ann Vasc Surg* 2003; **17**:650–55.

10 Mounier-Vehier C, Haulon S, Devos P, *et al.* Renal atrophy outcome after revascularization in fibromuscular dysplasia disease. *J Endovasc Ther* 2002; **9**:605–13.

11 van Jaarsveld BC, Krijnen P, Derkx FH, *et al.* Resistance to antihypertensive medication as predictor of renal artery stenosis: comparison of two drug regimens. *J Hum Hypertens* 2001; **15**:669–76.

12 van Jaarsveld BC, Krijnen P, Pieterman H, *et al.* The effect of balloon angioplasty on hypertension in atherosclerotic renal-artery stenosis. Dutch Renal Artery Stenosis Intervention Cooperative Study Group. *N Engl J Med* 2000; **342**:1007–14.

13 White CJ, Ramee SR, Collins TJ, Jenkins JS, Escobar A, Shaw D. Renal artery stent placement: utility in lesions difficult to treat with balloon angioplasty. *J Am Coll Cardiol* 1997; **30**:1445–50.

14 Blum U, Krumme B, Flugel P, *et al.* Treatment of ostial renal-artery stenoses with vascular endoprostheses after unsuccessful balloon angioplasty. *N Engl J Med* 1997; **336**:459–65.

15 Watson PS, Hadjipetrou P, Cox SV, Piemonte TC, Eisenhauer AC. Effect of renal artery stenting on renal function and size in patients with atherosclerotic renovascular disease. *Circulation* 2000; **102**:1671–77.

16 Harden PN, MacLeod MJ, Rodger RS, *et al.* Effect of renal-artery stenting on progression of renovascular renal failure. *Lancet* 1997; **349**:1133–36.

17 Bush RL, Najibi S, MacDonald MJ, *et al.* Endovascular revascularization of renal artery stenosis: technical and clinical results. *J Vasc Surg* 2001; **33**:1041–49.

18 Dorros G, Jaff M, Mathiak L, *et al.* Four-year follow-up of Palmaz-Schatz stent revascularization as treatment for atherosclerotic renal artery stenosis. *Circulation* 1998; **90**:642–47.

19 Henry M, Amor M, Henry I, *et al.* Stents in the treatment of renal artery stenosis: long-term follow-up. *J Endovasc Surg* 1999; **6**:42–51.

20 Iannone LA, Underwood PL, Nath A, Tannenbaum MA, Ghali MG, Clevenger LD. Effect of primary balloon expandable renal artery stents on long-term patency, renal function, and blood pressure in hypertensive and renal insufficient patients with renal artery stenosis. *Cathet Cardiovasc Diagn* 1996; **37**:243–50.

21 Rundback JH, Gray RJ, Rozenblit G, *et al.* Renal artery stent placement for the management of ischemic nephropathy. *J Vasc Interv Radiol* 1998; **9**:413–20.

22 Shannon HM, Gillespie IN, Moss JG. Salvage of the solitary kidney by insertion of a renal artery stent. *AJR Am J Roentgenol* 1998; **171**:217–22.

23 Leertouwer TC, Gussenhoven EJ, Bosch JL, *et al.* Stent placement for renal arterial stenosis: where do we stand? A meta-analysis. *Radiology* 2000; **216**:78–85.

24 Henry M, Klonaris C, Henry I, *et al.* Protected renal stenting with the PercuSurge GuardWire device: a pilot study. *J Endovasc Ther* 2001; **8**:227–37.

25 Guzman RP, Zierler RE, Isaacson JA, Bergelin RO, Strandness DE, Jr. Renal atrophy and arterial stenosis. A prospective study with duplex ultrasound. *Hypertension* 1994; **23**:346–50.

26 van de Ven PJ, Kaatee R, Beutler JJ, *et al.* Arterial stenting and balloon angioplasty in ostial atherosclerotic renovascular disease: a randomised trial. *Lancet* 1999; **353**:282–86.

CHAPTER 11

Aortoiliac occlusive disease

Eric Peden, Ruth L. Bush, Alan B. Lumsden

Following the introduction of transluminal angioplasty nearly four decades ago by Charles T. Dotter, endovascular techniques for the treatment of aortoiliac occlusive disease have rapidly evolved.[1] In an effort to deal with several of the limitations of transluminal angioplasty, including vessel wall recoil, dissection, and restenosis, researchers proposed the concept of intravascular stents as a means of maintaining vessel patency and improving the clinical outcome of balloon angioplasty. Since the first reported case of successful deployment of intravascular stents in canine femoral and popliteal arteries in 1969,[1] a variety of stent devices composed of various materials have been introduced.[2–4] Currently, intravascular stenting is recognized as a potentially effective modality in overcoming elastic recoil of the arterial wall, stabilizing intimal dissection at the site of angioplasty, and maintaining luminal patency of arteries with calcified and eccentric atherosclerotic plaques.

Traditional open surgical intervention for aortoiliac occlusive disease, aortobifemoral bypass grafting, has had excellent results with patency rates approaching 90% at 5 years and 70% at 10 years.[5] Aortobifemoral bypass grafting, although certainly a durable operation in properly selected patients, does have major morbidity associated with it even though mortality rates are usually less than 3%. The most common cause of both morbidity and mortality in patients undergoing this procedure is an adverse cardiac event including fatal and nonfatal myocardial infarction and arrhythmias. With the advent of endovascular interventions, these cardiac complications may be reduced by the avoidance of general anesthesia, less intraoperative blood loss, and a shorter procedural time, all resulting in a decrease in physiologic stress. Furthermore, the length of the hospital stay is shortened as are patient recovery times and return to functional status. Equally important, further endovascular and open surgical treatment options remain feasible for recurrent or progressive disease. Thus, endovascular treatment should be considered as first-line therapy for amenable lesions in patients with symptomatic aortoiliac occlusive disease.

Clinical presentation

Patients with aortoiliac occlusive disease present with a broad spectrum of symptomatology. The severity of presenting symptoms is related to the metabolic demand placed on the distal tissues, the amount of collateral flow compensation, the chronicity of the lesions, and the presence or absence of occlusive disease at other levels in the arterial tree. Unpredictably, patients with severe occlusive disease including complete obstruction can be entirely asymptomatic. If the occlusion is long-standing so that sufficient collaterals have developed and the metabolic demand is nominal, such as in a minimally ambulatory patient, symptoms may be mild if present at all. On the opposite end of the spectrum is critical limb ischemia with threatened limb loss. Critical limb ischemia, in the setting of rest pain or tissue loss, is essentially always associated with multilevel disease.

The most common presentation is that of claudication, cramping with activity that goes away at rest in a functional muscle group. Symptoms attributed to arterial insufficiency should be reproducibly provoked with exertion and relieved with rest. With aortoiliac occlusive disease, the claudication can affect the musculature of the buttock, hip, thigh, and calf. These symptoms can range from mild with prolonged exertion to extremely limiting with minimal activity leading to a severe impact on daily living as well as routine activities needed for independent living. Classically, patients with significant aortoiliac lesions have been described as presenting with Leriche syndrome. This specific presentation involves hip, thigh, and buttock claudication in combination with impotence and absent of palpable femoral pulses.[6] Aortoiliac lesions can also present with distal embolization and the "blue toe" syndrome.[7] In this process, distal atheroemboli cause severe pain and discoloration of the toes and forefoot that may lead to limb loss.

Diagnostic evaluation

As with any medical condition, evaluation begins with a good history and physical examination. Past history should focus on cardiovascular and atherosclerotic risk factors, previous cardiovascular events, and previous interventions and therapies. Attention to comorbidities is crucial because they impact both efficacy of revascularization as well as the patient's long-term survival. In terms of behavioral modification, smoking cessation is particularly important in promoting revascularization success, limb salvage, and survival.[8] Continued smoking negatively affects both endovascular and open surgical revascularization. Overall, the long-term survival of patients with peripheral vascular disease is markedly reduced compared with age-matched controls without vascular disease, thus preoperative health optimization is essential. The ankle brachial index (ABI) has been shown to be a strong predictor of survival in patients, with the presence of an ABI < 0.3 correlating with significantly poorer survival.[9] The implication of these observations is that patients with aortoiliac occlusive disease need investigation and treatment of their underlying risk factors and comorbidities in order to impact long-term survival.

The details of the presenting complaints should focus on the ischemic symptoms evoked and the disability that they cause. As with most other occlusive vasculopathies, the mere presence of a stenosis or occlusion in this region of the body is not a specific indication for intervention. The symptoms will frequently point to the level of occlusive disease. Just as superficial femoral artery disease leads to calf claudication, aortoiliac disease frequently causes pain in the hip, thigh, and buttocks. On examination, absent or weak femoral pulses are highly suggestive of significant aortoiliac occlusive disease. In obese patients or patients that have had previous groin surgery, such as femoral popliteal bypass grafting, the pulses can frequently be difficult to palpate. If distal pulses are present, significant aortoiliac disease is unlikely, although not impossible if the patient has had long-standing chronic disease with a slow progression of symptoms, thus, allowing for significant collateralization.

Following a physical examination, the next step in the evaluation of patients with suspected significant peripheral vascular disease affecting the legs should be noninvasive testing in the vascular lab. This allows confirmation of the physical findings and a baseline study for future comparison. Several parameters are possible to measure, including segmental pressures, pulse volume recordings, Doppler waveform analysis, and direct imaging with duplex ultrasound. Segmental pressures should be obtained from the upper thighs to the toes. This enables localization of disease to one or multiple segments. Normal segmental pressures commonly show high thigh pressures of 20 mm Hg or greater in comparison to the brachial artery pressures. The low thigh pressure should be equivalent to brachial pressures. Subsequent pressures should fall by no more than 10 mm Hg at each level. Pulse volume tracings are suggestive of proximal disease if the upstroke of the pulse is not brisk, the peak of the wave tracing is rounded, and there is disappearance of the dicrotic notch. Doppler waveform analysis can also indicate aortoiliac disease if the waveforms in the common femoral arteries are biphasic or monophasic as well as asymmetrical. The caveat to Doppler waveform analysis is meticulous technique by a certified vascular ultrasound technician, such that the appropriate 60° Doppler angle is maintained. Alteration of this angle can markedly alter waveform appearance and subsequent interpretation. Direct imaging of the stenotic vessels with duplex ultrasound is less reliable because of the difficulty in visualizing the vessels through overlying bowel. Patients that have convincing history for claudication and a normal vascular lab study should have the testing repeated with exercise. The vasodilatation produced by exercising leads to enhanced pressure drops and can uncover a significant iliac lesion missed on a resting study.

Suggestive findings on clinical evaluation and vascular lab studies typically prompt evaluation with angiography. Other choices include Magnetic Resonance Angiography (MRA) or Computed Tomography Angiography (CTA). MRA and CTA are both highly sensitive means to visualize the vessels and occlusive lesions. MRA avoids iodinated contrast agents but requires considerable time for imaging, which can be an issue for patients with claustrophobia. CTA is quicker than MRA and produces good images, but shares the potential complication with conventional angiography of contrast injection. Either of these two studies can confirm significant disease suspected from exam and Doppler findings and allow for further treatment planning. Neither method currently allows treatment at the same time as does conventional angiography. Ultimately, conventional angiography is required if the patient is to undergo endovascular treatment and frequently to investigate the possibility of endovascular versus open surgical revascularization.

Lesion classification

The most commonly quoted classification system of iliac lesions has been set forth by the TransAtlantic inter-Society Consensus (TASC) group with recommended treatment options.[10] As seen in Table 11.1, from the TASC review, type A lesions are treated preferentially by endovascular techniques and type D lesions are more suited for surgical treatment. There is currently no consensus as to recommendations for the best treatment of moderately severe iliac artery lesions, namely TASC type B and TASC type C lesions.

Angiographic technique

Assessment of the patient, prior to coming to the interventional suite, is performed to determine the renal function of the patient and to direct the sequence

Table 11.1 TASC morphologic stratification of iliac lesions.[10]

Type	Definition	Treatment choice
A	a. Single stenosis <3 cm in length (unilateral/bilateral) of the CIA or EIA	Percutaneous endovascular procedure
B	a. Single stenosis 3–10 cm in length, not extending into CFA b. Two stenosis of total <5 cm in length, not extending into CFA c. Unilateral CIA occlusion	Unresolved
C	a. Bilateral stenosis of the CIA and/or EIA, 5–10 cm in length and not extending into the CFA b. Unilateral EIA occlusion not extending into the CFA c. Unilateral EIA stenosis extending into CFA d. Bilateral CIA occlusion	Unresolved
D	a. Diffuse stenosis of CIA, EIA, and CFA of >10 cm in length b. Unilateral occlusion of CIA and EIA c. Bilateral EIA occlusion d. Iliac stenosis in conjunction with AAA or other lesion requiring operative intervention	Open surgery

CIA, common iliac artery; EIA, external iliac artery; CFA, common femoral artery; AAA, abdominal aortic aneurysm.

of the study, based on expected findings from both clinical and noninvasive evaluation. In general, preprocedure planning can greatly facilitate the study and result in the use of a lower contrast volume, the fewest number of access sites, and the smallest caliber of catheters. It is important not to bring the patient to the angiography suite in a dehydrated state, as the two principal risk factors for the development of contrast nephropathy are preexisting renal dysfunction and dehydration. For patients with a creatinine level greater than 1.2, pretreatment should be with intravenous hydration and acetylcysteine (Mucomyst®), based on published data.[11] Other options for avoiding iodinated contrast usage include carbon dioxide angiography or gadolinium.[12,13]

Initial access is routinely obtained with a retrograde common femoral artery access and rarely with a brachial artery puncture in the case of absent femoral pulses. The authors prefer to use a 4 or 5 Fr system for initial access and diagnostic angiography. A minor puncture in the artery leads to shorter compression times for hemostasis, less groin complications, and earlier ambulation. In the setting of unilateral disease, the femoral puncture is made on the side with the strongest pulse.

Assuming that renal function is adequate, a multiside hole catheter (pigtail catheter) is placed in the upper abdominal aorta at the level of the first lumbar vertebrae and serial images are performed. With digital subtraction angiography, a total volume of 20–30 mL of iodinated contrast is needed to visualize the aorta thoroughly. The catheter is then brought down to the level of the aortic bifurcation and the injection is repeated with a lesser volume for imaging of the pelvic vasculature. If iliac disease is suspected, but not seen on an anteriorposterior (AP) pelvic angiogram, oblique images should be obtained. The right iliac system is best visualized with a left anterior oblique projection at approximately 30°. This helps to separate the origins of the external and internal iliac arteries, such that their images are not superimposed. Similarly, the left iliac system is best visualized by a right anterior oblique angle.

Imaging of the infrainguinal arterial system ideally should be performed prior to any intervention, if the patient's renal function can accommodate the additional contrast necessary. Pressures across stenotic lesions should be determined if there is any doubt as to the hemodynamic significance of the lesion. A pressure gradient of at least 10 mm Hg is predictive of hemodynamic significance. Pressures also allow for comparison of pre- and posttreatment results.

Intravascular ultrasound (IVUS) is an alternative or additional imaging modality that may be used to assess the characteristics of the lesion and better assess the degree of stenosis. In our practice, we do not routinely utilize IVUS for initial diagnostic evaluation of aortoiliac occlusive lesions. We more commonly use IVUS to evaluate completeness of stent opposition. Buckley and colleagues reported that their iliac interventions have benefited from post-intervention interrogation from IVUS by more accurate angioplasty and stent deployment.[14]

As with any other occlusive lesion, the sequence for intervention is first to image the lesion, then to navigate a guidewire across the lesion, with subsequent intervention. A completion study is performed last to ensure a satisfactory result and to evaluate any complications, such as residual stenosis or thrombosis. Crossing a high-grade stenosis or occlusion can be challenging in the iliac arteries. There are several techniques to assist in difficult cases. First and foremost is to reimage the lesion. Another view or with a different angle of the image intensifier will frequently uncover the anatomic reason for difficulty. Frequently, the difficulty is from vessel tortuosity or aspect of the lesion not visualized or appreciated on the original view. Use of an angled hydrophilic guidewire and an angled catheter can also greatly assist in the management of a difficult lesion. In addition to providing directional capabilities, the catheter adds extra body and support to the wire trying to cross the lesion. Patience, persistence, and periodic reimaging will facilitate the crossing of a lesion in the great majority of cases.

Infrarenal aortic stenosis

Techniques used for angioplasty with or without stenting of the aorta and iliac segments are similar. While percutaneous transluminal angioplasty (PTA) has demonstrated excellent results in focal stenoses of the abdominal aorta and iliacs, primary stenting may reduce the degree of restenosis with PTA alone and decrease distal embolization.[15–19]

Focal aortic stenoses are treated by mounting a balloon-expandable stent on a larger caliber angioplasty balloon or using a large self-expanding stent. The role of covered stents, such as cuffs, made for endoluminal abdominal aortic aneurysm repair has not been rigorously studied. The aortic diameter should be sized with a calibrated catheter or by preintervention CT scanning to avoid undersizing. Balloon size will range from 12 to 18 mm in most cases. A single stent is generally required in most cases with no special technical requirements; large Palmaz-type stents (Palmaz XXL) have been successfully used and may be inflated up to 25 mm in diameter. Concentric aortic stenosis may encroach upon the inferior mesenteric artery and coverage of this vessel may be unavoidable. Furthermore, only midabdominal aortic lesion should be treated in this fashion. Different techniques, which are described below, are employed in the situation where the lesion involves the aortic bifurcation. For focal aortic stenoses, technical success, safety, and adequate patency rates have been reported with primary stent placement as already cited.[17,19–22] Durability remains satisfactory in properly selected patients.

Figure 11.1 is an example of a focal aortic stenosis that is well suited for endovascular intervention. Care should be taken to use low inflation pressures to avoid the potentially fatal complication of aortic rupture. The inflation pressures are generally kept at 3–4 mm Hg or less. Patient complaints of back or abdominal pain during balloon inflation should be taken seriously as they may suggest impending rupture. Many interventionalists reserve stenting for

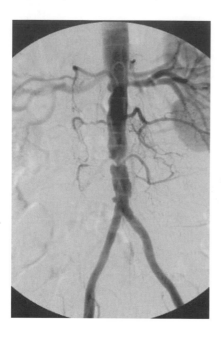

Figure 11.1 Aortogram reveals a focal aortic stenosis that is amenable to balloon-expandable stent placement.

suboptimal angioplasty results. These results that prompt stenting include residual stenosis of 30% or greater, persistent pressure gradient of 10 mm Hg or more, and dissection at the site of angioplasty.

Iliac artery stenosis

Patients with iliac lesions present with a wide spectrum of symptoms depending on the amount of involvement of the iliac arteries, whether the lesions are focal versus multisegment, and the degree, if any, of infrainguinal disease. As previously discussed, indications for intervention are severe disabling claudication, rest pain, tissue loss, or blue toe syndrome. Individual risk factors and possible adverse outcomes associated with each procedure must also be taken into consideration in deciding the best therapeutic treatment option. Whereas initially, iliac artery angioplasty with subsequent stent placement had been used for only focal lesions, with technological advances, more complex multisegment lesions are now approached endoluminally.

Once the lesion has been well imaged, a decision will have to be made to treat from an ipsilateral retrograde approach or a contralateral approach, crossing the aortic bifurcation. The decision is based typically on the location of the lesion. If the lesion to be treated is in the distal common iliac artery or external iliac artery, a contralateral approach can be utilized. Frequently, the diagnostic catheter has already been placed in the contralateral groin, so this approach can be done with a single puncture. If this approach is chosen, the diagnostic catheter should be used to cannulate across the aortic bifurcation and then a wire advanced to support the passage of a long sheath. With a sheath traversing the aortic bifurcation in place, diagnostic images can be obtained while maintaining position of the wires during crossing of the lesion and treatment, as well as after the intervention for a completion study.

If the lesion to be treated is in the common iliac artery or proximal external iliac artery, an ipsilateral retrograde femoral approach can be utilized. Imaging during this sequence is then performed either through a catheter placed through the other groin and positioned at the lower aorta or by retrograde injection from the ipsilateral sheath.

Intervention from the ipsilateral groin will require gaining access to the femoral artery in situations where little or no palpable pulse is present. Our preferred method of doing this is with ultrasound guidance and a micropuncture (0.014 in. wire) kit. The ultrasound probe is used to visualize the artery in a transverse plane with the vessel centered in the field of view. The micropuncture needle is then used to penetrate the skin in the middle of the probe. The needle or the tissue movement around the needle is then visualized and directed at the artery.

Other methods to puncture a pulseless femoral artery are possible as well. Sometimes, a calcified femoral artery can be palpated and the puncture directed at that structure. The medial third of the femoral head marks where the femoral artery is located, and this bony landmark can be a target for fluoroscopically guided puncture. Contrast can be injected from catheter on the other side and a puncture directed toward the column of dye. Additionally, a wire can be passed from the contralateral limb and the puncture can be directed at this fluoroscopic target. Alternatively, a Doppler needle can be used to direct the puncture.

Once the lesion of interest has been crossed, a decision will have to be made for primary stenting versus angioplasty with selective stenting. The Dutch iliac stent trial study group showed that primary stenting versus angioplasty with selective stenting had equal patency rates in both short- and long-term follow-up.[23] Importantly, patients in the selective stent group required subsequent stenting in nearly half of all cases. In general, indications for selective stenting following angioplasty are residual stenosis greater than 30%, persistent pressure gradient across the lesion, flow limiting dissection, and treatment of a total occlusion.

Although, simple iliac TASC type A lesions can be treated with angioplasty alone, it is more common to see more complex lesions and therefore, almost routinely primary stenting is employed. Additionally, there is some evidence that primary stenting yields better long-term results.[24] Once the lesion is traversed and necessary diagnostic imaging performed, stent diameter is estimated using either calibrated catheters or skin markers. It is a preferred practice to first perform balloon angioplasty, both to predilate the lesion as well as to appropriately size the vessel for subsequent stent placement. Both balloon expandable and self-expanding stents can be used in the iliac arteries. Balloon expandable stents are preferred if the positioning must be very exact. Self-expanding stents may be preferred if the section of iliac artery to be treated is very tortuous, or the lesion is in an area of movement such as the external iliac artery, since these stents tend to conform to the shape of the vessel.

Lesions involving the origin of the common iliac artery at the aortic bifurcation deserve extra consideration. Concern exists that intervening on one side may lead to compromise of the origin of the other iliac artery by movement of an eccentric plaque. One option is the kissing stent technique where stents are placed in bilateral iliac arteries and "kiss" in the lower aorta. Kissing stents are not routinely employed unless the lesion is bilateral or involves the very orifice of the common iliac artery.[25] A "protective" balloon inflation in the contralateral iliac is likewise rarely necessary and as long as wire access is across the iliac origin, it is unlikely that contralateral lumen compromise may be corrected with kissing balloons and/or stents. The need for additional treatment is based on the completion study after stent deployment. Figures 11.2 demonstrates a proximal left common iliac lesion that was then stented without a kissing balloon or stent with good technical result. Figure 11.3 shows a TASC type C lesion that was treated with kissing stent technique. Bilateral involvement in this case demanded kissing stent placement with a satisfactory radiographic result.

The role of stent grafts in aortoiliac occlusive disease has yet to be fully elucidated. A recent report suggested that the use of stent grafts can have a positive impact. TASC C and D lesions were treated with stent grafting with good results.[26] Atherectomy devices have been reported for use principally for recurrent stenosis, but their role in endovascular therapy for aortoiliac disease has not been established and is discussed elsewhere. Similarly, the interventional vascular community eagerly awaits the release of more data about drug-eluting stents in the periphery. A recent randomized trial of coated nitinol stents in the superficial femoral artery has thus far failed to show any benefit over bare metal stents.[27] There is limited experimental animal data

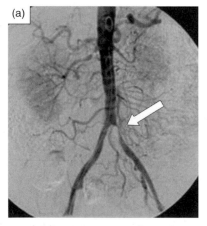
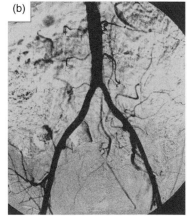

Figure 11.2 (a) A proximal left common iliac artery stenosis (arrow) which was treated with primary stent placement. (b) Completion angiogram demonstrating satisfactory results.

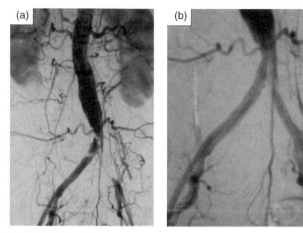

Figure 11.3 (a) A TASC type C lesion as evidenced by bilateral iliac artery lesions. (b) Following kissing stent placement, completion angiogram shows good technical result.

that looks promising and hopefully will be converted into a randomized trial in humans in the near future.[28] Controlled-release local delivery of sirolimus from a coated stent reduced neointimal formation in rabbit iliac arteries in a dose-dependent manner.

Results from clinical series

Multiple studies have documented excellent results following both focal and complex iliac artery stenting procedures with most reporting superior results over angioplasty alone.[3,4,15,24,29,30] Henry and colleagues reported the Palmaz stent application in 184 patients who received 230 iliac stent placements.[31] Mean follow-up was 35 months that consisted of angiography at 4–6 months following stent placement (in 98% of patients) and serial duplex scan studies. Similar to the study reported by Palmaz and colleagues,[32] the majority of patients (89%) included in this series were treated for claudication. Immediate clinical improvement was achieved in 91% of patients. The primary patency rates at 1-, 2-, and 3-years were 94%, 91%, and 86%, respectively, which were superior to those of balloon angioplasty. More than 70% of patients received one stent placement while the remaining patients had two or more Palmaz stents in the iliac artery. The restenosis rate in the iliac artery was 0.5% at 6 months. The authors reported predictors for success in iliac artery stenting, which included lesion length of less than 3 cm, artery diameter greater than 6 cm, and absence of secondary arterial lesions.[32]

Cikrit and colleagues reported their experience with Palmaz stent application in iliac artery disease with long-term follow-up.[33] In 39 iliac occlusive lesions, the placement of the Palmaz stent significantly decreased the intraluminal pressure gradient from 32 mm Hg to 1 mm Hg. Similar improvement of ankle/brachial pressure index was also noted following stent deployment, which increased from 0.53 to 0.8. Life-table analysis showed cumulative patency rates of 1-, 3-, and 5-years at 91%, 91%, and 86%, respectively.[33]

While iliac stent placement is traditionally reserved for situations of suboptimal or failed angioplasty results, the potential benefits of primary treatment of iliac lesions using the Palmaz stents have also been investigated. Early report by Bonn and colleagues noted that primary stenting using the Palmaz stents for iliac lesions had early technical success without incurring any additional complications compared with angioplasty alone.[34] A similar finding was also reported by Williams and colleagues.[35] In their study, 73 patients underwent a primary stenting procedure for aortoiliac lesions with an overall complication rate of 13%. The authors also demonstrated an initial cost savings of 25–66% compared with surgical interventions.

A prospective randomized multicenter trial comparing the results of primary Palmaz stenting versus angioplasty alone for iliac lesions was reported by Richter and colleagues.[36] Patients in both groups had similar mean transstenotic pressure gradients prior to the treatment. However, patients who were treated with primary Palmaz stenting had significantly less pressure gradients following the stent placement. At the 2 year follow-up, the restenosis rates in the angioplasty group and the stent group were 27% and 14%, respectively. Of the angioplasty group, 28% required additional intervention for iliac restenosis at 3 years, in contrast to 2% of the stent group who required reintervention. The improved patency rates and clinical outcomes of primary stent placement using the Palmaz stents have been further validated by other studies, including primary stenting of the infrarenal aorta.[16,19,35,37]

A study reported by Sullivan and colleagues examined the outcome of 424 limbs in 288 patients treated with balloon angioplasty and primary stenting for occlusive iliac lesions.[38] Palmaz stents were used in 86% of cases while Wallstents were used in the remaining 14% of cases. Angiographic patency at 1- and 2-years were 88% and 75%, respectively. The authors noted that factors that favorably affected clinical outcomes include younger age, higher degree of initial iliac stenosis, and patent ipsilateral superficial femoral artery.

The Wallstents has been studied extensively throughout Europe in the past decade, due in part to the collaborative effort of the European Wallstent Peripheral Artery Implant Study. In the initial series by Gunther and colleagues,[39] 31 patients with iliac artery disease including 16 iliac occlusions underwent Wallstent placement based on inadequate iliac angioplasty. Restenosis with stent occlusion occurred in one patient after 6 months. The benefit of stent placement in improving poor angioplasty results was highlighted by the authors. Martin and colleagues reported results of a multicenter trial of the Wallstent in the140 patients with iliac occlusive lesions.[40] The average length of iliac lesions was less than 10 cm. The 6-month angiographic patency was 93%. The results using the Wallstent were similar to those with the Palmaz stent in the treatment of iliac lesions. The primary patency rates at 1- and 2-years were 81% and 71%; and secondary patency rates were

91% and 86%, respectively. Murphy and colleagues reported their finding of using the Wallstent in treating 94 iliac artery lesions.[41] Indications for therapy included diffuse stenoses (>3 cm in length), chronic occlusions, failed angioplasty procedures, and dissections of the iliac arteries. Approximately half of the patients had claudication while the remaining had limb-threatening ischemia. Initial technical success was achieved in 91% of patients. Overall complication rate was 9%, which included iliac artery rupture, distal embolization, and groin hematoma. Primary patency rates at 1 and 2 years were 78% and 53%, respectively. Secondary patency rates were 86% and 82%, respectively. The limb salvage rate for patients with limb-threatening ischemia was 98% at a mean follow-up of 14 months.

Common problems and complications

The complication profile is similar for either aortic or iliac interventions. Since the deployment of a balloon-expandable stent requires the physical mounting of the stent on a balloon catheter, accidental dislodgment of the stent from the catheter delivery system may occur. Femoral puncture site complications are the most frequent problems.[42] Recurrent problems include bleeding, pseudoaneurysm formation, arteriovenous fistula, and thrombosis. These complications can largely be avoided by localizing the femoral head prior to percutaneous puncture and good manual compression. Should a puncture site complication be suspected, the best initial test is an ultrasound with duplex imaging.

Iliac stenting helped improve the technical results of iliac balloon angioplasty and avoided acute complications, such as acute occlusion. Use of stents helped extend the use of percutaneous techniques to cases that are otherwise limited to surgery. Potential problems in those patients seem more likely than in patients who are ideal candidates for balloon angioplasty alone.

The complication rate in iliac arteries after stenting is relatively uncommon. For the Wallstent in iliac stenoses the total complication rate was 6.8%, with a major complication rate of 3.4% that included subacute stent thrombosis.[24,31,33] Similar complications occur that are nonspecific for percutaneous procedures including complications related to the puncture sites, arterial dissection, and vessel rupture. Unlike the self-expanding stents, which are deformable and constantly exerts an outward radial force, external compression on the balloon-expandable stents due to vascular clamping injury can result in permanent stent deformity. While short-term failure is mainly thrombosis in the stented vessel, the long-term patency can be adversely affected by restenosis induced by intimal hyperplasia. Factors associated with stented artery thrombosis are iliac artery occlusion, multiple stent deployment, and hypercoagulable disorders. Stent placement in an occluded iliac artery is particularly prone to restenosis (Figure 11.4), due in part to the lack of an endothelial lining in the occluded vessel. Stent deployment may further denude the intimal lining, thereby reducing the protective antithrombotic function of endothelium.

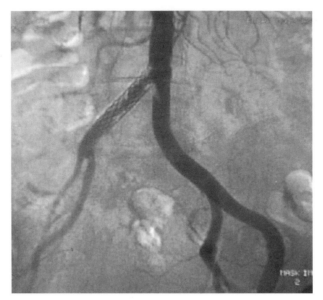

Figure 11.4 Aortogram revealing an in-stent stenosis within the common iliac artery stent.

Additionally, the incidence of distal embolization following the stent place-ment ranged between 2.4% and 7.8% (Plate 8, facing p. 80).[43] As with all radiographic intervention, transient contrast-induced nephropathy may occur following an interventional procedure.

Conclusions

Intravascular stent placement has proven to be an invaluable tool in both the primary treatment of aortoiliac occlusive disease and the management of com-plications of balloon angioplasty. Clinical application of iliac stents has also extended to the treatment of patients with total iliac occlusion and restenosis. Although balloon angioplasty has met with limited success in treating totally occluded iliac arteries, the use of intravascular stents has improved the success rate to approximately 80% at 3 years, with a late occlusion rate similar to that of stenotic lesions. The benefit of primary stenting of the iliac artery has been demonstrated in several series with a favorable 5-year patency rate of greater than 90%, which is comparable to conventional surgical reconstruction. The Achilles heel of intravascular stenting is the induction of intimal hyperplasia leading to restenosis. The incidence of restenosis that occurs within 1 year following the stent placement has been shown to occur in greater than 20% of cases. There are many areas in which future research may be focused in attempts to solve this dilemma. Promising future advances include the use of drug-eluting stents, vascular brachytherapy, cutting balloons, and aggressive antiplatelet regimens, which are being tested to improve clinical outcomes.

References

1 Dotter CT, Judkins MP. Transluminal recanalization in occlusive disease of the leg arteries. *GP* 1968; **37**:98–106.

2 Uren NG, Chronos NA. Intracoronary stents. *BMJ* 1996; **313**:892–93.

3 Sigwart U, Puel J, Mirkovitch V, Joffre F, Kappenberger L. Intravascular stents to prevent occlusion and restenosis after transluminal angioplasty. *N Engl J Med* 1987; **316**:701–6.

4 Onal B, Ilgit ET, Yucel C, Ozbek E, Vural M, Akpek S. Primary stenting for complex atherosclerotic plaques in aortic and iliac stenoses. *Cardiovasc Intervent Radiol* 1998; **21**:386–92.

5 Poulias GE, Doundoulakis N, Prombonas E, *et al.* Aorto-femoral bypass and determinants of early success and late favourable outcome. Experience with 1000 consecutive cases. *J Cardiovasc Surg (Torino)* 1992; **33**:664–78.

6 Mohler ER, III, Hiatt WR, Olin JW, Wade M, Jeffs R, Hirsch AT. Treatment of intermittent claudication with beraprost sodium, an orally active prostaglandin I2 analogue: a double blinded, randomized, controlled trial. *J Am Coll Cardiol* 2003; **41**:1679–86.

7 Wingo JP, Nix ML, Greenfield LJ, Barnes RW. The blue toe syndrome: hemodynamics and therapeutic correlates of outcome. *J Vasc Surg* 1986; **3**:475–80.

8 Schillinger M, Exner M, Mlekusch W, *et al.* Effect of smoking on restenosis during the 1st year after lower-limb endovascular interventions. *Radiology* 2004; **231**:831–38.

9 McDermott MM, Feinglass J, Slavensky R, Pearce WH. The ankle-brachial index as a predictor of survival in patients with peripheral vascular disease. *J Gen Intern Med* 1994; **9**:445–49.

10 Dormandy JA, Rutherford RB. Management of peripheral arterial disease (PAD). TASC Working Group. TransAtlantic Inter-Society Consensus (TASC). *J Vasc Surg* 2000; **31**:S1–S296.

11 Tepel M. Acetylcysteine for the prevention of radiocontrast-induced nephropathy Minerva Cardioangiol 2003; **51**:525–30.

12 Oliva VL, Denbow N, Therasse E, *et al.* Digital subtraction angiography of the abdominal aorta and lower extremities: carbon dioxide versus iodinated contrast material. *J Vasc Interv Radiol* 1999; **10**:723–31.

13 Sam AD, II, Morasch MD, Collins J, Song G, Chen R, Pereles FS. Safety of gadolinium contrast angiography in patients with chronic renal insufficiency. *J Vasc Surg* 2003; **38**:313–18.

14 Buckley CJ, Arko FR, Lee S, *et al.* Intravascular ultrasound scanning improves long-term patency of iliac lesions treated with balloon angioplasty and primary stenting. *J Vasc Surg* 2002; **35**:316–23.

15 Treiman GS, Schneider PA, Lawrence PF, Pevec WC, Bush RL, Ichikawa L. Does stent placement improve the results of ineffective or complicated iliac artery angioplasty? *J Vasc Surg* 1998; **28**:104–12; discussion 113–14.

16 Saha S, Gibson M, Torrie EP, Magee TR, Galland RB. Stenting for localised arterial stenoses in the aorto-iliac segment. *Eur J Vasc Endovasc Surg* 2001; **22**:37–40.

17 Eftekhar K, Young N, Fletcher J, Bester L, Wong L, Puttaswamy V. Clinical efficacy of metal stents for the treatment of focal abdominal aortic stenosis. *Australas Radiol* 2004; **48**:17–20.

18 Hallisey MJ, Meranze SG, Parker BC, *et al.* Percutaneous transluminal angioplasty of the abdominal aorta. *J Vasc Interv Radiol* 1994; **5**:679–87.

19 Nyman U, Uher P, Lindh M, Lindblad B, Ivancev K. Primary stenting in infrarenal aortic occlusive disease. *Cardiovasc Intervent Radiol* 2000; **23**:97–108.

20 Lim MC, Choo M, Tan HC. Stenting of stenosis of the abdominal aorta. *Singapore Med J* 1995; **36**:562–65.

21 McPherson SJ, Laing AD, Thomson KR, *et al.* Treatment of infrarenal aortic stenosis by stent placement: a 6-year experience. *Australas Radiol* 1999; **43**:185–91.

22 Stoeckelhuber BM, Meissner O, Stoeckelhuber M, Wiesmann M, Kueffer G. Primary endovascular stent placement for focal infrarenal aortic stenosis: initial and midterm results. *J Vasc Interv Radiol* 2003; **14**:1443–47.

23 Tetteroo E, van der Graaf Y, Bosch JL, *et al.* Randomised comparison of primary stent placement versus primary angioplasty followed by selective stent placement in patients with iliac-artery occlusive disease. Dutch Iliac Stent Trial Study Group. *Lancet* 1998; **351**:1153–59.

24 Bosch JL, Hunink MG. Meta-analysis of the results of percutaneous transluminal angioplasty and stent placement for aortoiliac occlusive disease. *Radiology* 1997; **204**:87–96.

25 Smith JC, Watkins GE, Taylor FC, Carlson LA, Karst JG, Smith DC. Angioplasty or stent placement in the proximal common iliac artery: is protection of the contralateral side necessary? *J Vasc Interv Radiol* 2001; **12**:1395–98.

26 Ali AT, Modrall JG, Lopez J, *et al.* Emerging role of endovascular grafts in complex aortoiliac occlusive disease. *J Vasc Surg* 2003; **38**:486–91.

27 Duda SH, Pusich B, Richter G, *et al.* Sirolimus-eluting stents for the treatment of obstructive superficial femoral artery disease: six-month results. *Circulation* 2002; **106**:1505–9.

28 Klugherz BD, Llanos G, Lieuallen W, *et al.* Twenty-eight-day efficacy and phamacokinetics of the sirolimus-eluting stent. *Coron Artery Dis* 2002; **13**:183–88.

29 Timaran CH, Ohki T, Gargiulo NJ, III, *et al.* Iliac artery stenting in patients with poor distal runoff: influence of concomitant infrainguinal arterial reconstruction. *J Vasc Surg* 2003; **38**:479–84; discussion 484–85.

30 Toogood GJ, Torrie EP, Magee TR, Galland RB. Early experience with stenting for iliac occlusive disease. *Eur J Vasc Endovasc Surg* 1998; **15**:165–68.

31 Henry M, Amor M, Ethevenot G, *et al.* Palmaz stent placement in iliac and femoropopliteal arteries: primary and secondary patency in 310 patients with 2–4-year follow-up. *Radiology* 1995; **197**:167–74.

32 Palmaz JC, Garcia OJ, Schatz RA, *et al.* Placement of balloon-expandable intraluminal stents in iliac arteries: first 171 procedures. *Radiology* 1990; **174**:969–75.

33 Cikrit DF, Gustafson PA, Dalsing MC, *et al.* Long-term follow-up of the Palmaz stent for iliac occlusive disease. *Surgery* 1995; **118**:608–13; discussion 613–14.

34 Bonn J, Gardiner GA, Jr., Shapiro MJ, Sullivan KL, Levin DC. Palmaz vascular stent: initial clinical experience. *Radiology* 1990; **174**:741–45.

35 Williams JB, Watts PW, Nguyen VA, Peterson CL. Balloon angioplasty with intraluminal stenting as the initial treatment modality in aorto-iliac occlusive disease. *Am J Surg* 1994; **168**:202–4.

36 Richter GM, Roeren T, Noeldge G, *et al.* Initial long-term results of a randomized 5-year study: iliac stent implantation versus PTA. *Vasa Suppl* 1992; **35**:192–93.

37 de Vries JP, van Den Heuvel DA, Vos JA, van Den Berg JC, Moll FI. Freedom from secondary interventions to treat stenotic disease after percutaneous transluminal angioplasty of infrarenal aorta: long-term results. *J Vasc Surg* 2004; **39**:427–31.

38 Sullivan TM, Childs MB, Bacharach JM, Gray BH, Piedmonte MR. Percutaneous transluminal angioplasty and primary stenting of the iliac arteries in 288 patients. *J Vasc Surg* 1997; **25**:829–38; discussion 838–39.

39 Gunther RW, Vorwerk D, Bohndorf K, Peters I, el-Din A, Messmer B. Iliac and femoral artery stenoses and occlusions: treatment with intravascular stents. *Radiology* 1989; **172**:725–30.

40 Martin EC, Katzen BT, Benenati JF, *et al.* Multicenter trial of the wallstent in the iliac and femoral arteries. *J Vasc Interv Radiol* 1995; **6**:843–49.

41 Murphy TP, Khwaja AA, Webb MS. Aortoiliac stent placement in patients treated for intermittent claudication. *J Vasc Interv Radiol* 1998; **9**:421–28.

42 McCann RL, Schwartz LB, Pieper KS. Vascular complications of cardiac catheterization. *J Vasc Surg* 1991; **14**:375–81.

43 Lin PH, Bush RL, Conklin BS, *et al.* Late complication of aortoiliac stent placement–atheroembolization of the lower extremities. *J Surg Res 2002*; **103**:153–59.

CHAPTER 12

Lower extremity arterial disease

Wei Zhou, Marlon A. Guerrero, Alan B. Lumsden

The symptoms of lower extremity occlusive disease are classified into two large categories: acute ischemia and chronic ischemia. Ninety percent of acute ischemia are either thrombotic or embolic. Frequently, sudden onset of limb-threatening ischemia may be the result of acute exacerbation of the preexisting atherosclerotic disease. Chronic ischemia is largely due to atherosclerotic changes of the lower extremity that manifests from asymptomatic to limb-threatening gangrene. As the population ages, the prevalence of chronic occlusive disease of the lower extremity is increasing and it significantly influences lifestyle, morbidity, and mortality. In addition, multiple comorbid conditions increase risks of surgical procedures. Endovascular interventions become an important alternative in treating lower extremity occlusive disease. However, despite rapid evolving endovascular technology, lower extremity endovascular intervention continues to be one of the most controversial areas of endovascular therapy.

Epidemiology

From extensive literature review, McDaniel and Cronenwett concluded that claudication occurred in 1.8% of patients under 60 years of age, 3.7% of patients between 60 and 70 years of age, and 5.2% of patients over 70 years of age.[1] Leng and his colleagues scanned 784 subjects using ultrasound in a random sample of men and women of ages between 56 and 77 years. Of the subjects that were scanned, 64% demonstrated atherosclerotic plaque.[2] However, a large number of patients had occlusive disease without significant symptoms. In a study by Schroll and Munck, only 19% of the patients with peripheral vascular disease were symptomatic.[3] Using ankle-brachial indices (ABIs), Stoffers and colleagues scanned 3171 individuals between the ages of 45 and 75 years, and identified that 6.9% of patients had ABIs <0.95, of whom only 22% had symptoms.[4] In addition, they demonstrated that the concomitant cardiovascular and cerebrovascular diseases were 3–4 times higher among the group with asymptomatic peripheral vascular diseases than those without peripheral vascular disease. Furthermore, they confirm that 68% of all peripheral arterial obstructive diseases were unknown to the primary care physician and this group mainly represented less-advanced cases of atherosclerosis. However, among patients with an ABI ratio <0.75, 42% were unknown to the primary physicians.

Clinical manifestation and classification

Lower extremity occlusive disease may range from exhibiting no symptoms to limb-threatening gangrene. There are two major classifications developed based on the clinical presentations.

The Fontaine classification uses four stages: Fontaine I is the stage when patients are asymptomatic; Fontaine II is when they have mild (IIa) or severe (IIb) claudication; Fontaine III is when they have ischemic rest pain; and Fontaine IV is when patients suffer tissue loss, such as ulceration or gangrene.[5]

The Rutherford classification has four grades (0–III) and seven categories (0–6). Asymptomatic patients are classified into category 0; claudicants are stratified into grade I and divided into three categories based on the severity of the symptoms; patients with rest pain belong to grade II and category 4; patients with tissue loss were classified into grade III and categories 5 and 6 based on the significance of the tissue loss.[6] These clinical classifications help to establish uniform standards in evaluating and reporting the results of diagnostic measurements and therapeutic interventions.

The most recent classification on lower extremity atherosclerotic disease was based on morphological characters of the lesions.[5] In 2000, TransAtlantic inter-Society Consensus (TASC) task force published a guideline separating lower extremity arterial diseases into femoropopliteal and infrapopliteal lesions. This guideline is particularly useful in determining intervention strategies based on the disease classifications.

Based on the guideline, femoropopliteal lesions are divided into four types: A, B, C, and D. Type A lesions are single focal lesions less than 3 cm in length and did not involve the origins of the superficial femoral artery (SFA) or the distal popliteal artery; type B lesions are single lesions 3–5 cm in length not involving the distal popliteal artery or multiple or heavily calcified lesions less than 3 cm in length; type C lesions are single lesions more than 5 cm in length, or multiple lesions between 3 and 5 cm in length with or without calcification; type D lesions were those with complete occlusion of common femoral artery (CFA), SFA, or popliteal artery.

In a similar fashion, infrapopliteal arterial diseases are classified into four types based on TASC guideline. Type A lesions are single lesions less than 1 cm in length not involving the trifurcation; type B lesions are multiple lesions less than 1 cm in length or single lesions shorter than 1 cm involving the trifurcation; type C lesions are those lesions that extensively involves trifurcation or those that are 1–4 cm stenotic or 1–2 cm occlusive lesions; type D lesions are occlusions longer than 2 cm or diffuse diseases.

Diagnostic evaluation

The diagnosis of lower extremity occlusive disease is often made based upon a focused history and physical examination, and confirmed by the imaging studies. A well-performed physical examination often reveals the site of lesions by detecting changes in pulses, temperature, and appearances. The bedside ABIs using blood pressure cuff also aid in diagnosis.

Noninvasive studies are important in documenting the severity of occlusive disease objectively. Ultrasound dopplers measuring ABIs and segmental pressures are widely utilized in North America and Europe. Normal ABI is greater than 1.0. In patients with claudication, ABIs decrease to 0.5–0.9 and to even lower levels in patients with rest pain or tissue loss.[7] Segmental pressures are helpful in identifying the level of involvement. Decrease in segmental pressure between two segments indicates significant disease. Ultrasound duplex scans are used to identify the site of lesion by revealing flow disturbance and velocity changes. A metaanalysis of 71 studies by Keolemay and associates confirmed that duplex scanning is accurate for assessing arterial occlusive disease in patients suffering from claudication or critical ischemia with an accumulative sensitivity of 80% and specificity of over 95%.[8] Adding an ultrasound contrast agent further increases sensitivity and specificity to ultrasound technology.[9] Other noninvasive imaging technologies, such as MRA and CTA, are rapidly evolving and gaining popularity in the diagnosis of lower extremity occlusive disease.

Contrast angiography remains the gold standard in imaging study. Using contrast angiography, interventionists can locate and size the anatomic significant lesions and measure the pressure gradient across the lesion, as well as plan for potential intervention. Angiography is, however, semiinvasive and should be confined to patients for whom surgical or percutaneous intervention is contemplated. Patients with borderline renal function may need to have alternate contrast agents, such as gadolinium or carbon dioxide, to avoid contrast-induced nephrotoxicity.

Treatment indications and strategies

Patients with vascular diseases frequently have complicated medical comorbidities. Careful patient evaluation and selection should be performed for any peripheral arterial vascular procedure. The fundamental principle is to assess not only the surgical risk from the peripheral arterial system but also the global nature of the atherosclerotic process. Full cardiac evaluations are often necessary due to the high incidence of concomitant atherosclerotic coronary arteries disease, resulting in a high risk for ischemic events. Hertzer and associates reviewed coronary angiographies on 1000 patients undergoing elective vascular procedure and identified 25% of concomitant correctable coronary artery disease including 21% in patients undergoing elective peripheral vascular intervention.[10] Conte and associates analyzed their 20-year experience in 1642 open lower extremity reconstructive surgeries and concluded that patients requiring lower extremity reconstruction presented an increasingly complex medical and surgical challenge compared with the previous decade in a tertiary practice setting.[11] With aging of the population, the growing number of vascular patients who have prohibitive medical comorbidities that are deemed high risk for open surgical repair. Endovascular intervention provides an attractive alternative.

As for open surgical repair, the clinical indications for endovascular intervention of lower extremity peripheral arterial diseases include lifestyle limiting claudication, ischemic rest pain, and tissue loss or gangrene. Importantly, endovascular procedures should be performed by a competent vascular interventionist who understands the vascular disease process and is familiar with a variety of endovascular techniques. In addition, certain lesions may not be amendable to endovascular treatment or may be associated with poor outcomes, such as long segment occlusion, heavily calcified lesion, orifice lesion, or lesions that cannot be traversed by a guidewire. A proper selection of patients and techniques are critical in achieving good long-term outcome.

Endovascular intervention for lower extremity occlusive disease is continuously evolving. Success and patency rates of endovascular intervention are closely related to the anatomic and morphological characters of the treated lesions. The TASC work group made recommendations on the intervention strategies of lower extremity arterial diseases based on the morphological characters. Based on TASC guideline, endovascular treatment is recommended for type A lesions, open surgery is recommended for type D lesions, and no recommendations were made for types B and C lesions. However, with rapid advancement in endovascular technologies, there are increased numbers of lesions amendable to endovascular interventions.

There is less literature support on infrapopliteal endovascular intervention due to higher complication and lower success rates. The treatment is restricted for patients with limb-threatening ischemia who lack surgical alternatives. However, with further advancement of endovascular technology and the development of new devices, endovascular intervention becomes an integral part of treatment. By itself or combined with open technique, percutaneous intervention plays an important role in therapeutic options for lower extremity occlusive disease. As described by TASC guideline, four criteria should be measured to evaluate the clinical success of the treatment: improvement in walking distance, symptomatic improvement, quality of life, and overall graft patency. These criteria should all be carefully weighed and evaluated for each individual prior to endovascular therapy.

Endovascular techniques and treatment outcomes

A sterile field is required in either an operating room or an angiography suite with image capability. The most common and safest access site is CFA via either retrograde or antegrade approach. For diagnostic angiography, arterial access should be contralateral to the symptomatic sides. For therapeutic procedures, location of the lesion and the anatomic structures of the arterial tree determine the puncture site. To avoid puncture iliac artery or SFA, the femoral head is located under the fluoroscopy and used as the guide for the level of needle entry. In addition, there are several useful techniques in help-ing access a pulseless CFA including ultrasound-guided puncture, utilizing micropuncture kit, and targeting calcification in a calcified vessel. Antegrade approach may be challenging particularly in obese patients. Meticulous tech-nique is crucial in preventing complications and bony landmark can be used as guidance to ensure CFA puncture.

We frequently used retrograde approach for lower extremity intervention. Vascular access is achieved using a standard seldinger technique. Familiarity with different types of wires and catheters is a fundamental step in successful endovascular intervention. The most commonly used starter wires are 0.035 in. Benson or "J" wires (Boston Scientific, Natick, MA). After the wire is secured in the aorta, a selective catheter is often used to help manipulate the wire across the aortic bifurcation when contralateral CFA approach is used. A long flexible guiding sheath across aortic bifurcation is helpful in maintaining target vessel access, stabilizing the wire and catheter, and minimizing blood loss. How-ever, in order to track a guiding sheath across aortic bifurcation, an exchange wire with relative stiff body is often required, such as Amplatz, Stiff Glide wire (Boston Scientific, Natick, MA). Once guiding sheath is secured in place, a contrast angiography is performed by injecting the contrast media through the side port of the sheath to further delineate the location and characteristics of the lesion.

Traversing the lesion with a wire is the most critical part of the procedure. Typically, 0.035 in. guidewires are used for femoropopliteal lesions and 0.014 or 0.018 in. guidewires are used for infrapopliteal access. Hydrophilic-coated wires, such as Glide wires, are useful in navigating through tight stenosis or occlusion. An angled-tip wire with a torque device may be helpful in crossing an eccentric lesion and a shaped selective catheter, such as Berenstein catheter or Angle Glide catheter (Boston Scientific, Natick, MA), is frequently used to help manipulate the wire across the lesion. The soft and floppy end of the wire is carefully advanced crossing the lesion under fluoroscopy and gentle force is applied while manipulating the wire. Once the lesion is traversed, one needs to pay particular attention on the tip of the wire to ensure a secure wire access and avoid vessel wall perforation or dissection.

Once the access to the diseased vessel is secured and the wire has suc-cessfully traversed the lesion, several treatment modality can be utilized, which are either used alone or in conjuction with others, namely angioplasty, stent or stent-graft placement, and atherectomy. The available angioplasty techniques are balloon angioplasty, cryoplasty, subintimal angioplasty, and cutting balloon. The most commonly used atherectomy techniques include percutaneous atherectomy catheter and laser atherectomy device.

Systemic anticoagulation should be maintained routinely during lower extremity arterial interventions to minimize the risk of pericatheter thrombosis. Unfractionated heparin (UFH) is the most commonly used agent, given on a weight-based formula. We typically used 80–100 mg/kg initial bolus for thera-peutic procedure to achieve the activated clotting time (ACT) above 250 s upon the catheter insertion and subsequent 1000 units for each additional hour of the procedure. Newer agents, such as low-molecular weight heparin, platelet IIb/IIIa inhibitor, direct thrombin inhibitor, or recombinant hirudin, have been available and can be used either alone or in conjunction with heparin particularly in patients sensitive to UFH. After these procedures, all patients are placed on antiplatelet therapy, such as aspirin. Additional antiplatelet agents, such as clopedigrol (Plavix), are given to selected patients with stent placement for at least 6 weeks after lower extremity interventions unless otherwise contraindicated.

Percutaneous angioplasty

After the lesion is crossed with a wire, an appropriated balloon angioplasty catheter is selected and tracked along the wire to traverse the lesion. The length of the selected catheter should be slightly longer than the lesion and the diameter should be equal to the adjacent normal vessel. The balloon tends to be approximately 10–20% oversized. The radiopaque markers of the balloon catheter are placed so that they will straddle the lesion. Then, the balloon is inflated with saline and contrast mixture to allow visualization of the insufflation process under the fluoroscopy (Figure 12.1). The patient may experience mild pain that is not uncommon. However, severe pain can be indicative of vessel rupture, dissection, or other complications. An angiography is crucial in confirming the intraluminal location of the catheter and absence of contrast extravasation. The inflation is continued until the waist of the atherosclerotic lesion is disappeared and the balloon is at the full profile. Frequently, several

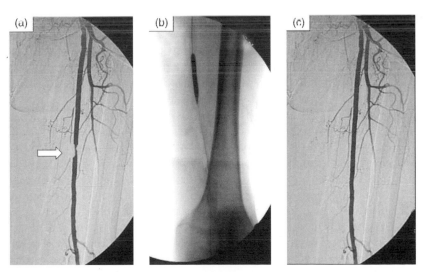

Figure 12.1 Balloon angioplaty of a focal superficial femoral artery. (a) Angiogram demonstrating a focal stenosis in the SFA (arrow). (b) This lesion was treated with balloon angioplasty. (c) Completion angiogram demonstrating satisfactory radiographic result.

inflations are required to achieve a full profile of the balloon. Occasionally, a lower profile balloon is needed to predilate the tight stenosis so that the selected balloon catheter can cross the lesion.

Besides length and diameter, the operators need to be familiar with several balloon characters. Noncompliant and low-compliant balloons tend to be inflated to their preset diameter and offer greater dilating force at the site of stenosis. Low-compliant balloons are the mainstay for peripheral intervention. A balloon with a low profile is used to minimize complication at the entry site and for crossing the tight lesions. Upon inflation, most balloons do not rewrap to their preinflation diameter and assume larger profile. Furthermore, trackability, pushability, and crossability of the balloon should be considered when choosing a particular type of balloon. Lastly, shoulder length is important characteristics when performing percutaneous angioplasty (PTA) to avoid injury to the adjacent arterial segments. After PTA, a completion angiogram is performed while the wire is still in place. Leaving the wire in place provides access for repeating the procedure if the result is unsatisfactory.

Percutaneous angioplasty is an established and effective therapy for select patients with lower extremity occlusive diseases. Studies have shown that PTA of femoropopliteal segment achieved over 90% technical success rate and 38–58% 5-year primary patency rate.[12-14] However, efficacy of PTA is highly dependent upon anatomic selection and patient condition.[5] PTA of lesions longer than 7–10 cm offer limited patency, while PTA of shorter lesions, such as less than 3 cm, have fairly good results. Lofberg and associates performed 127 femoropopliteal PTA procedures and reported primary 5-year success rate of 12% in limbs with occlusion longer than 5 cm versus 32% in limbs with occlusion less than 5 cm in length.[15] Initial technical success rates in occlusive lesions are worse than stenotic lesions. Concentric lesions respond better to PTA than eccentric lesions and heavy calcifications have a negative impact on success rates. A metaanalysis by Hunink and associates showed that adjusted 5-year primary patencies after angioplasty of femoropopliteal lesions varied from 12% to 68%, the best results being for patients with claudication and stenotic lesions.[16] Distal runoff is another powerful predictor of long-term success. Johnston analyzed 254 consecutive patients who underwent femoral and popliteal PTA and reported a 5-year patency rate of 53% for stenotic lesions and 36% for occlusive lesions in patients with good runoffs versus 5-year patency of 31% for stenotic lesions and 16% for occlusive lesions in patients with poor runoff.[12] Literature reviews showed that 5-year patency rates varied from 27% to 67% based on the runoff status.[16]

Due to limited success with infrapopliteal PTA, the indication for infrapopliteal artery PTA is stringent, reserved for limb salvage. Current patency rates from infrapopliteal PTA can be improved further by proper patient selection, ensuring straight-line flow to the foot in at least one tibial vessel, and close patient surveillance for early reintervention. Possible future advances including the use of drugeluting stents, cutting balloons, and atherectomy devices are being investigated to improve clinical outcomes following endovascular interventions on the tibial arteries. Varty and associates reported a 1-year limb salvage rate of 77% in patients with critical ischemia who underwent infrapopliteal PTA.[17] In patients with favorable anatomies, a 2-year limb salvage rate after infrapopliteal artery PTA is expected to exceed 80%.

Cryoplasty

Cryoplasty (CryoVascular Systems, Los Gatos, CA) is a new and promising approach in the treatment of PVD. It offers attractive advantages to endoluminal therapy. Although its profile and deployment process is similar to traditional angioplasty, cryoplasty has fundamental differences from angioplasty. First, the cryoplasty balloon is inflated with compressed liquid nitrous oxide (NO) instead of saline/contrast. Second, cryoplasty is designed to dilate and treat a disease vessel simultaneously by delivering cold thermal energy to vessel wall that potentially reduces the rate of restenosis (Figure 12.2). The balloon inflation is controlled by a battery-power inflation device provided by the manufacturer. The balloon surface temperature rapidly decreases to −2°C to −10°C upon decompression of liquid nitrous oxide, then allows it to return to body temperature. This process creates microfractures within the plaques that weakens the plaques and induces uniform dilation. The homogenous dilation subsequently leads to less dissection and less medial tearing. The cold thermal energy to the vessel wall created during insufflation process potentially reduces the magnitude of the inflammatory response associated

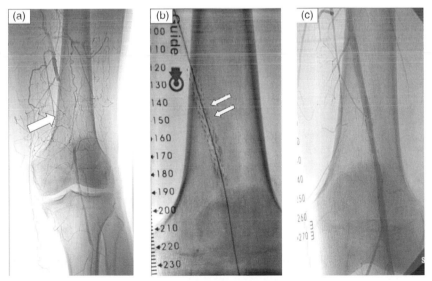

Figure 12.2 SFA occlusion. (a) Angiogram demonstrating a segmental occlusion in the distal SFA (single arrow). (b) This lesion was treated with cryoplasty that lowered the balloon catheter temperature to a temporary freezing state during the balloon angioplasty procedure (double arrows). (c) Completion angiogram demonstrated satisfactory result with no evidence of vessel dissection.

with balloon injury and induces apoptosis of smooth muscle cells. All of the abovementioned factors are known to contribute to the restenosis process, and each is favorably impacted by cryoplasty. *In vivo* studies have showed that cryoplasty-induced apoptosis in the injured lesion further reduced the rate of restenosis. Lastly, cryoplasty appears to alter the morphology of collagen and elastin fibers in a way that limits recoil without impairing the conduit function of the artery.

Several recent studies showed promising mid-term and short-term outcomes using cryoplasty for lower extremity atherosclerotic diseases. A pilot study by Fava and colleagues involving 15 patients with femoropopliteal diseases technically showed a success rate of 93% and a primary angiographic patency rate of 83.3% during 14 months of mean follow-up.[18] Their preliminary data was reconfirmed by Joye on treating 26 tibioperoneal lesions using cryoplasty, which showed a technical success rate of 95% and a 6-month limb salvage rate of 95%.[19] Another preliminary study, reported in the 14th Annual International Symposium on Endovascular Therapy, revealed promising outcomes with a restenosis rate of 20–30% in 1 year. However, further clinical trials are warranted to determine the efficacy of this technique. A multicenter, prospective registry using cryoplasty in patients with femoropopliteal lesions is ongoing and has completed enrollment in December 2002. Furthermore, a multicenter, prospective trial using cryoplasty for limb salvage has been initiated.[19] If proven successful, cryoplasty would address the shortfalls of angioplasty (dissection, elastic recoil, injury response) without leaving behind an implantable device such as a stent.

Cutting balloon angioplasty

Recently peripheral cutting balloon (Boston Scientific, Natick, MA) has become available and adds another viable angioplasty option to the endovascular armamentarium. The peripheral cutting balloon device features tiny, longitudinally mounted atherotomes (microsurgical blades) on the surface of an angioplasty balloon (Figure 12.3). As the balloon is expanded, the atherotomes scores the lesion, and thus changes the compliance of the diseased vessel that allows the balloon to dilate the vessel with less pressure and reduce the balloon trauma. Potentially, the cutting balloon prevents elastic recoil of the lesions and increases the precision of balloon deployment, which is particularly useful for recalcitrant restenotic lesions, bypass graft stenosis, or bifurcation lesions.

Cutting balloon angioplasty (CBA) was shown to be efficacious for complex lesions in the coronary literature. Long-term data on utilizing CBA for peripheral intervention are not yet available, while short-term and mid-term results are promising. Ansel and associates treated 93 infrapopliteal lesions in 73 patients who presented with limb-threatening ischemia and reported 89.5% of limb salvage rate during their mean 1-year follow-up.[20] A multiple center, prospective clinical trial on utilizing cutting balloon to treat stenotic or thrombosed hemodialysis graft has been initiated. The result from this trial can potentially impact the usage of cutting balloon in lower extremity intervention.

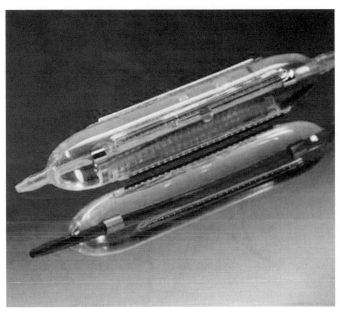

Figure 12.3 A cutting balloon catheter showing fine atherotomes embedded on the angioplasty balloon surface that potentially minimizes vessel trauma created by the balloon angioplasty procedure.

Subintimal angioplasty

The technique of subintimal angioplasty (SA) was first described in 1987 when successful establishment of flow was made by accidental creation of a subintimal channel during treatment of a long popliteal artery occlusion. Subintimal angioplasty is recommended for chronic occlusion, long segment of lesion, and heavily calcified lesions. In addition, this technique is applicable for vessels with diffuse diseases and for vessels that had previously failed intraluminal approach when it is difficult to negotiate the wire across the entire diseased segment without dissection. SA is also appropriate for flush occlusions when there is no "stump" for engaging a guidewire into the lumen.

The principle of this technique is to bypass the occlusion by deliberately creating a subintimal dissection plan commencing proximal to the lesion and continuing in the subintimal space before breaking back into the true lumen distal to the lesion. The occluded lumen is recanalized through the subintimal plan. SA can be performed through either ipsilateral antegrade or contralateral retrograde using the CFA approach. If selecting contralateral CFA puncture, a long guiding sheath is placed across the aortic bifurcation to provide access for the femoropopliteal and infrapopliteal vessels. The subintimal dissection is initiated at the origin of an occlusion by directing the tip of an angled guidewire, usually an angled hydrophilic wire, such as Glidewire. A supporting catheter is used to guide the tip of the guidewire away from the important collaterals. When the wire is advanced, a loop is naturally formed at the tip of the guidewire. Once the subintimal plan is entered, the wire tends to move freely in dissection space. Subintimal location of the wire and the catheter can be confirmed by injecting small amount of diluted contrast. At this point, the wire and the catheter are then advanced along the subintimal plan until the occlusion segment is passed. A loss of resistance is often encountered as the guidewire reenter the true lumen distal to the occlusion. Recanalization is confirmed by advancing the catheter over the guidewire beyond the point of reentry and obtaining an angiogram. This is followed by a balloon angioplasty. Occasionally, resistance may be encountered during wire advancement in the subintimal space. In such situations, a more stiff wire is helpful to overcome the resistance and better track the balloon catheter. However, a soft hydrophilic wire is preferred to complete the crossing and reenter the lumen of the distal artery. Once the entire lesion is crossed, an appropriate wire is placed in the subintimal plan through over-the-catheter exchange technique, following which a balloon catheter is exchanged over the wire for SA. It is important to pay special attention to the tip of the wire as maintaining the wire position is one of the most critical parts of the procedure. To confirm the patency, the completion angiogram is performed prior to withdrawing the catheter and wire. If flow is impaired, repeat balloon dilatation may be necessary. Frequently, a stent is required to maintain a patent lumen and treat residual stenosis if more than 30% luminal reduction is confirmed on completion angiogram.

Multiple studies have demonstrated the efficacy of SA. Bolia and his colleagues reported their extensive experiences on subintimal angioplasty for treating long segment occlusions of infrainguinal vessels.[21-23] They achieved a technical success rate of over 80% for both femoropopliteal and tibial arteries. One-year patency rates varied from 53% for infrapopliteal vessels to 71% for femoropopliteal segments. Limb salvage rates reached over 80% at 12 months. They also reported that the factors influencing patency are smoking, number of runoff vessels, and occlusion length. Studies by other groups showed similar results.[24,25] Treiman and colleagues treated 25 patients with 6–18 cm femoropopliteal occlusion and achieved a technical success rate of 92% and a 13-months primary patency rate of 92%,[25] while Lipsitz and associates reported a technical success rate of 87% in treating 39 patients and achieved a 12-months cumulative patency of 74%.[24] Additionally, Ingle and associates reported a technical success rate of 87% on 67 patients with femoropopliteal lesions and a 36-months limb salvage rate of 94%.[26] As demonstrated herein, although technical success rates are similar in most series, the patency rates vary widely in different studies. Patient selection, anatomic character, and lesion locations may account for the wide range of outcomes.

Endoluminal stent

Although suggested by Dotter during the late 1960s, the use of an endoluminal stent was not pursued until the limitations of PTA were widely recognized. There are several situations where stent placement is appealing. The primary

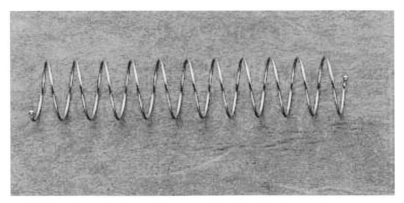

Figure 12.4 Intracoil stent that is an FDA approved stent for SFA placement.

indication is the potential salvage of an unacceptable angioplasty result. Stent placement is typically used when residual stenosis after PTA is 30% or greater. An endoluminal stent is also used for dissection, perforation, and other PTA complications. Primary stent placement has become a viable alternative for treating ulcerative lesions that may potentially be the source for embolization. Primary stent is also used to treat occlusive lesions that have a tendency of reocclusion and distal embolization after PTA. In addition, an endoluminal stent is potentially beneficial for early restenosis post-PTA. Drug-eluting stents are currently under investigation in the United States and may be promising in decreasing restenotic rates.

The balloon-expandable Palmaz® stent (Johnson & Johnson, Interventional Systems, Warren, NJ) and the self-expanding Wallstent® (Schneider Peripheral Division, Minneapolis, MN) are both approved by the Food and Drug Administration (FDA) for intraarterial usage, but only in the iliac arterial system. The IntraCoil® peripheral self-expanding stent (Sulzer Intra Therapeutic Inc., St. Paul, MN) has been approved by the FDA for femoropopliteal intervention (Figure 12.4). The IntraCoil stent is a coil-shaped stent mounted on the end of a delivery catheter. The catheter is tracked along the wire to the site of the lesion under fluoroscopy. Then, the deployment system is initiated. The coil releases and supports the lumen of the treated femoral and popliteal arteries.

Eventhough technical success rates are high, published series on femoropopliteal artery stents show that patency rates are comparable to PTA alone with primary patency rates varying from 18% to 72% at 3 years.[5,27] Gray and associates stented 58 limbs after suboptimal PTA for long SFA lesions and demonstrated 1-year primary patency rate of 22%.[28] However, Mewissen treated 137 limbs using self-expanding SMART nitinol stents in patients with TASC A, B, and C femoropopliteal lesions and reported 1-year primary patency of 76% and 24-month primary patency rate of 60%.[29] Patient selection and the anatomic character of the lesions may play important roles in the outcomes. Additionally, stent characteristics may contribute to the patency rate.

Several clinical studies have demonstrated the significant improvements of the new generation of nitinol stents for the SFA lesions: the German Multi-center Experience, the Mewissen trial, the BLASTER (Bilateral Lower Arterial Stenting Employing Reopro) Trial, and the SIROCCO trials.[30] The German Multicenter Experience was a retrospective review of 111 SFA stenting procedures and predicted that the 6-month patency rate for Smart stents was 82% versus 37% for the Wallstent. The BLASTER Trial evaluated the feasibility of utilizing nitinol stents with and without intravenous abciximab for the treatment of femoral artery disease and the preliminary results showed 1-year clinical patency rate of 83%.

Furthermore, drug-eluting stent, which showed effectively decreasing restenosis in coronary intervention, may offer another promising alternative in lower extremity diseases. The drug released over a period of time interferes with smooth muscle cell proliferation – the main cellular element and source of extracellular matrix – producing restenosis. The first clinical trial of a drug-eluting stent used Cordis Cypher SMART stents coated with sirolimus (SIROCCO trial).[31,32] The SIROCCO results showed binary in-lesion restenosis rates of 0% in the sirolimus-eluting group versus 23.5% in the noneluting group at 6-month follow-up angiography.

Stent graft

The concept of endobypass using stent graft in treating atherosclerotic SFA disease has been entertained. A stent graft is placed percutaneously across a long segment or multiple segments of lesions and is used to create a femoropopliteal bypass. Theoretically, endobypass has the potential of being as successful as surgical bypass graft by relining of the vessel wall in its anatomical position without the negative impact of anastomosis. Stent grafts can be divided into two categories: unsupported and fully supported. The unsupported grafts consist of segments of bypass graft, such as PTFE, with an expandable stent at one or both ends. The unsupported grafts are flexible with a low profile, but prone to external compression. The supported stent grafts consist of a metallic skeleton covered with graft fabric. The presence of a dense metal skeleton promotes an extensive inflammatory response and increases the risk of thrombosis. There is no FDA approved stent graft for peripheral intervention. However, Viabahn (WL Gore, CA) is the most commonly used device in the United States, which is composed of an ultrathin PTFE graft externally supported by self-expanding nitinol meshwork. The Viabahn device has a specific delivery mechanism by pulling back the attached string that results in proximal-to-distal delivery of the endoprosthesis.

Although it is an intriguing concept, data on endobypass results is limited and graft thrombosis rate is high. Additionally, covering major collateral vessels can potentially jeopardize the viability of the limb if stent-graft occlusion occurs. Bauermeister treated 35 patients with Hemobahn and reported 28.6% of occlusion rate on an average 7-month follow-up.[33]

Atherectomy

The basic principle of atherectomy is to remove the atheroma from obstructed arterial vessels. There are currently five atherectomy devices approved by the FDA: Simpson AtheroCath (DVI, Redwood City, CA), Transluminal Extraction Catheter (Interventional Technologies, San Diego, CA), Theratec recanalization arterial catheter (Trac-Wright), Auth Rotablator (Heart Technologies, Redmond, WA), and SilverHawk system (FoxHollow Technologies, Redwood City, CA). These devices either cut and remove or pulverize the atheroma plaques.

The Simpson AtheroCath has a directional cutting element that is exposed to one-third of the circumference of the arterial wall. The atheroma protruding into the window is excised and pushed into the collection chamber. The Transluminal Extraction Catheter has an over-the-wire nondirectional cutter mounted on the distal end of a torque tube. The excised atheroma is simultaneously removed by aspiration through the torque tube. The Theratec recanalization arterial catheter is a nondirectional, noncoaxial, atheroablative device. The rotating cam tip pulverizes the atheromatous lesion into minute particles. The Auth Rotablator is a nondirectional, coaxial, atheroablative device with a metal burr embedded with fine diamond chips. Lastly, the SilverHawk device, approved by FDA for peripheral use in 2003, is a monorail catheter designed to overcome the drawback of directional artherectomy catheter (Figure 12.5). The working end consists of a hinged housing unit containing a carbide cutting blade. The blade is activated from the motor drive unit and the catheter is then advanced through the length of the lesion. Once each pass is completed, the cutter then packs the tissue into the distal end of the nosecone to maximize collection capacity. The SilverHawk can then either be removed or torqued to treat a different quadrant in the same lesion or other lesions.

Despite the promising early technical and clinical success, the mid- and long-term results have been disappointing due to high incidence of restenosis.

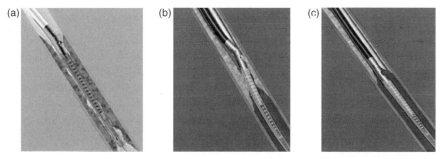

Figure 12.5 The SilverHawk arthrectomy device. (a) The arthrectomy device is first advanced through the artery to the site of the blockage. (b) Once the SilverHawk catheter is at the site of the blockage, a tiny rotating blade is activated that permits the catheter to shave plaque off the artery wall. (c) The plaque collects in the tip of the catheter and then is completely removed from the body.

For this reason, atherectomy devices have not been popularized. TALON registry designed to track outcomes after treatment with the SilverHawk System showed improved outcome recently. The registry provides both site-specific and aggregate data on the acute and long-term results of plaque excision in the femoral–popliteal and tibial–peroneal arteries. Excised plaque from each enrolled patient is collected to allow for histologic evaluation and genomic research. Results from TALON registry can potentially help elucid-ate whether this technique is a feasible alternative in treating lower extremity arterial disease.

Laser atherectomy and angioplasty

Since laser atherectomy was reported in the 1960s, a variety of innovative approaches have been developed trying to overcome the limitation of laser angioplasty. Recent developments in Excimer laser technology have led to increased optimism regarding the ability to safely deliver laser energy. Excimer laser atherectomy (LA) approved by FDA for peripheral artery intervention employs precision laser energy control (shallow tissue penetration) and safer wavelengths (ultraviolet as opposed to the infrared spectra in older laser technology), which decreases perforation and thermal injury to the treated vessels.

An Excimer laser atherectomy catheter, with diameters varying from 0.9 to 2.5 mm, is tracked over the guidewire to the desired target. Once activated, the Excimer laser utilizes ultraviolet energy to ablate the lesion and create a non-thrombogenic arterial lumen. This lumen is further dilated by an angioplasty balloon. Because the Excimer laser can potentially reduce the rate of distal embolization by evaporating the lesion, it may be used as an adjunct tool for ostial lesions and lesions that can be traversed by a wire but not an angioplasty balloon catheter.

Several studies regarding the use of Excimer laser atherectomy combined with balloon angioplasty on lower extremity occlusive disease have showed promising clinical outcomes.[34-36] Peripheral Excimer Laser Angioplasty (PELA) trials involves 318 patients with chronic SFA occlusion, and achieved a technical success rate of 83.2%, 1-year primary patency rate of 33.6%, and an assisted primary patency rate of 65%.[37] Steinkamp and his colleagues treated 127 patients with long-segment of popliteal artery occlusion using laser atherectomy followed by balloon angioplasty and reported a 3-year primary patency rate of 22%.[36] The clinical trial evaluating the use of Laser Angioplasty for Critical limb Ischemia (LACI) is ongoing in the United States, and the pilot study reported a 6-month primary patency rate of 33% and clinical improvement up to 89%.[38]

Common problems and complications

Angioplasty-related complications

Complications related to PTA vary widely including dissection, rupture, embolization, pseudoaneurysms, restenosis, hematoma, and acute occlusion secondary to thrombosis, vasospasm, or intimal injury.[39] Clark and associates analyzed the data from 205 patients in the SCVIR Transluminal Angioplasty and Revascularization (STAR) registry and reported a complication rate of 7.3% for patients undergoing femoropopliteal angioplasty.[40] Minor complications accounted for 75% of the cases including distal emboli (41.7%), puncture site hematomas (41.7%), contained vessel rupture (8.3%), and vagal reactions (8.3%). In another study, Axisa and colleagues reported an overall rate of significant complications for patients undergoing PTA of the lower extremities as 4.2% including retroperitoneal bleeding (0.2%), false aneurysm (0.2%), acute limb ischemia (1.5%), and vessel perforation (1.7%).[41]

Complications limiting the application of SA are parallel to those of PTA. A study investigating the use of SA in 65 patients with SFA occlusion found that complications developed in 15% of patients.[42] These complications included significant stenosis (44%), SFA rupture (6%), distal embolization (3%), retroperitoneal hemorrhage (1.5%), and pseudoaneurysm (1.5%). Additional complications reported consist of perforation, thrombosis, dissection, and extensions beyond the planned reentry site.[43] Importantly, damage to significant collateral vessels may occur in 1–1.5% of patients who underwent SA. If a successful channel is not achieved in this situation, the patient may have a compromised distal circulation that necessitates distal bypass.

Cryoplasty is a modified form of angioplasty and long term results on lower extremity intervention are not yet available. Fava and associates treated 15 patients with femoropopliteal disease and had a 13% complication rate involving guidewire dissection and PTA-induced dissection of a tandem lesion remote to the cryoplasty zone.[18]

Endoluminal stent and stent-graft related complications

In addition to the aforementioned complications as with angioplasty, endoluminal stent is associated with the risk of stent fraction and deformity. The adductor canal has nonlaminar flow dynamics, especially with walking. The forces exerted on the SFA include torsion, compression, extension, and flexion. These forces exert significant stress on the SFA and stents. In addition, the lower extremity is subject to external trauma, which further increases the risk of stent deformity and fracture (Figure 12.6). SIROCCO study showed that stent fracture, although not associated with clinical symptoms, occurs in 18.2% of the procedures involving both drug-eluting stents and control stents.[32]

Stent grafts may present additional complication of covering important collaterals that results in compromise distal circulation. A prospective study evaluating hemobahn stent grafts in the treatment of femoropopliteal arterial occlusions demonstrated a 23% immediate complication rate including distal embolization (7.7%), groin hematoma (13.5%), and arteriovenous fistula (1.9%).[44]

Atherectomy-related complications

Overall complication rates associated with atherectomy range from 15.4% to 42.8%, including spasm, thrombosis, dissection, perforation, distal emboli,

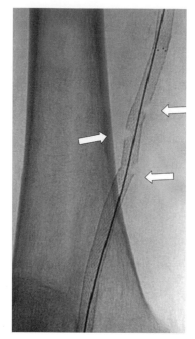

Figure 12.6 Stent fracture is a known complication due in part to the constant external force exerted on the stent and the artery.

no reflow, and hematoma.[45-47] Jahnke and associates conducted a prospective study evaluating high-speed rotational atherectomy in 15 patients with infrapopliteal occlusive disease. They yielded a 94% technical success rate, but was complicated by vessel rupture (5%), distal embolization (5%), and arterial spasm (5%).[48] Although the excimer laser atherectomy reduces embolic events by evaporating the lesion, embolization still remain a problematic complication. Studies show that distal embolic events occur in 3–4% of procedures,[49] and perforation in 2.2–4.3% of cases.[50,51] Other complications compromising laser atherectomy therapy include acute reocclusion, vasospasm, direct vessel injury, and dissection.

References

1 McDaniel MD, Cronenwett JL. Basic data related to the natural history of intermittent claudication. *Ann Vasc Surg* 1989; **3**:273–77.

2 Leng GC, Papacosta O, Whincup P, *et al*. Femoral atherosclerosis in an older British population: prevalence and risk factors. *Atherosclerosis* 2000; **152**:167–74.

3 Schroll M, Munck O. Estimation of peripheral arteriosclerotic disease by ankle blood pressure measurements in a population study of 60-year-old men and women. *J Chronic Dis* 1981; **34**:261–69.

4 Stoffers HE, Rinkens PE, Kester AD, *et al*. The prevalence of asymptomatic and unrecognized peripheral arterial occlusive disease. *Int J Epidemiol* 1996; **25**:282–90.

5 Dormandy JA, Rutherford RB. Management of peripheral arterial disease (PAD). TASC Working Group. TransAtlantic Inter-Society Concensus (TASC). *J Vasc Surg* 2000; **31**:S1–S296.

6 Rutherford RB. Standards for evaluating results of interventional therapy for peripheral vascular disease. *Circulation* 1991; **83**:I6–11.

7 Ouriel K. Peripheral arterial disease. *Lancet* 2001; **358**:1257–64.

8 Koelemay MJ, den Hartog D, Prins MH, *et al.* Diagnosis of arterial disease of the lower extremities with duplex ultrasonography. *Br J Surg* 1996; **83**:404–9.

9 Eiberg JP, Hansen MA, Jensen F, *et al.* Ultrasound contrast-agent improves imaging of lower limb occlusive disease. *Eur J Vasc Endovasc Surg* 2003; **25**:23–28.

10 Hertzer NR, Beven EG, Young JR, *et al.* Coronary artery disease in peripheral vascular patients. A classification of 1000 coronary angiograms and results of surgical management. *Ann Surg* 1984; **199**:223–33.

11 Conte MS, Belkin M, Upchurch GR, *et al.* Impact of increasing comorbidity on infrainguinal reconstruction: a 20-year perspective. *Ann Surg* 2001; **233**:445–52.

12 Johnston KW. Femoral and popliteal arteries: reanalysis of results of balloon angioplasty. *Radiology* 1992; **183**:767–71.

13 Gallino A, Mahler F, Probst P, Nachbur B. Percutaneous transluminal angioplasty of the arteries of the lower limbs: a 5 year follow-up. *Circulation* 1984; **70**:619–23.

14 Hunink MG, Donaldson MC, Meyerovitz MF, *et al.* Risks and benefits of femoropopliteal percutaneous balloon angioplasty. *J Vasc Surg* 1993; **17**:183–92; discussion 192–94.

15 Lofberg AM, Karacagil S, Ljungman C, *et al.* Percutaneous transluminal angioplasty of the femoropopliteal arteries in limbs with chronic critical lower limb ischemia. *J Vasc Surg* 2001; **34**:114–21.

16 Hunink MG, Wong JB, Donaldson MC, *et al.* Patency results of percutaneous and surgical revascularization for femoropopliteal arterial disease. *Med Decis Making* 1994; **14**:71–81.

17 Varty K, Bolia A, Naylor AR, *et al.* Infrapopliteal percutaneous transluminal angioplasty: a safe and successful procedure. *Eur J Vasc Endovasc Surg* 1995; **9**:341–45.

18 Fava M, Loyola S, Polydorou A, *et al.* Cryoplasty for femoropopliteal arterial disease: late angiographic results of initial human experience. *J Vasc Interv Radiol* 2004; **15**:1239–43.

19 Joye JD. An overview of cryoplasty. *Endovascular Today* 2004; **54**–56.

20 Ansel GM, Sample NS, Botti IC, Jr., *et al.* Cutting balloon angioplasty of the popliteal and infrapopliteal vessels for symptomatic limb ischemia. *Catheter Cardiovasc Interv* 2004; **61**:1–4.

21 Bolia A, Bell PR. Femoropopliteal and crural artery recanalization using subintimal angioplasty. *Semin Vasc Surg* 1995; **8**:253–64.

22 London NJ, Srinivasan R, Naylor AR, *et al.* Subintimal angioplasty of femoropopliteal artery occlusions: the long-term results. *Eur J Vasc Surg* 1994; **8**:148–55.

23 Nydahl S, Hartshorne T, Bell PR, *et al.* Subintimal angioplasty of infrapopliteal occlusions in critically ischaemic limbs. *Eur J Vasc Endovasc Surg* 1997; **14**:212–16.

24 Lipsitz EC, Ohki T, Veith FJ, *et al.* Does subintimal angioplasty have a role in the treatment of severe lower extremity ischemia? *J Vasc Surg* 2003; **37**:386–91.

25 Treiman GS, Whiting JH, Treiman RL, *et al.* Treatment of limb-threatening ischemia with percutaneous intentional extraluminal recanalization: a preliminary evaluation. *J Vasc Surg* 2003; **38**:29–35.

26 Ingle H, Nasim A, Bolia A, *et al.* Subintimal angioplasty of isolated infragenicular vessels in lower limb ischemia: long-term results. *J Endovasc Ther* 2002; **9**:411–16.

27 Becquemin JP, Favre JP, Marzelle J, *et al*. Systematic versus selective stent placement after superficial femoral artery balloon angioplasty: a multicenter prospective randomized study. *J Vasc Surg* 2003; **37**:487–94.

28 Gray BH, Sullivan TM, Childs MB, *et al*. High incidence of restenosis/reocclusion of stents in the percutaneous treatment of long-segment superficial femoral artery disease after suboptimal angioplasty. *J Vasc Surg* 1997; **25**:74–83.

29 Mewissen MW. Self-expanding nitinol stents in the femoropopliteal segment: technique and mid-term results. *Tech Vasc Interv Radiol* 2004; **7**:2–5.

30 Laird JR. Interventional options in SFA. *Endovascular Today* 2004; 9–12.

31 Duda SH, Poerner TC, Wiesinger B, *et al*. Drug-eluting stents: potential applications for peripheral arterial occlusive disease. *J Vasc Interv Radiol* 2003; **14**:291–301.

32 Duda SH, Pusich B, Richter G, *et al*. Sirolimus-eluting stents for the treatment of obstructive superficial femoral artery disease: six-month results. *Circulation* 2002; **106**:1505–9.

33 Bauermeister G. Endovascular stent-grafting in the treatment of superficial femoral artery occlusive disease. *J Endovasc Ther* 2001; **8**:315–20.

34 Gray BH, Laird JR, Ansel GM, Shuck JW. Complex endovascular treatment for critical limb ischemia in poor surgical candidates: a pilot study. *J Endovasc Ther* 2002; **9**:599–604.

35 Schneider PA, Caps MT, Ogawa DY, Hayman ES. Intraoperative superficial femoral artery balloon angioplasty and popliteal to distal bypass graft: an option for combined open and endovascular treatment of diabetic gangrene. *J Vasc Surg* 2001; **33**:955–62.

36 Steinkamp HJ, Rademaker J, Wissgott C, *et al*. Percutaneous transluminal laser angioplasty versus balloon dilation for treatment of popliteal artery occlusions. *J Endovasc Ther* 2002; **9**:882–88.

37 Scheinert D, Laird JR, Jr., Schroder M, *et al*. Excimer laser-assisted recanalization of long, chronic superficial femoral artery occlusions. *J Endovasc Ther* 2001; **8**:156–66.

38 Gray BH, Laird JR, Ansel GM, Shuck JW. Complex endovascular treatment for critical limb ischemia in poor surgical candidates: a pilot study. *J Endovasc Ther* 2002; **9**:599–604.

39 Silva MB, Jr., Hobson RW, 2nd, Jamil Z, *et al*. A program of operative angioplasty: endovascular intervention and the vascular surgeon. *J Vasc Surg* 1996; **24**:963–71; discussion 971–73.

40 Clark TW, Groffsky JL, Soulen MC. Predictors of long-term patency after femoropopliteal angioplasty: results from the STAR registry. *J Vasc Interv Radiol* 2001; **12**:923–33.

41 Axisa B, Fishwick G, Bolia A, *et al*. Complications following peripheral angioplasty. *Ann R Coll Surg Engl* 2002; **84**:39–42.

42 Yilmaz S, Sindel T, Yegin A, Luleci E. Subintimal angioplasty of long superficial femoral artery occlusions. *J Vasc Interv Radiol* 2003; **14**:997–1010.

43 Desgranges P, Boufi M, Lapeyre M, *et al*. Subintimal angioplasty: feasible and durable. *Eur J Vasc Endovasc Surg* 2004; **28**:138–41.

44 Jahnke T, Andresen R, Muller-Hulsbeck S, *et al*. Hemobahn stent-grafts for treatment of femoropopliteal arterial obstructions: midterm results of a prospective trial. *J Vasc Interv Radiol* 2003; **14**:41–51.

45 Grubnic S, Heenan SD, Buckenham TM, Belli AM. Evaluation of the pullback atherectomy catheter in the treatment of lower limb vascular disease. *Cardiovasc Intervent Radiol* 1996; **19**:152–59.

46 Henry M, Amor M, Ethevenot G, *et al*. Percutaneous peripheral atherectomy using the rotablator: a single-center experience. *J Endovasc Surg* 1995; **2**:51–66.

47 Savader SJ, Venbrux AC, Mitchell SE, *et al*. Percutaneous transluminal atherectomy of the superficial femoral and popliteal arteries: long-term results in 48 patients. *Cardiovasc Intervent Radiol* 1994; **17**:312–18.

48 Jahnke T, Link J, Muller-Hulsbeck S, *et al.* Treatment of infrapopliteal occlusive disease by high-speed rotational atherectomy: initial and mid-term results. *J Vasc Interv Radiol* 2001; **12**:221–26.

49 Scheinert D, Laird JR, Jr., Schroder M, *et al.* Excimer laser-assisted recanalization of long, chronic superficial femoral artery occlusions. *J Endovasc Ther* 2001; **8**:156–66.

50 Steinkamp HJ, Werk M, Haufe M, Felix R. Laser angioplasty of peripheral arteries after unsuccessful recanalization of the superficial femoral artery. *Int J Cardiovasc Intervent* 2000; **3**:153–60.

51 Steinkamp HJ, Wissgott C, Rademaker J, *et al.* Short (1–10 cm) superficial femoral artery occlusions: results of treatment with excimer laser angioplasty. *Cardiovasc Intervent Radiol* 2002; **25**:388–96.

CHAPTER 13

Arteriovenous graft interventions

Joseph J. Naoum, Wei Zhou, Eric Peden

The prevalence of renal failure has increased and more autogenous and prosthetic graft placements and revisions are necessary to obtain access for hemodialysis. The population with renal failure undergoing hemodialysis is older and has comorbidities such as hypertension and diabetes. A hemodialysis access that remains patent and free of infection is critical to ensure adequate treatment for those with end-stage renal disease. Unfortunately, graft failures contribute to multiple hospital admissions, invasive studies and interventions, and add to the overall morbidity associated with hemodialysis. In up to 20% of all dialysis, patient admissions are related to access site problems and the most common complication leading to failure of vascular access site is thrombosis. Ballard and colleagues found that 18% of the total surgical caseload was related to the treatment of dialysis access complications in a 4-year single institution review of angioaccess procedures.[1] Thus, a large portion of the cost of hemodialysis treatment goes to providing, preserving, and maintaining permanent vascular access, which requires a reported 0.41 to 2.5 access interventions per dialysis year.[2,3]

The type and management of hemodialysis access greatly influences the long-term care and quality of life of patients undergoing treatment. Multiple factors are involved in arteriovenous (AV) access thrombosis and failure. These factors include adequacy of the patient's arteries and veins, actual access site and anatomic configuration, intrinsic coagulation state, systemic blood pressure, cardiac output, comorbidites, and choice of prosthetic material if used.[3] The Kidney Disease Outcomes Quality Initiative (K/DOQI) guidelines for vascular access recommend primary placement of native or autogenous hemodialysis fistulas in preference to polytetrafluoroethylene (PTFE) or Dacron grafts because the former has fewer complications and longer durability.[4,5] However, the secondary patency rates tend to be higher as a result of multiple revisions in attempts to maximize the life of each individual access. In a cohort of 1574 prosthetic AV access out of 2247 newly placed accesses, there was a 41% greater risk of failure than with autogenous AV access and a 91% higher chance of needing revision. PTFE grafts had a 2-year primary patency rate of 24.6% (versus 39.8% for autogenous AV access, $p < 0.001$) and equivalent secondary patency rates (64.3% versus 59.5%).[6]

Thrombosis of autogenous AV access is most often due to a stenosis within 2 to 3 cm from the arteriovenous anastomosis in 64% of radiocephalic fistulas and

24% of brachiobasilic fistulas.[2,3] Stenosis at the cephalic arch of brachiocephalic fistulas occurs in 30 to 55 % of dysfunctional AV access.[2,7] Thrombosis of prosthetic AV grafts is most often due to venous anastomotic outflow stricture at or near the venous anastomosis in 75–93% of cases.[7,8] The K/DOQI also recommends early detection and treatment of stenosis within a poorly functioning hemodialysis access to extend its lifespan. To prolong graft life and decrease the frequency of interventions, graft surveillance within dialysis units may be performed. Measurements of venous resistance, defined by various clinical and hemodialysis recirculation parameters, can lead to recognition of a problem before thrombosis occurs making correction easier and more expedient for the patient and physician. Clinical screening methods include loss of a palpable graft thrill, pulsatility of the graft, increased venous pressures during hemodialysis, reduced dialysis flow rates, and prolonged needle site bleeding. In a retrospective study of a single dialysis unit graft surveillance policy by Roberts and associates, patients in whom early intervention was undertaken had a better graft survival (15.8 versus 6.3 months, $p < 0.01$) than patients who were treated after prosthetic AV graft thrombosis had occurred.[9] However, in a study by Lumsden and associates, all patients in a single dialysis unit were surveyed with duplex ultrasound and those with a stenosis >50% within the graft were randomized to percutaneous transluminal angioplasty (PTA) treatment or observation.[10] There were no significant differences in 6 and 12-month patency rates between the two groups. They concluded that a policy of duplex ultrasound graft surveillance is expensive and does not lead to improved patency.

The high cost of hospitalization and treatment of dysfunctional or thrombosed AV access requires effective and less invasive outpatient procedures. The advent of improved endovascular techniques for the treatment of AV access has been associated with a low morbidity. These procedures are rapid, safe, effective, and allow dialysis to be performed immediately after the procedure.

Endovascular treatment strategies

Percutaneous techniques have become commonplace in the management of thrombosed AV access. These endovascular maneuvers need to be applied in grafts that have formerly functioned. Contraindications to endovascular treatment include coagulopathy, infection, existing contraindication to the use of iodinated contrast or thrombolysis, and the need for urgent dialysis.

Diagnostic angiography

The patient is placed on a radiolucent operating table. There should be unimpeded fluoroscopy from the distal limb to the junction of the superior vena cava and the right atrium; thus, permitting evaluation of both the venous outflow tract and arterial inflow. The entire limb is prepped into the surgical field.

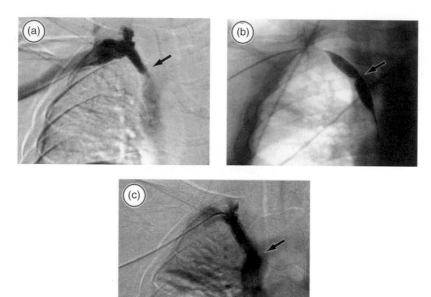

Figure 13.1 Venogram of a patient with a thrombosis dialysis access, who had a history of subclavian vein dialysis catheter placement. (a) A subclavian vein stenosis (arrow) is likely the result of previous dialysis catheter insertion. (b) This lesion can be successfully treated with balloon angioplasty. (c) Completion venogram demonstrates good radiographic results.

The procedure is commonly performed under local anesthesia with lidocaine and supplemental intravenous sedation as needed.

The venous outflow tract is examined first. A venogram must be performed to document patency of the runoff veins or collateral channels before thrombectomy commences. A Berenstein catheter (Angiodynamics, Inc., Queensbury, NY) is advanced over a guidewire past the venous anastomosis and the central veins including the superior vena cava are evaluated. Stenosis is a common occurrence along the outflow tract of hemodialysis accesses, especially if internal jugular or subclavian dialysis catheters have been previously inserted. If a stenosis is identified, it must be treated first (Figure 13.1). If a central stenosis does not respond to treatment, efforts to restore flow through the access will likely be futile.

After establishing adequate patency of the venous outflow tract, the graft is addressed. The elements of a complete study include first examining the venous outflow anastomosis, followed by the access in its entire length, and the arterial inflow last. This is usually achieved by introducing two sheaths, one directed toward the venous outflow and a second toward the arterial inflow. Several strategies exist for thrombectomy and treatment of clotted or dysfunctional hemodialysis access. Digital substraction, road mapping, and image sequencing functions are helpful, but not necessary.

Stenoses greater than 50% that hinder dialysis or threaten patency are considered significant. The presence of upstream collateral branches is a hint that a stenosis is present and should stimulate a more detailed search. When there is no obvious stenosis on the angiogram despite clinical abnormalities, complex angled views may be necessary and pullback pressure measurements from the superior vena cava to the arterial anastomosis may be needed.

Pharmacological thrombolysis and thromboembolization

In 1985, Zeit and Cope first described the use of thrombolytic agents in thrombosed prosthetic AV access.[11] Twenty-six patients were treated 33 times with a streptokinase dilution introduced into the graft via multiple needle puncture sites. A functioning shunt was obtained in 73%, though surgical correction of a stenosis or pseudoaneurysm was necessary in 30%. Subsequently, pulse-spray thrombolysis was introduced in 1989 with urokinase (Abbott Laboratories, Abbott Park, IL).[12]

In a study that included 29 thrombosed dialysis AV grafts, infusion catheters were inserted by crossing catheters, one directed towards the arterial anastomosis and the other directed toward the venous anastomosis, which ensured that the entire graft was treated.[12] A starting bolus of 250,000 U of urokinase was used, mixed with heparin; additional dosing was performed on a need-be basis for residual clot. This technique of thrombolysis would reveal venous stenoses that were then dilated and the arterial plug was macerated with a balloon catheter. In these patients, a 100% technical success rate was achieved. Flow was restored in 19 min and time for total lysis was 49 min. Roberts and colleagues performed a larger review of the pulse-spray technique in 1993.[9] He reviewed 209 thrombosed grafts treated with crossing catheters and found 99% to be patent and functioning at the conclusion of the procedure. The average procedural duration was 40 min. Thus, this treatment option was felt to be safe, expeditious, and effective.

Cynamon later popularized the "lyse and wait" technique in 1997.[13] The graft was instilled with lytic agent initially 250,000 U urokinase through sheaths that could tolerate high flow rates (500+ ml/min) so that the patient could undergo immediate hemodialysis without waiting for puncture site hemostasis, and the patient waited in the interventional preoperative area. Thus, the angiography suite was available for use while allowing time for lysis. Overall, with the "lyse and wait" technique, operator, room, and fluoroscopy times are all greatly reduced.

Pharmacological declotting has been studied with both urokinase, and after this lytic agent was removed from the market, with of recombinant tissue plasminogen activator.[13–15] Many, who use tissue plasminogen activator for peripheral thrombolysis, have noticed its propensity for creating bleeding complications.[14,15] In a review of graft declotting in 20 patients treated with tissue plasminogen activator (tPA) compared to 20 historic controls treated with urokinase, Vogel and associates reported a mean total procedure time of 74 min after the administration of 250,000 U urokinase and 103 min after the administration of 4 mg tPA.[15] To perform this technique, a 5000 U heparin and lytic agent mixture was prepared and instilled into the graft via an 22-gauge needle or if necessary a 5-Fr micropuncture introducer system (Cook, Bloomington, IN) with an assistant compressing both the arterial and venous outflow over 2 min. The graft angiogram, via the existing access, was performed only when an interventional suite became available between other cases. A venous angioplasty was performed at the discretion of the operator, the arterial plug was removed with a 5-Fr Fogarty catheter (Baxter, Santa Ana, CA), and any residual thrombus was mobilized or fragmented with balloon maneuvers. Technical and clinical success, as defined by the ability to undergo hemodialysis, was achieved in 95% of cases.[15]

Poulain and associates demonstrated that using 20-gauge needles for antegrade and retrograde graft puncture followed by infusion of thrombolytics for a period of 2 h and aspiration of the thrombus through an 8-Fr catheter, a hemodialysis access could be routinely declotted successfully.[16] Trerotola and colleagues popularized a technique without using urokinase in which the venous anastomosis of the graft is first dilated after administering systemic heparin only.[17] A Fogarty catheter is inflated within the graft and pushed toward the venous outflow in order to the clear the clot from the graft. Then, a Fogarty balloon is advanced through the arterial anastomosis, inflated, and pulled back to remove the arterial plug and once again flushed through the venous outflow into the lungs. Proponents of this technique argue that the pulmonary emboli are of small volume and do not cause significant hemodynamic changes. However, the long-term sequela and potential development of pulmonary hypertension still needs to be elucidated.

These techniques were the standard for treatment of thrombosed PTFE grafts, until the advent and widespread use of mechanical thrombectomy devices in more recent years.

Percutaneous mechanical thrombectomy

There are some general principles for treating patients with thrombosed prosthetic AV access. The age of the thrombus is of particular importance, as acute, fresh (<3 day old) thrombus is much more successfully removed than chronic, organized, fibrosed clot. However, adjunctive thrombolytic agent may facilitate removal. There is no data to support the addition of thrombolytics to percutaneous mechanical thrombectomy (PMT); nonetheless, intuitively this combined approach makes sense. Also, as the device is extended past the graft into the native vessels, damage to wall on contact may occur.

The AngioJet® rheolytic catheter (Possis Medical, Inc., Minneapolis, MN) is a mechanical thrombectomy system that fits through a 6-Fr sheath and over a 0.035 in. guidewire. The theoretical principle of this device is based on the Venturi effect and performs a hydrodynamic thrombectomy (Figure 13.2). Rapidly flowing multiple saline jets (8000 psi) are directed backward from

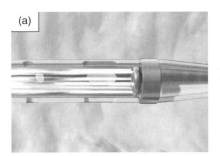
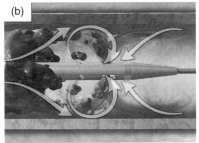

Figure 13.2 The AngioJet thrombectomy catheter uses a hydrodynamic principles to remove thrombus. (a) Multiple high saline jets are emitted backward from the tip of the catheter to create a suctioning force. (b) This creates a Venturi's effect, which draws thrombus into the jet stream and is evacuated out of the catheter.

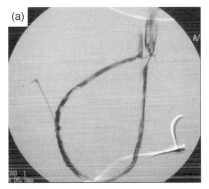
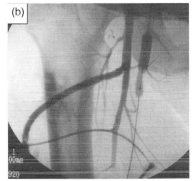

Figure 13.3 A thrombosed AV graft is treated with the AngioJet catheter. (a) Venogram demonstrates significant amount of thrombus. (b) Following the AngioJet thrombectomy, the completion venogram demonstrates a patent dialysis AV graft.

the tip of the device, rather than outward to the vessel wall, which reduces intimal injury. The thrombus is drawn into the vacuum created by these rapidly flowing jets and then out of the catheter to a collection bag (Figure 13.3). The remaining arterial plug is removed at the end of graft declotting with a standard Fogarty embolectomy catheter and treated with the device. In a prospective, randomized trial comparing surgical thrombectomy with AngioJet thrombectomy in thrombosed hemodialysis grafts, 153 patients were studied with follow-up to 6 months.[14] There was no difference between the groups in their ability to undergo hemodialysis treatment, nor was there any difference in the primary patency rates. However, the surgical group did have more major complications, primarily wound related. Another similar study noted the clinical benefit of AngioJet thrombectomy in thrombosed dialysis access when compared to open thrombectomy.[18] The Oasis Thrombectomy System (Boston Scientific, Quincy, MA) works on the same principle. However, instead of having multiple jets, it creates a single high-velocity jet stream. The power of the venturi effect is less than the AngioJet device but appears adequate for most uses.[19]

The Arrow-Trerotola™device (Arrow International, Reading, PA) is basically an over-the-wire rotating fragmentation basket, which macerates the clot that is then removed via an aspiration port. The remaining arterial plug is removed at the conclusion of graft declotting with a standard Fogarty embolectomy catheter. Rocek and associates evaluated this type of "mechanical thrombolysis" in a preliminary report of only 7 patients.[20] The procedures took an average of 126 min, there were no major complications, and the primary patency at 6-months was 60%. The authors concluded that this technique was rapid and effective, however, they tested it in autogenous native fistula, which most likely accounts for the above average primary patency rate. Additionally, Lazarro and colleagues studied a much larger group (50 patients) prospectively out to 3 months after using the Arrow-Trerotola catheter solely (they also removed the arterial plug with this device) in thrombosed grafts.[21] These authors used historical controls for comparison in which the Fogarty catheter portion of the procedure was performed. They demonstrated no differences in either technical success or 3-month patency rates; thus showing that the additional catheter maneuver was not necessary for sufficient functioning of this device.

The Amplatz Thrombectomy Device (ATD; Microvena Corp., White Bear Lake, MN) is a gas-powered impeller enclosed within a cage at the end of a 6- or 8-Fr catheter that rotates and creates a vortex that fragments clot into small pieces. The liquefied clot can then be aspirated or embolized. Sofocleous and associates evaluated the Amplatz thrombectomy device and compared it to pulse-spray thrombolysis.[22] In 126 episodes of graft occlusion in 79 patients, the patients were divided almost equally between the two treatment modalities. Though the technical success rates were similar, the Amplatz device was associated with a significantly higher local complication rate. This fact, along with the technical difficulties the authors cite in using the 8-Fr device led to conclusions limiting its use.

AKónya Eliminator™ (Idev Technologies, Inc., Houston, TX) is a nonmotor driven mechanical thrombectomy device intended for the declotting of synthetic dialysis grafts. The wire thrombectomy basket can be manipulated to accommodate various dialysis graft sizes up to 8 mm. Axial and rotational movements provide the mechanism of action for thrombus maceration and allow the liquefied clot to be aspirated or embolized.

The advantages of these devices over local thrombolysis are a more rapid establishment of a patent lumen, only a single catheterization session, fewer laboratory tests for monitoring the fibrinolytic effect, and decreased chance of remote bleeding. In addition, with the use of fluoroscopic guidance and the ability to perform immediate arteriography, percutaneous correction of the underlying lesion, which causes the thrombosis, is possible.

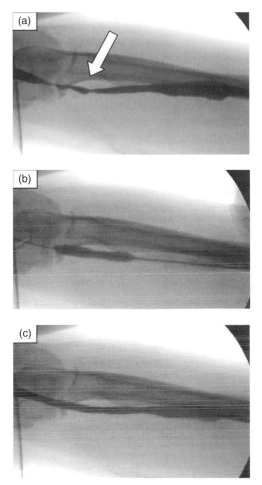

Figure 13.4 A thrombosed AV graft caused by venous anastomotic stenosis. (a) A high-grade stenosis is seen at the venous anastomotic site (arrow). (b) A high-pressure balloon angioplasty catheter is used to treat this stenosis. (c) Completion venogram demonstrates a satisfactory radiographic result.

Balloon angioplasty

Percutaneous transluminal angioplasty (PTA) of venous outflow tract and especially the venous anastomosis relies on stretching the characteristic tough and rubbery neointimal hyperplastic lesion. Considerable resistance to dilatation may exist and with focal lesions a persistent luminal narrowing will be visible under fluoroscopy with the balloon inflated. High-pressure balloons should be available to treat lesions that resist conventional balloon angioplasty (Figure 13.4). Ross and associates have reported their experience of over 100 successful cases in which a Conquest angioplasty balloon (Bard Peripheral,

Tempe, AZ) with a bursting pressure of 30 atm in the treatment of severe venous stenosis.[23] In a report by Trerotola and associates, seven of 87 PTA procedures with conventional high-pressure angioplasty were unsuccessful requiring aggressive balloon inflation over 30 atm to achieve 100% technical success.[24] Balloon inflation should last between 45 s and 5 min and can be repeated. A final procedure fistulogram is essential because it usually allows enough delay to reveal venous elastic recoil that can occur even shortly after an apparent successful angioplasty and can result in failure to restore proper access function. Lesions in which a localized area of waist narrowing is identified and successfully treated, usually respond well without elastic recoil. Lesions prone to failure after PTA are usually long and >2 cm. Extreme care must be exercised when dilating a recently operated segment. Fibrosis around the anastomosis is yet not complete, offering little resistance to rupture, hematoma, or pseudoaneurysm formation.

Stenting

Stainless steel alloy balloon-expanded stents are deployed by a coaxial balloon and fixed to the access or vessel wall by friction and subsequent endothelialization. External or mechanical forces that exert compression may render the stent susceptible to deformation and a decrease in the luminal diameter. A recent development in stent technology has been the manufacture of nitinol stents made with an alloy composed of nickel and titanium. These stents self-expand to their nominal diameter when deployed.[25] The equilibrium between the elastic recoil of the access or vessel and the radial expansion force of the stent determines the luminal diameter of the stent.[25] Self-expanding stents are capable of recovering their original shape or diameter once an applied external force is removed.

Stent placement is probably indicated in patients in whom multiple endovascular and surgical procedures have failed, are high risk, or a lesion is identified in a surgically inaccessible location. Persistent recoil following PTA can be treated by stenting (Figure 13.5). Acute dilatation induced rupture or access site aneurysmal formation can be alternatively treated successfully by placing a PTFE covered stent.[7]

Contraindications to stent placement include infection or inability to dilate and treat a lesion with a high-pressure angioplasty balloon catheter. Also stents should not be deployed if it jeopardizes important venous collaterals or is in an area where it will be punctured through for hemodialysis.

Results from clinical series

Central venous stenoses

Haage and associates analyzed the effectiveness of Wallstent (Boston Scientific, Natick, MA) placement for the treatment of brachiocephalic and subclavian venous obstruction in 50 patients with shunt dysfunction.[26] Stent deployment

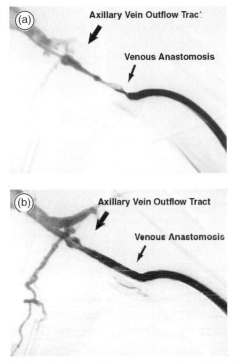

Figure 13.5 A high-grade stenosis at the axillary venous anastomosis treated with stent placement. (a) A thrombosed AV graft caused by a high-grade venous anastomotic lesion near the axillary vein (arrow). (b) The venous stenosis was successfully treated with stenting.

was successful in all patients with 26% necessitating additional stent placement. Primary patentcy rates at 3, 6, 12, and 24 months were 92%, 84%, 56%, and 28% respectively. Cumulative overall patency was 97% after 12 months and 81% after 24 months. Verstandig and colleagues treated 10 patients with shunt thrombosis, dysfunction, or arm swelling associated with brachiocephalic or subclavian stenosis or occlusion using Wallstents.[27] Stent deployment was successful in all cases. A second stent was required in 70% of cases. Primary patency rates at 6, 12, and 24 months were 66%, 25%, and 0%. Secondary patency rates at 6, 12, and 24 months were 100%, 75%, and 57%.

Stent placement in the central veins of patients on hemodialysis results in symptomatic relief and preservation of access. However, repeat interventions are required to maintain patency.

Native arteriovenous fistulas

Rajan and associates reviewed their treatment experience with balloon angioplasty of 94 radiocephalic and 57 brachiocephalic dysfunctional, native or autogenous hemodialysis fistulas.[2] Radiocephalic primary patency rates at 3, 6, and 12 months were 85%, 75%, and 62% respectively. Secondary patency rates for the same time intervals were 91%, 88%, and 86%, respectively. Brachiocephalic primary patency rates at 3, 6, and 12 months were 73%, 51%, and 39%. The difference in primary patency rates between the two types of fistula following angioplasty were significant ($p = 0.004$); however, secondary patency rates were essentially the same. Location of the lesions did not affect primary or secondary patency rates, and no factors were found to influence secondary patency in this study.

In a cohort study of 53 dysfunctional no-thrombosed native hemodialysis radiocephalic, brachiocephalic, or brachiobasilic fistulas, Clark and associates reported a primary patency rate at 6 and 12 months of 55% and 26%, respectively.[3] Secondary patency rates were both 82% at 6 and 12 months.[3] They identified several prognostic factors of restenosis. Lesions >2 cm in length were five times more likely to have loss of patency than those <2 cm. The risk of patency loss also doubled if at least one comorbid factor such as diabetes, coronary artery disease, or peripheral vascular disease was present.

PTA can achieve high secondary patency rates in dysfunctional native arteriovenous fistulas and safely prolong their use for hemodialysis.

Synthetic arteriovenous grafts

Fifty-nine patients who were randomized to endovascular therapy by Marston and associates had graft function restored.[28] Eighty-two percent underwent mechanical thrombectomy and 18% pharmacological thrombectomy all followed by percutaneous angioplasty. Primary patency rates at 6 and 12 month were 11% and 9%, respectively. Dougherty and associates treated 39 patients over a 4-year period with pharmacological thrombectomy followed by angioplasty in 92% of cases.[8] The primary patency rate at 12 months was $13.7\% \pm 6.6\%$ and an assisted 12-month primary patency rate of $21.4\% \pm 7.7\%$. The median time for graft rethrombosis was 6 months, similar to a retrospective review showing a patency rate following angioplasty of 5.5 months, but with a shorter procedure time and length of hospital stay.[29]

Percutaneous stenting represents an attempt to improve the preservation of hemodialysis grafts. In cases of inadequate angioplasty, stents can be placed to treat thrombosed prosthetic dialysis grafts. Kolakowski and associates described the use of stents, following failure of angioplasty described as a >30% residual stenosis in 23 forearm grafts and 38 upper arm grafts.[30] Cumulative primary patency rates at 3, 6, and 12 months were 36.4%, 15.6%, and 0% for forearm grafts, which were inferior to the 59.5%, 34%, and 17% rates observed for upper arm grafts ($p = 0.03$). Secondary patency rates were 40.9%, 40.9%, and 30.7%, respectively for forearm grafts, and 64.9%, 42.3%, and 19.7% for upper arm grafts ($p = $ ns). The authors concluded that sustained patency was better for upper arm grafts than for forearm grafts.

Quinn and associates reported their findings of using 25 self-expanding stents in 19 patients with AV graft dysfunction, and they reported a technical success rate of 90%.[31] Primary patency rate at 2 years was 25% with a secondary patency of 34%. Vorwerk demonstrated grafts with stents placed to have a 76% patency at 3 months dropping to 31% at 1 year.[32] With repeat interventions, the patency rates improved to 86% at 1 year. Zaleski and associates reviewed the success of metallic Wallstents in the treatment of intragraft stenoses in patients with synthetic hemodialysis grafts, who had experienced multiple episodes of graft thrombosis, had very limited vascular access for hemodialysis, and were considered poor surgical candidates.[33] Primary patency rates were 36% at 6 months and 12% at 12 months. Secondary patency rates were 91% at 6 months and 71% at 12 months. The authors concluded that metallic stent deployment can salvage synthetic AV grafts by alleviating intragraft stenoses.

A prospective, randomized trial that included 16 centers and 190 patients, compared the use of Fluency (Bard Peripheral Vascular, Tempe, AZ) covered stents to angioplasty for the treatment of ≤7 cm stenosis in failing synthetic grafts. Ninety-seven patients received the covered-stent graft and 93 patients underwent PTA alone. Venographic assessments were done up to 6 months. The anatomic success rate defined as a <30% residual stenosis was 94% for stent grafting and 73% for PTA ($p < 0.001$). The primary patency rates at 6 months were 48.5% for the covered-stent grafts and 32% for PTA ($p = 0.009$). The investigators concluded that PTFE covered-stent grafts were safe and provided a 6-month patency rate superior to PTA in the treatment of AV access venous anastomotic strictures.

Overall, stenoses in vascular grafts tend to recur and contribute to the difficulty in maintaining a functioning graft. Furthermore, repeated needle punctures during hemodialysis treatments may render the graft's inner surface nonhomogeneous and perhaps more prone to thrombosis and failure. However, percutaneous thrombectomy and balloon angioplasty demonstrates the ability to extend graft function.

Complications

The overall complication rate of dialysis graft thrombectomy and intervention is reported to be between 0 and 35%.[1,34] In a retrospective review of 579 thrombosed hemodialysis grafts, 48 complications occurred.[22] Sofocleous and associates found an overall technical success rate of 81%. Primary and secondary patency rate at 6 months were 36% and 67%, respectively.[22] The authors concluded that the majority of complications occurring during percutaneous thrombolysis or thrombectomy of thrombosed grafts can be treated at the same sitting, allowing the same access to be used for hemodialysis.

Graft rupture during thrombectomy or PTA is identified as contrast extravasation from the site (Figure 13.6). Several techniques are available to deal with this problem and include digital compression, prolonged inflation of an angioplasty balloon to approximately 4 atm to achieve tamponade, or deployment of a bare metal or covered stent. Pseudoaneurysms limit available puncture sites, and predispose patients to infection and rupture. Pseudoaneurysm formation associated with introducer sheath access site can be

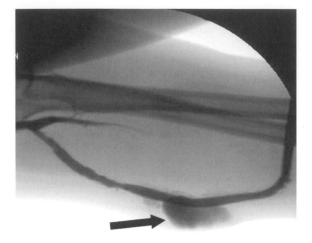

Figure 13.6 Rupture of an AV graft can occur as a complication of balloon angioplasty, which is evidenced by the contrast extravasation at the site of intervention (arrow).

avoided by cutting down to the dialysis graft and primarily closing the defect with a 5-0 or 6-0 prolene. Pseudoaneurysms can be treated by exclusion with a covered self-expandable stent. Complications associated with stent placement include thrombosis, access site rupture, stent migration, stent fragmentation, obstruction of important venous outflows, and misplacement.

Bleeding from previous hemodialysis puncture sites following thrombectomy and restoration of blood flow and hematoma formation at the procedure-catheter entry sites can be easily controlled with gentle focal pressure, hemostatic pledgets, or skin suturing without involving the access itself. Skin infection at procedure entry points can compromise the function and availability of the graft. Careful attention to sterile technique is important.

Care must be taken when approaching the arterial anastomosis. Arterial embolization can result from clot fragmentation or dislodgement of the arterial plug, and intimal dissection can be observed due to wire or thrombectomy device vessel damage.

Even in the face of complications inherent to any interventional technique, graft patency can be successfully managed and prolonged immediately during endovascular interventions.

Conclusions

Frequent hospital admissions are necessary for thrombectomy or graft revisions. The endovascular approach for graft thrombectomy and revision is minimally invasive, allows remote lesions to be addressed within the outflow tract, and visualizes the entire graft. Percutaneous management of dysfunctional or thrombosed, autogenous or synthetic dialysis fistulas can successfully and safely extend the functional lifespan of dialysis access and preserve valuable veins for future use.

References

1 Ballard JL, Bunt TJ, Malone JM. Major complications of angioaccess surgery. *Am J Surg* 1992; **164**:229–32.

2 Rajan DK, Bunston S, Misra S, Pinto R, Lok CE. Dysfunctional autogenous hemodialysis fistulas: outcomes after angioplasty – are there clinical predictors of patency? *Radiology* 2004; **232**:508–15.

3 Clark TW, Hirsch DA, Jindal KJ, Veugelers PJ, LeBlanc J. Outcome and prognostic factors of restenosis after percutaneous treatment of native hemodialysis fistulas. *J Vasc Interv Radiol* 2002; **13**:51–59.

4 Eknoyan G, Levin NW, Eschbach JW, *et al*. Continuous quality improvement: DOQI becomes K/DOQI and is updated. National Kidney Foundation's Dialysis Outcomes Quality Initiative. *Am J Kidney Dis* 2001; **37**:179–194.

5 Eknoyan G, Levin N. NKF-K/DOQI Clinical Practice Guidelines: Update 2000. Foreword. *Am J Kidney Dis* 2001; **37**:S5–6.

6 Gibson KD, Gillen DL, Caps MT, Kohler TR, Sherrard DJ, Stehman-Breen CO. Vascular access survival and incidence of revisions: a comparison of prosthetic grafts, simple autogenous fistulas, and venous transposition fistulas from the United States Renal Data System Dialysis Morbidity and Mortality Study. *J Vasc Surg* 2001; **34**:694–700.

7 Turmel-Rodrigues L, Pengloan J, Baudin S, *et al*. Treatment of stenosis and thrombosis in haemodialysis fistulas and grafts by interventional radiology. *Nephrol Dial Transplant* 2000; **15**:2029–36.

8 Dougherty MJ, Calligaro KD, Schindler N, Raviola CA, Ntoso A. Endovascular versus surgical treatment for thrombosed hemodialysis grafts: a prospective, randomized study. *J Vasc Surg* 1999; **30**:1016–23.

9 Roberts AC, Valji K, Bookstein JJ, Hye RJ. Pulse spray pharmacomechanical thrombolysis for treatment of thrombosed dialysis access grafts. *Am J Surg* 1993; **166**:221–5; discussion 225–26.

10 Lumsden AB, MacDonald MJ, Kikeri D, Cotsonis GA, Harker LA, Martin LG. Cost efficacy of duplex surveillance and prophylactic angioplasty of arteriovenous ePTFE grafts. *Ann Vasc Surg* 1998; **12**:138–42.

11 Zeit RM, Cope C. Failed hemodialysis shunts. One year of experience with aggressive treatment. *Radiology* 1985; **154**:353–56.

12 Bookstein JJ, Fellmeth B, Roberts A, Valji K, Davis G, Machado T. Pulsed-spray pharmacomechanical thrombolysis: preliminary clinical results. *AJR Am J Roentgenol* 1989; **152**:1097–100.

13 Cynamon J, Lakritz PS, Wahl SI, Bakal CW, Sprayregen S. Hemodialysis graft declotting: description of the "lyse and wait" technique. *J Vasc Interv Radiol* 1997; **8**:825–29.

14 Duszak R, Jr., Sacks D. Dialysis graft declotting with very low dose urokinase: is it feasible to use "less and wait?" *J Vasc Interv Radiol* 1999; **10**:123–28.

15 Vogel PM, Bansal V, Marshall MW. Thrombosed hemodialysis grafts: lyse and wait with tissue plasminogen activator or urokinase compared to mechanical thrombolysis with the Arrow-Trerotola percutaneous thrombolytic device. *J Vasc Interv Radiol* 2001; **12**:1157–65.

16 Poulain F, Raynaud A, Bourquelot P, Knight C, Rovani X, Gaux JC. Local thrombolysis and thromboaspiration in the treatment of acutely thrombosed arteriovenous hemodialysis fistulas. *Cardiovasc Intervent Radiol* 1991; **14**:98–101.

17 Trerotola SO, Lund GB, Scheel PJ, Jr., Savader SJ, Venbrux AC, Osterman FA, Jr. Thrombosed dialysis access grafts: percutaneous mechanical declotting without urokinase. *Radiology* 1994; **191**:721–26.

18 Bush RL, Lin PH, Lumsden AB. Management of thrombosed dialysis access: thrombectomy versus thrombolysis. *Semin Vasc Surg* 2004; **17**:32–39.

19 Lee MS, Singh V, Wilentz JR, Makkar RR. AngioJet thrombectomy. *J Invasive Cardiol* 2004; **16**:587–91.

20 Rocek M, Peregrin JH, Lasovickova J, Krajickova D, Slaviokova M. Mechanical thrombolysis of thrombosed hemodialysis native fistulas with use of the Arrow-Trerotola percutaneous thrombolytic device: our preliminary experience. *J Vasc Interv Radiol* 2000; **11**:1153–58.

21 Lazzaro CR, Trerotola SO, Shah H, Namyslowski J, Moresco K, Patel N. Modified use of the arrow-trerotola percutaneous thrombolytic device for the treatment of thrombosed hemodialysis access grafts. *J Vasc Interv Radiol* 1999; **10**:1025–31.

22 Sofocleous CT, Cooper SG, Schur I, Patel RI, Iqbal A, Walker S. Retrospective comparison of the Amplatz thrombectomy device with modified pulse-spray pharmacomechanical thrombolysis in the treatment of thrombosed hemodialysis access grafts. *Radiology* 1999; **213**:561–67.

23 Ross JR. Ultra high-pressure PTA for hemodialysis. *Endovasc Today* 2003; **3**:1–4.

24 Trerotola SO, Stavropoulos SW, Shlansky-Goldberg R, Tuite CM, Kobrin S, Rudnick MR. Hemodialysis-related venous stenosis: treatment with ultrahigh-pressure angioplasty balloons. *Radiology* 2004; **231**:259–62.

25 Leung DA, Spinosa DJ, Hagspiel KD, Angle JF, Matsumoto AH. Selection of stents for treating iliac arterial occlusive disease. *J Vasc Interv Radiol* 2003; **14**:137–52.

26 Haage P, Vorwerk D, Piroth W, Schuermann K, Guenther RW. Treatment of hemodialysis-related central venous stenosis or occlusion: results of primary Wallstent placement and follow-up in 50 patients. *Radiology* 1999; **212**:175–80.

27 Verstandig AG, Bloom AI, Sasson T, Haviv YS, Rubinger D. Shortening and migration of Wallstents after stenting of central venous stenoses in hemodialysis patients. *Cardiovasc Intervent Radiol* 2003; **26**:58–64.

28 Marston WA, Criado E, Jaques PF, Mauro MA, Burnham SJ, Keagy BA. Prospective randomized comparison of surgical versus endovascular management of thrombosed dialysis access grafts. *J Vasc Surg* 1997; **26**:373–80; discussion 380–81.

29 McCutcheon B, Weatherford D, Maxwell G, Hamann MS, Stiles A. A preliminary investigation of balloon angioplasty versus surgical treatment of thrombosed dialysis access grafts. *Am Surg* 2003; **69**:663–67; discussion 668.

30 Kolakowski S, Jr., Dougherty MJ, Calligaro KD. Salvaging prosthetic dialysis fistulas with stents: forearm versus upper arm grafts. *J Vasc Surg* 2003; **38**:719–23.

31 Quinn SF, Schuman ES, Hall L, *et al.* Venous stenoses in patients who undergo hemodialysis: treatment with self-expandable endovascular stents. *Radiology* 1992; **183**:499–504.

32 Vorwerk D, Guenther RW, Schurmann K. Stent placement on fresh venous thrombosis. *Cardiovasc Intervent Radiol* 1997; **20**:359–63.

33 Zaleski GX, Funaki B, Rosenblum J, Theoharis J, Leef J. Metallic stents deployed in synthetic arteriovenous hemodialysis grafts. *AJR Am J Roentgenol* 2001; **176**:1515–19.

34 Silas AM, Bettmann MA. Utility of covered stents for revision of aging failing synthetic hemodialysis grafts: a report of three cases. *Cardiovasc Intervent Radiol* 2003; **26**:550–53.

CHAPTER 14

Venous insufficiency and varicose veins

Panagiotis Kougias, Patrick E. Duffy, E. John Harris, Jr

Varicose veins consist of tortuous superficial veins with incompetent valves, and represent a point in the continuum of changes that occur in the lower extremities of patients suffering from chronic venous insufficiency. Varicosities are most often associated with incompetence of the greater saphenous vein (GSV). The entire GSV from the saphenofemoral junction (SFJ) to the ankle may be involved or there may be segments with isolated incompetence, often associated with incompetent perforating veins. There may also be duplicated saphenous veins and one or both trunks may be incompetent. The disease is particularly prevalent in western societies and is associated with a substantial social and financial impact.[1-3] Recurrent (or persistent) varicose veins are a significant problem, occurring in 20–40% of patients who have had varicose vein surgery.[4] Clinical examination alone is not sufficient to document recurrence of varicose veins after intervention. Duplex ultrasonography is able to characterize the presence and type of recurrent varicose veins.[5] Surveillance following interventions for primary venous insufficiency should use objective criteria and must be extended beyond short-term follow-up as the risk for recurrence increases with time.

Various surgical and endovascular approaches have been devised to correct the underlying pathophysiologic derangements that lead to varicosities, all of which are related to various degrees of recurrence and patient discomfort. These include traditional surgical and more recently introduced endovenous techniques, for which an overview is provided in this chapter.

Diagnosis and preoperative evaluation

A thorough history of the patient is of paramount importance. Pain, easy fatigability, heaviness, recurrent superficial thrombophlebitis, and bleeding from skin erosion as well as cosmetic issues are common complaints among patients with varicose veins that constitute indications for intervention. The need for a detailed physical examination cannot be overemphasized. This can reveal varicosities, or the presence of more advanced associated lesion of chronic venous insufficiency, such as lower extremity edema, pigmentation, lipodermatosclerosis or other skin changes, and healed or active ulceration.

A continuous wave handheld Doppler is a necessary adjunct that can document the presence of reflux at the bedside, and is the only test needed in patients with telangiectasias or those who are elderly or too sick to undergo operative intervention. This test has essentially replaced more traditional clinical tests such as the Trendelenburg's or Perthe's tests.

Patients with symptomatic varicose veins should have further evaluation with duplex imaging. All three anatomic venous components of the lower extremity – superficial, deep, and perforators – can be assessed by duplex, which provides information on vein patency, wall characteristics, valve morphology, and competence, as well as qualitative information on the presence of reflux and obstruction. For quantitative information on reflux and obstruction, plethysmography can be used, and is particularly useful when both reflux and obstruction are elicited on duplex studies, in which case it helps to identify the predominant pathophysiologic component.

The introduction of duplex imaging has revolutionized our understanding and management of venous insufficiency. Prior to the widespread use of duplex, the diagnosis of venous reflux was mainly clinical, and the treatment was that of a "blind stripping" of the clinically enlarged varicosities. Improper preoperative diagnosis and absent intraoperative imaging were associated with high recurrence rates that plagued the treatment of varicose veins for several years. In many instances, GSV is not the primary culprit responsible for the venous reflux condition. Anterolateral tributary veins, posteromedial tributary veins, or even small groin veins, such as epigastric veins, can be the source.[6] If a surgeon identifies the correct vein prior to treatment, be it surgical stripping or endovenous ablation, the immediate recurrence rate is extremely low. Recurrences, in contemporary series, come from neovascularization and/or progression of disease; not from improper diagnosis and treatment. It should be emphasized that ultrasound technicians are often unfamiliar with superficial venous anatomy and its many variations. The treating physician must therefore be self-sufficient with regard to handling an ultrasound probe and recognizing the nuances of venous anatomy.

Finally, venography is needed when complex reconstruction procedures are planned in patients with obstruction (ascending venography is appropriate by injecting contrast in a dorsal foot vein) or incompetence (descending venography is indicated with contrast injection into the external iliac via a contralateral approach) of the deep venous system.

Overview of surgical treatment for varicose veins

General considerations

Standard indications for intervention include cosmesis, itching, pain, leg heaviness and fatigue, external bleeding, and superficial thrombophlebitis. In addition, surgery is indicated when varicose veins are part of more extensive venous disease as manifested by ankle hyperpigmentation, lipodermatosclerosis, atrophic leg changes, and venous ulcer.[7] Unfortunately, physician perception regarding availability and efficacy of treatment of varices may deny the patient the precise care sought.[8] Small telangiectasias may be as symptomatic as larger varicosities, mainly because of pressure on somatic nerves by the dilated veins. Approximately 50% of patients with telangiectasias will have symptoms, and 85% will be relieved of them by appropriate therapy.[9] General objectives of treatment should be ablation of the hydrostatic forces of axial reflux and removal of the hydrodynamic forces of perforator vein reflux. The selection of the most appropriate procedure is then individualized.

Great saphenous vein ablation

Surgical or endovascular ablation of the GSV is indicated when incompetence at the SFJ is present. Surgical ablation in the form of stripping has been considered the "gold standard" against which the less invasive newly introduced endovenous ablation techniques are now compared.[10,11] Stripping below the knee is usually avoided because the calf perforators are not directly connected to the saphenous vein at that level. It is also associated with a higher incidence of saphenous nerve injury. The below-knee saphenous segment can be stripped if it is grossly dilated. For incompetence at the SFJ, simple GSV ligation has been performed in an effort to preserve the vein for subsequent arterial bypass. However, this procedure does not address the underlying pathophysiologic derangements and does not treat reflux.[12]

External GSV wrapping

This technique is an alternative recommended, when preservation of the GSV conduit for use in a future arterial reconstruction procedure is essential, as is the case, for instance, in diabetics and heavy smokers with anticipated severe peripheral vascular or coronary disease. The procedure is indicated for such a patient who on the preoperative evaluation demonstrates mobile cusps of the terminal and subterminal valve of GSV or lesser saphenous vein, a vessel diameter less than 12 mm, and has mild to moderate GSV incompetence. In addition, vessel size greater than 5 mm is desirable since valve incompetence in a smaller vessel usually indicates a primary valve defect as cause of the reflux, less likely to respond favorably to external wrapping.[13] With careful patient selection this technique has results that compare favorably to those of stripping,[14] although more long-term follow-up is needed before definitive conclusions are made.

Endovenous treatments for varicose veins

Sclerotherapy
General considerations
The aim of injection sclerotherapy is to introduce a small volume of sclerosant in a vein, empty of blood, and then appose the vein walls by firm compression. High-quality foam can be produced with two disposable syringes and a three-way tap using the detergent agent sodium tetradecyl sulfate (STS) or

pilodocanol in the method described by Tessari and associates.[15] Repeated pulling and release of the pistons will mix the chemical agent with sterile air producing compact foam with very small bubble diameter. Other methods that involve the same principle of mixing sclerosing agent with air have also been described and include the use of osmotic solutions such as hypertonic saline or the use of chemical irritants such as chromated glycerine.[16]

Knowing the physics of sclerosing foam injection is important in understanding the pathophysiology of sclerosis. The foam is made of very small bubbles of gas covered by liquid with high surface tension. The quantity of sclerosing drug in any given volume of foam is related to the size of bubbles: with little bubbles, the foam will be highly active because of high agent concentration; large bubbles form poorly active foam. Sclerosis with foam is an active dynamic process since the interaction of foam with endothelium forms links with cell membranes. The higher the concentration of drug in the foam, the greater the number of links that would occur between the sclerosing foam and endothelium. Large bubbles of foam, even if it seems to last more *in vitro*, has a weaker effect because there is less sclerosing drug available for this linkage. Endothelial cells demonstrate similar biologic response to sclerosing agent injection irrespective of vein size and there are reports of saphenous veins 6–10 mm in diameter that have been successfully treated with low-concentration foam of purified STS.[16]

After injection the foam adheres to the inner venous wall and with proper maneuvers it is possible to be advanced in collaterals and close to veins of the deep system. When the size of the bubble is sufficiently small, no (or poor) mixing with blood occurs in the vein immediately after the injection; this results in a closer relationship between the injected dose and the final result. The durability of the foam is related to bubble size, the tensio-activity of the liquid solution, and the conditions in which the foam is generated and kept. The foam is visible under ultrasound, and the air it contains explains this property. This is an important consideration when performing duplex-guided sclerotherapy, because it gives an enhanced view of the process, facilitates the identification of the injected flow, and allows injection of the foam in a safer way near the SFJ or sapheno–popliteal junction, or within the collaterals under direct visualization. A substantial contraction can take place during foam injection and can significantly alter the vein diameter. Dramatic changes from 15 to 3 mm have been reported.[16] Finally, creation of the foam results in a net reduction of sclerosing drug doses and 0.4–0.5 ml of liquid solution can be transformed into 2–2.5 ml of foam. Higher amounts of foam can be produced from the same quantity of liquid according to the volume of air used, but the optimal dilution varies depending on the method used for foam production. For instance, with the Tessari method it has been reported to be 1 : 4 to 1 : 5.[16]

Principles of surgical treatment

The principal indication for sclerotherapy has been symptom relief and improved cosmesis in patients with telangiectasias, reticular veins, and venulactases. Sclerotherapy is an adequate treatment for nonsaphenous local varicose veins, varicose tributaries of the saphenous trunk without saphenous insufficiency, postoperative residual veins, and recurrent varicosities.[17] In addition, sclerotherapy had been utilized as a temporary palliative treatment in older patients with SFJ reflux who are too sick to undergo definitive treatment and present with an emergency such as bleeding from the varicosities.

More recently, ultrasound guidance and improved foam quality have expanded the traditional indications of sclerotherapy to include treatment of an incompetent saphenous trunk. It was originally thought that a diameter of less than 8 mm at the SFJ was a requirement for successful treatment.[18] Very recently, however, it was shown that ultrasound-guided foam sclerotherapy can be appropriate even if the diameter of the GSF at the SFJ is greater than 20 mm in size.[19] This is a relatively new indication and further long-term follow-up data are necessary before it can be widely recommended.

Technique

No universally accepted sclerotherapy technique exists. The French school advocates a proximal to distal technique. Others, treat the largest vein first in order to eliminate pressure transmission to smaller vessels, and this may imply a distal-to-proximal sequence if a perforator is the source of the venous hypertension. Effort should be made that the sclerosant stays within the vein that needs to be treated. The veins need to be kept empty of blood during and after the injection. The most dilute solution that can accomplish the desirable effect needs to be used, with the use of only small amounts of sclerosant agent at a give site, generally no more than 0.5 1 ml per site to minimize the risk of complications.[20] Simple telangiectasias require even smaller volumes. The length of postoperative compression also varies depending on the vein size, and may be only 1 day for small varicosities or 1–2 weeks for large clusters of varicose veins. Rapid ambulation is important as it decreases the concentration of the sclerosant and therefore diminishes its effect on the deep venous system.

Outcomes

Complications of sclerotherapy are infrequent. Anaphylaxis occurs in less than 0.3% of patients and may be fatal. A small test dose is therefore recommended prior to initiating full treatment. Minor allergic reactions can also occur up to 48 h after the injection. Ulceration may follow extravascular injection that manifests as blanching of the skin immediately after the injection due to intense vasoconstriction. Immediate treatment options include injecting the skin with normal saline or local anesthetic, or rubbing the skin surface with nitrate. In a number of cases, an ulcer will ultimately form, that is painful and heals slowly over 6–8 weeks. Arterial injection is a rather serious complication that necessitates hospital admission and the immediate administration of heparin. The posterior tibial artery at the ankle appears to be the most frequently involved artery. Brown pigmentation due to hemosiderin deposition occurs in 1–30% of cases, but usually resolves without further treatment. Superficial thrombophlebitis may occur due to inadequate compression. The risk of deep venous thrombosis is minimized if the patient ambulates promptly. Finally, nerve damage may occur due to close injection or a bandage that has been placed very tight.

Frullini and colleagues reported their 3 year experience in treating 453 patients with foam sclerotherapy using two different techniques for foam production and stated that their average success rate was 88.1–93.3% depending on technique for a follow-up period from 20–180 days.[16] The authors treated small telangiectasias as well as medium to large varicosities. Side effects they encountered included malaise, phlebitis, transient visual disturbance, deep venous thrombosis, lymphedema, pigmentation, and skin necrosis. Overall incidence of complications was approximately 8%. Barret and associates reported a 100% clinical success rate after STS injection for incompetent GSV for diameters even greater than 20 mm.[21] After a 2-year follow-up they noticed a recurrence rate of 4% and 6% for patients with initial GSV greater than or smaller than 10 mm respectively. The authors describe a detailed treatment protocol that includes sclerosing foam generation from STS with the Tessari method at a 1 : 3 STS to air ratio. They also used polidocanol for small visible varicosities. Ambulation was mandatory immediately after the procedure. All the patients were placed in 30–40 mm Hg graduated compression stockings for at least 2 weeks and were advised to avoid strenuous physical activity for at least 3 weeks to minimize valsava maneuvers that may contribute to recanalization.

Radiofrequency ablation
General considerations

Although high ligation and stripping of the GSV has been well accepted by most vascular surgeons, the postoperative morbidity, mostly pain and bruising, and recommended activity limitations are less than ideal from a patient's perspective and leave ample room for improvement. In this high-tech era, where less invasive techniques are perceived as more desirable, new or revisited therapies for minimally invasive obliteration of the GSV have attracted attention. It is in this context that the VNUS Closure® catheter (VNUS Medical Technologies, Inc., Sunnyvale, CA) was developed to control saphenous vein reflux with minimal patient discomfort and early return to full activity. In fact, controlled collagen denaturation of incompetent superficial veins to ablate or reduce venous luminal diameter is not a new idea.[22,23] However, the use of radiofrequency-resistive heating of the vein wall, controlled by vein-wall temperature and impedance feedback, is a novel idea. A concept central in the radiofrequency-induced venous ablation is that of thermal damage to collagen. Skin can withstand temperature rises for very short exposure times and the response appears to be logarithmic as the exposure times become shorter. For instance, an increase in body temperature to 60°C will produce cell destruction if the exposure is longer than 10 s. Tissues, however, can withstand temperatures up to 70°C if the duration of the exposure is maintained less than 1 s. Tissue injuries from brief exposure to temperatures less than 50°C

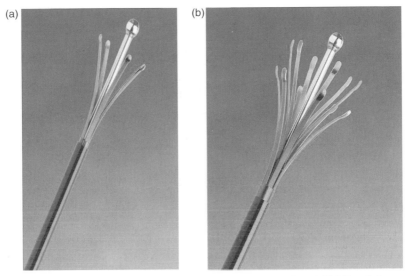

Figure 14.1 The VNUS Closure catheter. Close-up view of the (a) 6 Fr and (b) 8 Fr radiofrequency catheter system.

would be expected to be reversible. Typically, the temperature used during radiofrequency ablation (RFA) reaches 85°C.

Technique

The VNUS radiofrequency catheter was first introduced in Europe in 1998, and received Australian and US Food and Drug Administration (FDA) approval in March of 1999 (Figure 14.1). It consists of a dedicated, microprocessor-controlled, bipolar generator and catheters with collapsible electrodes that are introduced into the vein lumen. Once introduced, the electrodes are energized to destroy the intima and contract the vein wall so that it will undergo fibrous obliteration.[6] This system offers two sheathable electrode catheters, 1.7 mm (6 Fr) and 2.7 mm (8 Fr), which allow radiofrequency obliteration of veins from 2 to 12 mm in diameter. These catheters provide rings of resistive vein-wall heating of 6–8 mm in length and measured withdrawal of the catheter along the length of the vein at the recommended rate of 3 cm/min will affect closure. The operator selects the treatment temperature, typically 85°C, and the generator monitors the catheter-vein wall impedance to maintain that temperature.

The catheter can be inserted into the saphenous vein through a venipuncture sheath either antegrade at the medial calf or retrograde at the SFJ and either percutaneously or through open exposure of the vein. A micropuncture introducer system can be used for this purpose. Proper positioning of the catheter can be determined by palpation or fluoroscopy, but most operators preferentially use ultrasonic imaging. The limb to be treated is then elevated and

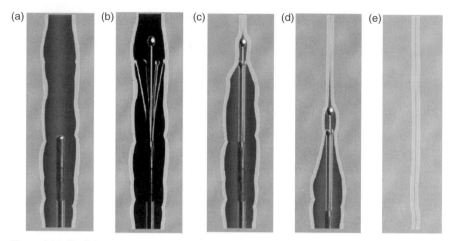

Figure 14.2 Radiofrequency venous ablation procedure. (a) The Closure catheter is first inserted in the reflux saphenous vein. (b) Once the catheter is appropriately positioned, the electrodes are deployed. (c) Radiofrequency energy is activated through the catheter electrodes which contact vein wall. (d) The catheter is slowly withdrawn which cause vein closure. (e) The denuded vein cause complete closure of the refluxing vein.

exsanguinated with a bandage applied from toes to the groin. The electrodes are then unsheathed and catheter-vein wall impedance assessed to assure proper vein-wall contact in the compressed saphenous vein (Figure 14.2). Subcutaneous infiltration of either normal saline or local tumescent anesthetic is essential to prevent skin burns when the treated vein is very superficial. In most procedures, completion ultrasound imaging is performed to identify areas with persistent flow that can be retreated.[6]

Results of radiofrequency saphenous vein ablation

It is clear that the radiofrequency ablation method is well tolerated with minimal short and long-term morbidity.[24] Main complications include paresthesias, superficial thrombophlebitis, local hematomas, and thermal skin injury. Patients treated with this method enjoy early return to full activity with minimal restrictions. Radiofrequency saphenous obliteration is mainly directed at patients with minimal venous insufficiency, CEAP clinical classes 0, 1, and 2 predominantly (CEAP classification is based on clinical signs [C], cause [E], anatomic distribution [A], and pathophysiologic condition [P]). One would expect good clinical results as assessed by symptom severity scores in this subset of patients, and indeed excellent outcomes have been reported. Greater than 90% of patients have improved symptom severity scores and patient satisfaction with the procedure is 96% at 1 year, albeit with limited follow-up at this interval from the total registry enrollment. These results are not dissimilar from those of high saphenous ligation combined with sclerotherapy in which 92 patients reported 90% satisfaction at 3 years, even though objective Doppler ultrasound confirmed recurrent or persistent reflux in 50% of these patients.[25]

The VNUS clinical registry was established in 1998, and several centers around the world are now contributing data. Data derived from this registry suggest the durability of endovenous radiofrequency ablation. For instance, 94% of limbs that were free of reflux at 1 year remained reflux free at subsequent follow-up. Absence of reflux by duplex ultrasound was 91.4, 90.1, 86.3, and 86.1% at 1, 2, 3, and 4 years, respectively. In the VNUS registry, 94% of the ablated veins are invisible by ultrasound examination after the second year of treatment.

A number of randomized trials compare radiofrequency ablation to vein stripping. Rautio and associates randomized 28 patients to receive either radiofrequency obliteration or vein stripping and reported significantly less postoperative pain, less postoperative analgesia requirements, and faster recovery in the radiofrequency group.[26] The EVOLVeS study was a multicenter, prospective, randomized study, comparing quality-of-life factors between radiofrequency ablation and vein stripping.[27] In all outcome variables, radiofrequency ablation superceded venous stripping: faster recovery, less postoperative pain, fewer adverse events, and superior quality-of-life score. Follow-up at 2 years on EVOLVeS patients demonstrated the same treatment efficacy between the radiofrequency ablation and the vein stripping groups with 91.2% versus 91.7% of limbs free of reflux, respectively. Additional European data indicate that the patient self-perceived quality-of-life and the postoperative pain were better at 2 years for radiofrequency ablation over vein stripping.

Endovenous laser ablation
General considerations
Endovenous laser treatment allows delivery of laser energy directly into the blood vessel lumen to produce endothelial and vein-wall damage with subsequent fibrosis. It is presumed that destruction of the GSV with laser is a function of thermal destruction of both the vein and red blood cells.[28,29] The wavelength of the laser beam correlates with the extent of thermal injury to tissue, which is also strongly dependent on the amount and duration of heat to which the tissue is exposed. Another possible mechanism of action of endovenous laser treatment is that postulated for radiofrequency closure, namely, collagen contraction. Collagen has been noted to contract at about 50°C whereas necrosis occurs between 70 and 100°C.[30] It is possible that collagen contraction, thermal damage, or a combination of these two effects is responsible for destruction and resorption of the GSV.

Technique
Endovenous laser treatment, which received approval from the US FDA in January 2002, allows delivery of laser energy directly into the blood vessel lumen. Nonthrombotic vein occlusion is accomplished by heating the vein

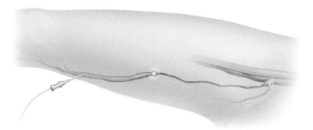

Figure 14.3 In endovenous laser venous ablation, an introducer sheath is inserted in the distal thigh through which the laser catheter is inserted and positioned just distal to the SFJ.

wall with 810-nm-wavelength laser energy delivered via a 600-μm laser fiber (Diomed, Andover, MA). The technique of using this laser ablation system is not substantially different from that used for RFA. Varicose veins are marked with the patient standing. A small amount of tumescent anesthetic is injected in the distal thigh and the GSV is accessed percutaneously with a 21 G needle under ultrasound guidance just proximal to the knee level. A microintroducer guidewire is inserted, followed by the introducer and then by a 0.035 guidewire. A 5 Fr sheath is then inserted over the 0.035 guidewire. Through this sheath, the laser fiber will be placed protected within a separate introducer sheath. The tip of the laser fiber is positioned 1 cm distal to the SFJ (Figure 14.3). The area surrounding the GSV and distal tributaries to be treated is infiltrated with tumescent anesthesia. Injecting tumescent anesthetic after the laser fiber and the sheath have been inserted into the vein facilitates their visualization with ultrasonography. The introducer sheath is then retracted 2 cm to prevent inadvertent laser exposure to the sheath. A helium–neon aiming beam that is continuously illuminated when the laser is on, ensures that the laser fiber is distal to the SFJ. Ultrasonography can also be used to confirm the position of the introducer sheath whose end needs to be just proximal to the SFJ (Figure 14.4). The laser is then set at the appropriate level of power, and the laser fiber is withdrawn at a rate of 1 mm/s after the laser is activated, which effectively achieves saphenous vein ablation (Figure 14.5). After the saphenous obliteration is complete smaller varicose tributaries are treated with intravascular laser or removed with a standard ambulatory phlebectomy technique. The treated leg is then wrapped in gauze to absorb the tumescent fluid and then with a short stretch overlying compression bandage. Recommendations for length of postoperative extremity compression vary, but most authors agree that graduated stockings need to be used for at least 1–2 weeks postoperatively.[28,31] Early ambulation is encouraged.

Results of laser saphenous vein ablation

Although most patients experience some degree of postoperative ecchymosis and discomfort, no other major complications have been reported. The lack

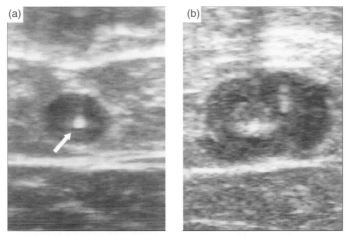

Figure 14.4 Duplex ultrasound is used to demonstrate the appearance of GSV before and after proper delivery of tumescent anesthesia. (a) Intraluminal position of laser catheter (arrow) within an enlarged GSV; (b) tumescent anesthesia delivered adjacent to laser fiber and catheter with fluid surrounding the compressed GSV.

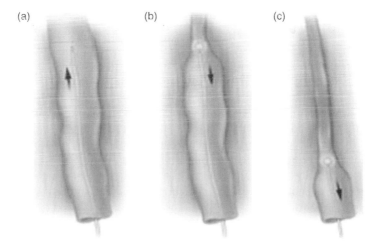

Figure 14.5 Endovenous laser venous ablation procedure. (a) The laser catheter is first advanced toward the SFJ. (b) Laser energy is activated and the catheter system is slowly withdrawn. (c) The laser energy effectively causes closure of the refluxing vein and achieves complete venous ablation.

of significant heating of perivenous tissues owing to the effect of perivascular lidocaine fluid probably explains the low complication rate found and argues well for the continued lack of significant complications. Patients treated with endovenous laser treatment with an 810-nm diode laser have shown an increase in posttreatment purpura and tenderness compared to radiofrequency closure. Most of the patients do not return to complete functional normality for 2–3 days as opposed to the 1-day "downtime" with radiofrequency closure of the GSV. Because the anesthetic and access techniques for the two procedures are identical, it is likely that nonspecific perivascular thermal damage is the probable cause for this increased tenderness. Some complications appear to be related to the properties of the laser used. Pulsed 810-, 940-, and 980-nm diode laser treatment seems to have an increased risk of vein microperforation, as opposed to continuous treatment with a 1040- and 1340-nm diodes that do not have intermittent vein perforations.[31] Wavelength, overall energy transmitted, and the time of exposure to the energy can all be associated with the perforation rates. Of note, thermal damage can be transmitted through blood components to sites remote to the intervention and accounts for postoperative pain and discomfort, induration along the vein side, paresthesias, and superficial thrombophlebitis.[32]

Min and associates presented 3-year data on 499 limbs treated for incompetent GSV.[33] At 1 month follow-up, successful endovenous laser treatment, defined as use of 810-nm diode laser energy delivered intraluminally, was observed in 490 of 499 limbs treated (98%). Posttreatment follow-up demonstrated continued GSV closure in 99.3% (444 of 447 limbs) at 3 months, 98.5% (390 of 396 limbs) at 6 months, 97.8% (351 of 359 limbs) at 9 months, 97.5% (310 of 318 limbs) at 1 year, and 93.4% (113 of 121 limbs) at 2 years. There were no recurrences in the 40 limbs followed out to 3 years. All recurrences in this series were noted before 9 months, with the majority seen by 3 months. Goldman and colleagues reported their experience using a 1340-nm diode electrode and did not have any recurrences in their initial short 6-month follow-up.[31] Theoretically, a longer wavelength will bypass the problems of hemoglobin absorption of energy, and therefore minimize the incidence of distal thermal damage from the moving red blood cells. Navarro and associates reported their 4-year follow-up on 200 limbs treated with endovenous laser at the 2003 UIP World Congress in San Diego and showed success rates approaching 95%.[34] They commented that their recurrences were due to recanalization as opposed to neovascularization, and occasionally due to progressive involvement and incompetence of SFJ branches left untreated.

Issues and perspective on endovenous treatment of varicose veins

Tumescent anesthesia

Tumescent is an adjective derived from the Latin tumescere (meaning to begin to swell) that describes something that is swollen and firm. Tumescent technique for local anesthesia refers to the technique of injecting large volumes of very dilute lidocaine and epinephrine in the subcutaneous tissue and was originally used to achieve local anesthesia prior to liposuction. Pure tumescent anesthesia is now recognized for its safety and ability to produce satisfactory anesthesia of skin, subcutaneous fat, and subjacent muscle. The tumescent solution contains lidocaine 0.5–1.0 gm/L and epinephrine 0.5–1.0 mg/L (1 : 2,000,000 to 1 : 1,000,000 dilution). Sodium bicarbonate can be added (10 MEq/L) to reduce the acidic pH of the anesthetic solution. Injection of the solution should be in the subfascial plane around the saphenous vein. A number of techniques have been described and automated pumps and injection systems are commercially available to maximize precision of the injection and patient comfort. After completion of the infiltration process, the injected areas appear swollen and firm and overlying skin is blanched. "Detumescence" occurs in approximately 20–30 min, however the profound local anesthetic and vasoconstrictive effect persists for several hours. A safe lidocaine dose should be no more than 35 mg/kg. The patient should be questioned on taking medications (ketoconazole, itroconazole, erythromycin, clarithromycin, certraline to mention a few) that interfere with the cytochrome P450 microsomal enzyme system that can lead to alteration of lidocaine metabolism with subsequent toxicity.

In the early days of radiofrequency ablation, patients were sometimes left with skin burns or paresthesias. Tumescence is beneficial during endovenous treatment for several reasons. First, it creates a reservoir of fluid surrounding the vein that acts as a heat sink. When heat is placed inside the vein during the venous ablation, it is quickly dissipated through the wall of the vein precluding any heat-related injury of surrounding tissue. As a result, the rate of skin burns and the paresthesias has been reduced to less than 1% in experienced hands. In addition, the tumescent fluid compresses the vein. This allows satisfactory treatment of even the most aneurysmal veins, even up to 30 mm in size. Furthermore, the tumescent solution provides effective analgesia and eliminates the hemodynamic risks of sympathectomy associated with a conduction block (epidural or spinal anesthetic), and the cardiac and pulmonary risks associated with general endotracheal anesthesia.

Adverse effects

The main advantage of endovenous techniques is avoiding the groin altogether and preserving venous drainage from the abdominal wall. Hematomas, wound infection from groin incisions, and neovascularization are all diminished with the endovenous techniques. With thermal ablation of the GSV, mild ecchymosis and a "pulling" sensation in the thigh are seen frequently after treatment. However, complications of paresthesia, hematoma, wound infection, and deep vein thrombosis would be considered rare. Patient selection appears to be sometimes an important predictor of specific complications. For instance, for veins located just below the surface of the skin, endovenous treatment may result in an unsatisfactory cosmetic result because the patient will experience a stain and palpable cord on the skin of the medial thigh and leg. Resolution of this problem is spontaneous, usually within a year. Vein tortuosity can be a cause of venous trauma since guidewire navigation is difficult and may require multiple entry sites to treat the lesions successfully. Finally, patients who are only poorly ambulatory have a higher risk for developing deep venous thrombosis and deserve special attention.

Neovascularization

Recurrence rates for saphenous reflux following stripping of the GSV have traditionally been reported over longer intervals of follow-up than those reported by the VNUS registry. Five-year results of a randomized trial of high ligation and GSV stripping with high ligation of the SFJ alone were compared. The results showed recurrent saphenofemoral incompetence in 29% of 52 limbs following high ligation and stripping and in 71% of 58 limbs following SFJ high ligation alone.[35] Neovascularization of the SFJ was the predominant cause of recurrent reflux, and was more common when a residual patent GSV segment remained in the high-ligation group (52%) than in the stripping group without a residual patent GSV (23%).[35] Neovascularization refers to the growth of new blood vessels in the groin, often after vein stripping, resulting in high recurrence rates.

It is suggested that scarring associated with surgical dissection incites neovascularization and that the RFA technique, without high ligation of the SFJ, avoids this stimulus for neovascularization at the SFJ. To further support this, in a study[36] carried out to 39 years, neovascularization was seen in 60% of groins after surgical ligation and stripping, of which 30% required additional treatment. Furthermore, Pichot and associates reported their experience on clinical and duplex findings on 63 limbs, 2 years after GSV radiofrequency ablation and noted that there was no neovascularity in any groin.[37] Unfortunately, these encouraging data lack consistency. In another study, among 49 limbs undergoing high ligation of the SFJ, in addition to radiofrequency ablation of the GSV, there was a 2% rate of saphenofemoral reflux at 6 months. In contrast, among 97 limbs undergoing radiofrequency ablation of the GSV without high ligation of the SFJ at the same centers during the same time period, an 8% rate of saphenofemoral reflux was noted by 6 months.[38] Although small numbers in this last series likely prevented this difference from being statistically significant, this observation certainly questions the suggestion that high ligation is unnecessary. It is possible that with longer follow-up and increasing recanalization over time, recurrent saphenous reflux will become significant in patients 5 years after the RFA procedure and perhaps adjunctive high ligation of the SFJ will be reconsidered.

Endovenous failure

Like any new technology, a learning curve has a confounding effect on the early treatment outcomes. It is intuitive that the patients with the longest follow-up were those treated early, and endovenous outcome data are therefore, a "moving target." Several modifications in the originally described endovenous techniques have been now well established and include the introduction of tumescent anesthesia, as well as aggressive early treatment of dilated tributary veins. In addition, technological advances have made possible changes in the equipment design and the delivery of thermal energy from the catheter to the vessel under treatment. The early literature reports failure rates of approximately 10%, using either radiofrequency or laser ablation, which have now been reduced as operators have gained more experience and the technique and equipment have been refined. Failure of endovenous treatments is defined as the reopening (partial or full) of any ablated vein, based on examination by ultrasound imaging. In most of the reported series, the failures seem to occur during the first year. It is still difficult to pinpoint a single etiology for this recurrence; however there is evidence that vein size is not much of an issue. Leaving untreated large tributaries or perforating veins seems to be more important. Authors, who aggressively treat all perforating and refluxing tributaries at the time of the initial ablation operation, have anecdotally reported 1-year closure rates between 97–99%. Longer follow-up is necessary to provide a sound basis for comparison of outcomes between endovenous and traditional open surgery for varicose veins.

As 59% of patients in the VNUS registry had adjunctive phlebectomy, varicosity free rates are not a true marker for failure of the RFA procedure and more likely reflects technical error and incomplete phlebectomy than failure of the technique to prevent varicosity recurrence.[24] Untreated thigh perforators may be another potential source of recurrent varices.[39] Phlebographic investigations have documented that as many as 60% of normal patients have mid-thigh perforators and 30% have distal thigh perforators that communicate with the GSV.[40] In a series of 128 limbs evaluated varicographically for recurrent varicose veins after varicose vein surgery involving a groin incision, 35% of the recurrences were in patients with obliterated saphenofemoral complexes. Of these nonsaphenofemoral recurrences, 91% were related to persistent thigh perforator reflux, and of these, 61% had a residual GSV segment into which the thigh perforator refluxed.[4]

It is obvious that a number of questions regarding the long-term fate of the obliterated saphenous vein and the associated patterns of treatment failure remain unanswered. How does the VNUS Closure® technique fare in patients with a significant number of incompetent thigh perforators? Will pressure transmitted from these incompetent perforators stimulate recanalization of the obliterated, yet connected, saphenous vein segment? Are these the patients who are recanalizing at 6 months or 1 year? The most current VNUS registry report includes 53 patients with CEAP clinical class 4, 5, or 6;[24] yet we do not know how this subset of patients, likely to have incompetent thigh perforators and saphenous incompetence, compared to the overall results.

Long-term fate of the ablated saphenous vein

The promise of the radiofrequency ablation technique centers upon a central question; is saphenous obliteration permanent? Unfortunately, in comparing reports from the VNUS registry, the number of durable saphenous vein occlusions appears to decrease with experience and extended follow-up. In the first registry report, 7.2% of successfully treated saphenous veins partially or totally recanalized by 4.9 months of follow-up.[41] In the most recent registry report, 14.3% of successfully treated saphenous veins partially or totally recanalized by 6 months of follow-up, and in the smaller group of 107 patients followed for 12 months, 12% of successfully treated saphenous veins were partially or totally recanalized.[24] The importance of any distinctions between complete occlusion, near complete occlusion, and recanalization for the RFA technique remain unclear, yet may become more important with increasing follow-up. A 94% freedom from saphenous reflux at 12 months after radiofrequency ablation regardless of the technical outcome has been reported, suggesting that both near complete and complete occlusion of the saphenous vein prevent reflux.[24]

Conclusions

Sclerotherapy, radiofrequency ablation, and laser ablation have revolutionized the management of patients with venous insufficiency. Recent data have demonstrated the safety and efficacy of these techniques, as well as their potential superiority to venous stripping in the areas of neovascularization and improved patient comfort. Continuous refinement of these methods allows for improving results with an associated decrease in the number of observed complications. Long-term data, however, are not yet available to fairly compare these modalities to the traditional great saphenous stripping, or to each other, and this represents a field open to future investigation. In addition, effort should be made towards standardizing the existing endovenous treatment protocols to allow for a more uniform approach and easier comparison of outcomes between patients with venous disease.

References

1 Bosanquet N. Costs of venous ulcers: from maintenance therapy to investment programmes. *Phlebology* 1992; **7**:44–46.
2 Smith JJ, Garratt AM, Guest M, Greenhalgh RM, Davies AH. Evaluating and improving health-related quality of life in patients with varicose veins. *J Vasc Surg* 1999; **30**:710–19.
3 Callam MJ. Epidemiology of varicose veins. *Br J Surg* 1994; **81**:167–73.
4 Stonebridge PA, Chalmers N, Beggs I, Bradbury AW, Ruckley CV. Recurrent varicose veins: a varicographic analysis leading to a new practical classification. *Br J Surg* 1995; **82**:60–62.
5 Bradbury AW, Stonebridge PA, Callam MJ, *et al.* Recurrent varicose veins: assessment of the saphenofemoral junction. *Br J Surg* 1994; **81**:373–75.
6 Harris EJ. Radiofrequency ablation of the long saphenous vein without high ligation versus high ligation and stripping for primary varicose veins: pros and cons. *Semin Vasc Surg* 2002; **15**:34–38.
7 Bergan JJ, Kumins NH, Owens EL, Sparks SR. Surgical and endovascular treatment of lower extremity venous insufficiency. *J Vasc Interv Radiol* 2002; **13**:563–68.
8 Weiss RA, Weiss MA, Goldman MP. Physicians' negative perception of sclerotherapy for venous disorders: review of a 7-year experience with modern sclerotherapy. *South Med J* 1992; **85**:1101–6.

9 Weiss RA, Weiss MA. Resolution of pain associated with varicose and telangiectatic leg veins after compression sclerotherapy. *J Dermatol Surg Oncol* 1990; **16**:333–36.

10 Rautio T, Ohinmaa A, Perala J, *et al.* Endovenous obliteration versus conventional stripping operation in the treatment of primary varicose veins: a randomized controlled trial with comparison of the costs. *J Vasc Surg* 2002; **35**:958–65.

11 Rautio TT, Perala JM, Wiik HT, Juvonen TS, Haukipuro KA. Endovenous obliteration with radiofrequency-resistive heating for greater saphenous vein insufficiency: a feasibility study. *J Vasc Interv Radiol* 2002; **13**:569–75.

12 Fligelstone L, Carolan G, Pugh N, Shandall A, Lane I. An assessment of the long saphenous vein for potential use as a vascular conduit after varicose vein surgery. *J Vasc Surg* 1993; **18**:836–40.

13 Reuther T NR, El Gammal C et al. Diameter of the long saphenous vein at the saphenofemoral junction comparing normal and primary varicose veins. *Phlebologie* 1999; **28**:48–52.

14 Lane RJ, Cuzzilla ML, Coroneos JC. The treatment of varicose veins with external stenting to the saphenofemoral junction. *Vasc Endovascular Surg* 2002; **36**:179–92.

15 Tessari L. Nouvelle technique d' obtention de la sclero-mousse. *Phlebologie* 2000; **53**:129.

16 Frullini A, Cavezzi A. Sclerosing foam in the treatment of varicose veins and telangiectases: history and analysis of safety and complications. *Dermatol Surg* 2002; **28**:11–15.

17 Kern P. Sclerotherapy of varicose leg veins. Technique, indications and complications. *Int Angiol* 2002; **21**:40–45.

18 Kanter A, Thibault P. Saphenofemoral incompetence treated by ultrasound-guided sclerotherapy. *Dermatol Surg* 1996, **22**:648–52.

19 Barrett JM, Allen B, Ockelford A, Goldman MP. Microfoam ultrasound-guided sclerotherapy treatment for varicose veins in a subgroup with diameters at the junction of 10 mm or greater compared with a subgroup of less than 10 mm. *Dermatol Surg* 2004; **30**:1386–90.

20 Weiss RA WM. Varicose Veins in *Cutaneous Surgery* In: RG W, ed: WB Saunders, 1994. Orlando, FL.

21 Barrett JM, Allen B, Ockelford A, Goldman MP. Microfoam ultrasound-guided sclerotherapy treatment for varicose veins in a subgroup with diameters at the junction of 10 mm or greater compared with a subgroup of less than 10 mm. *Dermatol Surg* 2004; **30**:1386–90.

22 Politowski M, Zelazny T. Complications and difficulties in electrocoagulation of varices of the lower extremities. *Surgery* 1966; **59**:932–34.

23 O'Reilly K. A technique of diathermy sclerosis of varicose veins. *Aust N Z J Surg* 1981; **51**:379–82.

24 Merchant RF, DePalma RG, Kabnick LS. Endovascular obliteration of saphenous reflux: a multicenter study. *J Vasc Surg* 2002; **35**:1190–96.

25 Rutgers PH, Kitslaar PJ. Randomized trial of stripping versus high ligation combined with sclerotherapy in the treatment of the incompetent greater saphenous vein. *Am J Surg* 1994; **168**:311–15.

26 Rautio T, Ohinmaa A, Perala J, *et al.* Endovenous obliteration versus conventional stripping operation in the treatment of primary varicose veins: a randomized controlled trial with comparison of the costs. *J Vasc Surg* 2002; **35**:958–65.

27 Lurie F, Creton D, Eklof B, *et al.* Prospective randomized study of endovenous radiofrequency obliteration (closure procedure) versus ligation and stripping in a selected patient population (EVOLVeS Study). *J Vasc Surg* 2003; **38**:207–14.

28 Perkowski P, Ravi R, Gowda RC, *et al.* Endovenous laser ablation of the saphenous vein for treatment of venous insufficiency and varicose veins: early results from a large single-center experience. *J Endovasc Ther* 2004; **11**:132–38.

29 Proebstle TM, Lehr HA, Kargl A, *et al.* Endovenous treatment of the greater saphenous vein with a 940-nm diode laser: thrombotic occlusion after endoluminal thermal damage by laser-generated steam bubbles. *J Vasc Surg* 2002; **35**:729–36.

30 Min RJ, Zimmet SE, Isaacs MN, Forrestal MD. Endovenous laser treatment of the incompetent greater saphenous vein. *J Vasc Interv Radiol* 2001; **12**:1167–71.

31 Goldman MP, Mauricio M, Rao J. Intravascular 1320-nm laser closure of the great saphenous vein: a 6- to 12-month follow-up study. *Dermatol Surg* 2004; **30**:1380–85.

32 Proebstle TM, Sandhofer M, Kargl A, *et al.* Thermal damage of the inner vein wall during endovenous laser treatment: key role of energy absorption by intravascular blood. *Dermatol Surg* 2002; **28**:596–600.

33 Min RJ, Khilnani N, Zimmet SE. Endovenous laser treatment of saphenous vein reflux: long-term results. *J Vasc Interv Radiol* 2003; **14**:991–96.

34 Navarro L. BC. Endolaser: four year follow-up evaluation (Abstract). UIP Congress 2003.

35 Dwerryhouse S, Davies B, Harradine K, Earnshaw JJ. Stripping the long saphenous vein reduces the rate of reoperation for recurrent varicose veins: five-year results of a randomized trial. *J Vasc Surg* 1999; **29**:589–92.

36 Fischer R, Linde N, Duff C, Jeanneret C, Chandler JG, Seeber P. Late recurrent saphenofemoral junction reflux after ligation and stripping of the greater saphenous vein. *J Vasc Surg* 2001; **34**:236–40.

37 Pichot O, Kabnick LS, Creton D, Merchant RF, Schuller-Petroviae S, Chandler JG. Duplex ultrasound scan findings two years after great saphenous vein radiofrequency endovenous obliteration. *J Vasc Surg* 2004; **39**:189–95.

38 Chandler JG, Pichot O, Sessa C, Schuller-Petrovic S, Osse FJ, Bergan JJ. Defining the role of extended saphenofemoral junction ligation: a prospective comparative study. *J Vasc Surg* 2000; **32**:941–53.

39 Bergan JJ. Saphenous vein stripping and quality of outcome. *Br J Surg* 1996; **83**:1027–7.

40 Tung KT, Chan O, Lea Thomas M. The incidence and sites of medial thigh communicating veins: a phlebographic study. *Clin Radiol* 1990; **41**:339–40.

41 Chandler JG, Pichot, O., Sessa C. Treatment of primary venous insufficiency by endovenous saphenous vein obliteration. *Vasc Surg* 2000; **34**:211–14.

CHAPTER 15

Ileofemoral deep venous thrombosis

James P. Gregg, Esteban A. Henao, Alan B. Lumsden

Deep venous thrombosis (DVT) is estimated to affect 20–30% of all major surgical patients, and as a result of pulmonary embolism, is responsible for more than 60,000 deaths annually in the United States.[1,2] The annual incidence of venous thromboembolism is close to 0.1% and increases from 0.01% in early adulthood to approximately 1% among patients greater than 60 years old.[3,4] Venous thrombosis may occur in any vein in the body but is most commonly seen in the lower extremities. Superficial vein thrombosis in the leg frequently occurs in varicosities and is usually benign and self-limiting. Involvement of the deep veins of the leg is a more serious condition, with thrombi in the proximal veins (popliteal, femoral, or iliac veins) more often associated with pulmonary emboli than the deep veins of the calf. Accurate diagnosis and prompt therapy are important to minimize the risk of fatal pulmonary embolism. Postthrombotic syndrome and recurrent thromboembolism are important long-term complications, which warrant a high index of suspicion in the clinician's mind when treating DVT.

The pathogenesis of venous thrombosis involves Virchow's triad: damage to the vessel wall, venous stasis, and hypercoagulability. The cause of venous thromboembolism is multifactorial and often results from a combination of risk factors including inherited conditions, acquired conditions, and hereditary, environmental, or idiopathic conditions.[5] DVT typically originates in the venous sinuses of the calf muscles but may originate in the proximal veins due to trauma or surgery.[6] Signs and symptoms result from venous outflow obstruction and from inflammation of the vessel wall and perivascular tissue.[5] Calf vein thrombi often undergo spontaneous thrombolysis and rarely result in symptomatic pulmonary embolism.[7] Approximately 25% of untreated calf thrombi extend into the proximal veins, usually within a week after presentation.[8] The risk of pulmonary embolism (either symptomatic or asymptomatic) with proximal vein thrombosis is approximately 50%, and most fatal emboli usually originate from proximal thrombi.[9,10] Rarely, venous thrombosis can become massive and result in severe symptoms such as phlegmasia cerulea dolens or phlegmasia alba dolens. In phlegmasia cerulea dolens, the thrombosis extends to collateral veins, which can lead to massive fluid sequestration. Clinical symptoms include significant swelling of leg, bluish discoloration, and pain (Figure 15.1). Phlegmasia alba dolens presents as a large, swollen,

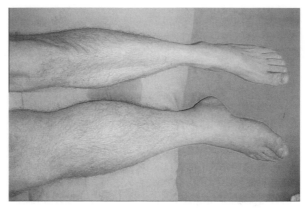

Figure 15.1 Severe DVT in the right lower leg. Note the increased right calf swelling compared to the left calf.

and painful limb made pale by severe edema. In this condition, the thrombosis involves major deep venous channels of the extremity, therefore sparing collateral veins. The venous drainage is decreased but still present. There is frequently an associated lymphangitis.

The initial therapy for DVT typically includes heparin or low molecular weight heparin followed by oral warfarin for 3–6 month.[11] Although anticoagulation therapy for iliofemoral DVT may be effective in inhibiting further clot propagation and prevent pulmonary embolism, it may not relieve thrombus burden and thus prevent chronic postthrombotic complications. The delayed complications of DVT are due to valvular damage from chronic thrombus and scarring. There has been increasing interest in thrombolysis or mechanical thrombectomy of acute DVT. Venous thrombolysis has been a controversial treatment option for deep-vein thrombosis. Thrombolytic therapy leads to a more rapid and complete dissolution of clot compared with heparin treatment alone, however, the optimal treatment for DVT is not completely clear. While the occlusive effects of DVT can quickly and effectively be treated with thrombolytic therapy, bleeding complications are significantly increased. Whether thrombolytic therapy lessens the destructive effects of DVT on valve function and leads to significantly improved clinical outcome is the crucial question that remains to be answered. Endovascular management, utilizing percutaneous mechanical thrombectomy alone or in combination with pharmacological thombolytic agents is safe and effective in the relief of thrombus burden. Along with the possible preservation of venous valve function, inciting anatomic lesions may be treated simultaneously.

Pathogenesis

Venous thrombi arise in the large venous sinuses in the calf, in valve cusp pockets in the deep veins of the calf, or at sites of vessel damage, and thrombosis occurs when activation of blood coagulation exceeds the ability of the natural anticoagulant mechanisms and the fibrinolytic system to prevent fibrin formation. The pathogenesis of venous thromboembolism involves Virchow's triad, demonstrated by the following: (1) damage to the vessel wall prevents the endothelium from inhibiting coagulation and initiating local fibrinolysis; (2) venous stasis, due to immobilization or venous obstruction, inhibits the clearance and dilution of activated coagulation factors; and (3) congenital or acquired thrombophilia promote coagulation.[5]

Thrombogenic factors include the activation of blood coagulation, venous stasis, and vessel wall damage. Coagulation proteins circulate as inactive precursors or zymogens. Each zymogen is converted into an active enzyme that then activates the next zymogen in the coagulation cascade pathway. Coagulation cascade is initiated via the extrinsic pathway by activating the tissue factor–factor VIIa complex, which is the only coagulation factor that normally circulates in its enzyme form. Coagulation is activated by: (1) contact of factor XII with collagen on exposed subendothelium of damaged vessels or by contact with prosthetic surfaces; (2) exposure of blood to tissue factor made available locally as a result of vascular wall damage; (3) activation of endothelial cells by cytokines; and (4) by activated monocytes that migrate to areas of vascular injury.[12,13] Factor X can be activated directly by extracts of malignant cells that contain a cysteine protease, which may be one of the mechanisms of thrombosis induction with malignant disease.[14] Clinical risk factors that predispose to venous thromboembolism by activating blood coagulation include malignancy, extensive surgery, trauma, burns, myocardial infarction, and local hypoxia produced by venous stasis.[12,13] Venous stasis allows the accumulation of activated coagulation factors and leads to local hypoxia, a fact that stimulates endothelial cell to release an activator of factor X. Venous stasis is produced by immobility, venous obstruction, increased venous pressure, venous dilation, and increased blood viscosity.[12,13] Vessel wall damage from vascular injury leads to expression of tissue factor, either directly by endothelial cells or by monocytes that are attracted to the site of damage, and exposure of blood to subendothelium leads to platelet adhesion and aggregation.[13]

Thrombosis occurs when coagulation overwhelms the natural anticoagulant mechanisms and fibrinolytic system. Endothelial protective mechanisms include: thrombomodulin, which binds to thrombin, creating a conformational change that alters thrombin's capability to activate platelets, convert fibrinogen to fibrin, and activate factors V, VIII, and XIII; generation of plasminogen activators by cells of vascular wall to limit fibrin deposition; and platelet aggregation inhibition by the release of prostacyclin and endothelium-derived nitric oxide.[13] Blood coagulation factors are inhibited naturally by: antithrombin that inhibits thrombin and factor Xa mainly, and also inactivates factors XIIa, XIa, and IXa; protein C that inactivates factors Va and VIIIa on the platelet and endothelial cell surface and stimulates fibrinolysis; protein S that is a cofactor for activated protein C; and heparin cofactor II that complexes and inactivates thrombin.[13] The plasma fibrinolytic system is the conversion of plasminogen to the active enzyme plasmin, which hydrolyzes fibrin, fibrinogen, and factors V and VIII. Two endogenous plasminogen activators, tissue plasminogen activator (tPA) and urokinase, are synthesized by and released from endothelial cells.[12]

Rationale for treatment

Untreated or inadequately treated venous thrombosis is associated with a high recurrence rate, and can be associated with clinically detectable pulmonary embolism.[8,15] Those individuals with preexisting risk factors, such as prolonged immobilization or malignancy are at an even higher risk.[12] In contrast, if patients are treated to a therapeutic level at presentation, and are subsequently followed with oral anticoagulation or subcutaneous unfractionated heparin, they have a significantly diminished chance of recurrence, and its associated complications.[15,16]

Heparinization, followed by oral coumadin therapy is the cornerstone of initial therapy in those without contraindication to its administration (Table 15.1). Low molecular weight heparins are effective in preventing recurrent thrombosis, demonstrate more predictable dose response, cause less bleeding, and can be used effectively as outpatient therapy.[5,17] The duration of therapy should be balanced against the risk of hemorrhage. Treatment duration of 3 months is generally considered sufficient for thrombosis associated with a major transient risk factor.[18]

Endovascular treatment strategies

The consequences of chronic deep venous insufficiency, the postthrombotic or postphlebitic syndrome, is a major medical problem and often results in

Table 15.1 Contraindications to systemic anticoagulation.

Absolute contraindications
- Severe bleeding
- Severe bleeding diathesis or platelet count $<20,000/mm^3$
- Neurosurgery, ocular surgery, or intracranial
  bleeding within the past 10 days

Relative contraindications
- Mild to moderate bleeding diathesis or thrombocytopenia
- Brain metastases
- Recent major trauma
- Major abdominal surgery within the past 2 days
- Gastrointestinal or genitourinary bleeding within the past 14 days
- Endocarditis
- Severe hypertension (systolic blood pressure
  >200 mm Hg, diastolic blood pressure
  >120 mm Hg) at presentation

a significant compromise of lifestyle for an affected patient.[19,20] DVT can render the venous valves incompetent, resulting in a spectrum of clinical presentations ranging from varicose veins through chronic lower extremity pain, and edema to venous skin changes and ulceration. Chronic venous insufficiency (CVI) secondary to postphlebitic syndrome occurs in 66% of patients following an episode of DVT and accounts for up to 75% of all cases of venous ulcerations.[21–23] Following extensive lower extremity deep venous thrombosis, the postphlebitic syndrome may manifest immediately or take several months or years to full patient debilitation.[24]

This complex entity occurs secondarily as a result of chronic venous hypertension and venous valvular insufficiency and reflux. Hemodynamic derangements may result from a combination of abnormalities: valvular incompetence, venous obstruction with flow diversion through high resistance collaterals, or residual venous stenoses causing flow resistance.[22,25] Techniques aimed at valve preservation and restoration of venous patency should theoretically decrease venous hypertension, reducing the incidence and degree of postthrombotic symptoms. Improvements in venous hemodynamics should lead to overall improved clinical symptoms. Venous valvular reflux is the dominant cause of chronic venous insufficiency.[23] This valvular incompetence has been shown to result directly from DVT. Furthermore, patients with deep venous obstruction have more severe valvular insufficiency, calf muscle pump dysfunction, and ambulatory venous hypertension than patients without evidence of obstruction.[26] The ability of interventions such as anticoagulation therapy, thrombolytic therapy, and surgical/endovascular thrombectomy to restore venous patency, alleviate obstruction, and ultimately decrease reflux in a diseased extremity can be used to return patients to their normal way of life free of pain, swelling and ulceration and, in the ideal case, free of the need for elastic support.

Catheter-directed thrombolysis

The delivery of a pharmacologic thrombolytic agent directly into an existing venous thrombosis has overtaken systemic thrombolysis, due in part to more complete clot lysis combined with a lower rate of bleeding complications. By using one of the many commercially available infusion catheters for thrombolytic agent delivery, high drug concentrations are able to be concentrated at the location of the thrombus. Catheter-directed thrombolysis has been advocated because of its theoretical advantage of complete and rapid clot dissolution. Multiple studies have documented the efficacy of several thrombolytic agents in the treatment of acute DVT, with total infusion times needed for thrombus removal ranging from hours to days.[27–30] An association between time to lysis and the development of venous reflux was evaluated in patients using serial duplex scans following a DVT episode.[31] With the exception of the posterior tibial vein, early lysis and rapid venous recanalization appears to protect valve integrity in the lower extremity. Though thrombolytic therapy for DVT has

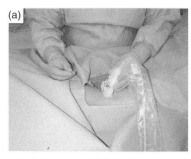 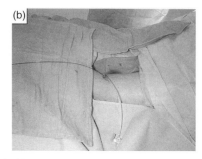

Figure 15.2 Ileofemoral DVT can be approached with endovascular intervention via a popliteal vein access. (a) Percutanous access should be performed under ultrasound guidance. (b) Following successful cannulation of the popliteal vein, an introducer sheath is placed.

excellent outcomes with thrombus clearance and thus, perhaps may lower the incidence of postphlebitic syndrome by preservation of valvular function,[27] the complication profile of the treatment secondary to the thrombolytic agent and the infusion times may be limitations for its widespread use.

Technique for venous lysis and angioplasty

The approach to thrombolytic therapy in the lower leg is best done via a popliteal vein access with the patient in a prone position. It is extremely helpful to perform the puncture with ultrasonic guidance (Figure 15.2). A 21-gauge micropuncture needle is used for entry, followed by an 0.014 in. wire. A microsheath is advanced, and the system is exchanged for a standard 0.035 in. wire and access sheath. Venography can then be performed to delineate the lesion and its related landmarks for possible intervention. In general, it is essential that the lesion in question be crossable with a wire prior to intervention. This maneuver is then followed by placement of a Katzen wire and Mewissen catheter for infusion of thrombolytic agents. The lesion is pulse sprayed slowly over 20–40 min with a bolus of 1–2 mg of tPA, or 250,000 U of urokinase. The infusion system is then secured to the patient, and thrombolytic therapy is continued for 12–24 h. Heparin is also infused through the access sheath during the duration of therapy. The patient's fibrinogen levels are closely followed vigilantly to avoid systemic thrombolytic infusion. Angiography is repeated after this period for reevaluation of the lesion. Any residual areas may be treated with angioplasty, with the possibility of stenting.

Mechanical thrombectomy systems

Relief of clot burden by directly extracting thrombus surgically or via thrombolytic dissolution can potentially decrease the risk of pulmonary embolism (PE) and also that of postphlebitic syndrome. Primarily because of the bleeding risks of catheter-directed thrombolysis, mechanical thrombectomy has

Table 15.2 Commercially available thrombectomy devices.

Catheter name (manufacturer)	Mechanism of clot extraction
AngioJet (Possis, Inc.)	Thrombus Aspiration
Hydrolyser (Cordis, Inc.)	Thrombus Aspiration
Oasis (Boston Scientific/Meditech)	Thrombus Aspiration
Amplatz (Microvena)	Microfragmentation
Helix (EV3)	Microfragmentation
Treretola (Arrow International)	Microfragmentation
Casteñeda and Cragg Brush (Micro Therapeutics)	Microfragmentation
Trellis infusion catheter (Bacchus Vascular)	Microfragmentation

emerged as an advantageous option for the treatment of acute DVT. Table 15.2 summarizes various thrombectomy catheters and the mechanisms of clot removal. A full discussion of each of the catheters is beyond the scope of this chapter. Based on the mechanism of thrombus removal, these catheters can be grouped into one of the two categories: microfragmentation or thrombus aspiration. The former mechanism involves a direct mechanical fragmentation of the thrombus using the thrombectomy device itself. The latter mechanism utilizes the principles of the Venturi's effect, in which the catheter creates a high velocity fluid stream that results in a correspondingly low-pressure zone in the area adjacent to the catheter. This creates a suctioning force, which can result in thrombus aspiration. Several mechanical thrombectomy catheters may be used in combination with adjunctive thrombolytic agents for more complete and rapid thrombus removal with lower mean thrombolytic infusion doses and durations. Reducing the dosage and/or time for complete thrombolysis should translate into cost savings and decreased bleeding complications. Furthermore, inciting lesions leading to thrombosis may be unmasked with mechanical thrombectomy with or without adjunctive lysis. Venous stenoses could be treated following thrombectomy in the same operative setting, resulting in more efficient patient care.

Several authors have evaluated multiple thrombectomy catheters in the treatment of DVT. However, to date, there is no prospective, randomized trial data available. In one review, Vedantham *et al.* used percutaneous mechanical thrombectomy (several devices tested including Amplatz Thrombectomy Device, Microvena, White Bear Lake, MN; AngioJet®, Possis Medical Inc., Minneapolis, MN; Trerotola Percutaneous Thrombectomy Device, Arrow International, Reading, PA; Oasis, Boston Scientific/Meditech, Natick, MA) for the treatment of lower extremity DVT.[32] Procedural success was achieved in 82% with underlying culprit stenoses uncovered and stented in 15 patients (18 limbs). These authors reported substantial thrombus removal with the two techniques combined, compared to either alone. In another study reported by Delomez and associates, which used the Amplatz thrombectomy device, researchers noted successful recanalization of the thrombosed segment in 83% of patients with proximal DVT.[33] At 29.6 months follow-up, 10 patients had minimal symptoms relating to the episode and only one patient had developed postthrombotic sequelae.

A retrospective clinical study of interventional management of DVT utilizing the AngioJet (Possis Medical Inc, Minneapolis, MN) thrombectomy system demonstrated its clinical efficacy in thrombus removal, venous patency restoration, and symptom relief.[34] The AngioJet rheolytic thrombectomy system is designed to produce an area of extremely low pressure at the catheter tip by controlled high velocity saline jets. Via this mechanism, thrombus surrounding the catheter tip is macerated and rapidly evacuated via an effluent lumen into a collection chamber. In this study, only four (23.5%) patients achieved >90% thrombus clearance with mechanical thrombectomy alone. Adjunctive thrombolytic agents were used in 9 of 17 patients, those that had a lesser amount of clot extracted with the use of the mechanical thrombectomy catheter. Often the thrombolytic catheter was left in place and the average duration of thrombolytic therapy was 20.2 h. Clinical symptomatic improvement was seen in 82% over a follow-up time frame of 11 months.[34] Another clinical study that evaluated the utility of the AngioJet thrombectomy combined with thrombolytic therapy in DVT was reported by our group recently. In this study, thrombolytic agents, including either urokinase, tPA, or reteplase, was added in the infusion saline, which was delivered via the AngioJet thrombectomy catheter system.[35] Complete thrombus removal was achieved in two-third of patients with symptomatic iliofemoral DVT, and partial resolution was achieved in one-third of patients. Overall, immediate (<24 h) improvement in clinical symptoms was noted in 74% of patients. There were no complications related to either mechanical thrombectomy or the short duration of thrombolytic agent infusion. This study concluded that addition of thrombolytic agent to mechanical thrombectomy facilitates thrombus extraction, decreases overall interventional treatment time, and improves patient outcomes.[35]

AngioJet rheolytic thrombectomy system

The AngioJet rheolytic thrombectomy system consists of three components: a single-use catheter, a single-use pump set, and a pump drive unit. The 6 Fr Xpeedior catheter has a working length of 60, 100, or 120 cm, is introduced via a percutaneous approach (6 Fr sheath) and operates over a 0.035 in. guide wire. The dual lumen catheter design consists of one lumen supplying pressurized saline to the distal catheter tip, and a second lumen incorporating the first lumen, guide wire, and thrombus particulate debris. The drive unit/pump generates high pressure (~10,000 psi) pulsatile saline flow that exits the catheter tip through multiple retrograde-directed jets. These high velocity jets create a localized low-pressure zone (Bernoulli effect) for thrombus aspiration and maceration. The jets also provide the driving force for evacuation of thrombus particulate debris through the catheter. The Xpeedior catheter design also has a means for radially directed low velocity fluid recirculation to assist with dislodgment from the vessel wall and direction to the catheter tip for evacuation. The AngioJet system works in an isovolumetric manner: the saline infusion flow rate (60 cc/min) is in balance with the evacuation rate of thrombus particulate debris.

Technique of pharmacomechanical thrombolysis for the treatment of DVT

One advantage of the AngioJet thrombectomy system is that it permits the infusion of the thrombolytic agent to create a condition called the pharmacomechanical thrombolysis (PMT). The initial setup for PMT is identical to the standard AngioJet thrombectomy therapy. After access is established with micropuncture and a sheath is inserted, a 0.035 in. wire is used to cross the lesion. After standard activation of the unit, 12 cc of normal saline (NS) prime is pumped out. Then, the NS bag is exchanged for 250,000 U of urokinase or 20 mg of tPA in 50 cc of NS. Next a stopcock is added to the outflow channel, which shuts off the outflow port. This effectively turns the AngioJet thrombectomy catheter into a mechanical infusion mode (Figure 15.3). During this infusion mode, one pedal tap is equal to one pump stroke for 0.6 ml of thrombolytic agent infusion. The catheter is advanced slowly at 0.5–1.0 mm increments until the lesion is crossed, then the agent is allowed to sit for approximately 20 min. Then, the stopcock is opened and the thrombolytic infusion bag is exchanged with the saline bag. The catheter is readvanced in thrombectomy mode across the lesion. A post thrombectomy angiogram is then performed. Further treatment may include traditional catheter-directed lysis, angioplasty, and stenting.

With this method, venous patency should be able to be restored, obviating the need for intensive care unit stays or multiple trips for repeat venography. Furthermore, in our experience, lower total doses of thrombolytic agent are used than with catheter-directed thrombolysis. This translates into lower overall cost and a reduction in potential hemorrhagic complications. Adjunctive endovascular techniques, such as balloon angioplasty with or

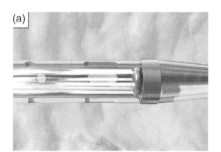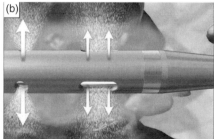

Figure 15.3 The AngioJet mechanical thrombectomy system. (a) Multiple high saline jets are emitted backward from the tip of the catheter to create a suctioning force, which removes thrombus. (b) With the outflow channel closed, this creates an infusion mode, which permits local delivery of thrombolytic agents into the thrombus.

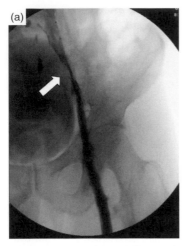 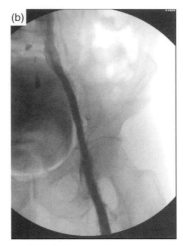

Figure 15.4 Compression of the left iliac vein by the overlying iliac artery, also know as the May–Thurner syndrome, which can be a cause of DVT. (a) Venogram demonstrates the venous compression (arrow). (b) Successful treatment is achieved following iliac venous stent placement.

without stent placement, may be performed in the same setting of pharma-comechanical thrombectomy. A common anatomical cause of DVT is known as the May–Thurner syndrome, which is due to the compression of the left iliac vein by the right iliac artery. Successful treatment of the iliac vein compression can be achieved with balloon angioplasty and stent placement (Figure 15.4).

Complications

Complications with the treatment of DVT include bleeding from antico-agulation (cerebral hemorrhage, gastrointestinal bleeding, and ecchymosis), catheter-related complications (hematoma, wound infection and inadequate therapy), and nonhemorrhagic complications including heparin-induced thrombocytopenia (HIT) and osteoporosis.

The diagnosis of HIT is based on characteristic clinical events and concurrent laboratory detection of HIT antibodies in the setting of recent heparin therapy. The central feature of HIT is thrombocytopenia that typically occurs 5–10 days after heparin exposure. HIT may develop more rapidly in patients previously exposed to heparin within the preceding 100 days.[36] Thrombosis is a common complication and is more frequently venous than arterial. The treatment of HIT includes the discontinuing and avoiding of additional heparin, and including heparin-coated central venous catheters. An anticoagulant other than heparin is recommended and the options include direct thrombin inhibitors lepirudin and argatroban. Warfarin therapy should be delayed until resolution of the thrombocytopenia.

Osteoporosis is another long-term complication of heparin therapy. Long-term heparin therapy may be associated with substantial bone loss. The condition is most likely to occur in patients receiving protracted therapy for venous thromboembolism associated with malignancy or pregnancy.[36] Symptomatic vertebral fracture and significant reduction in bone density may present with the condition. Treatment with low molecular weight heparin is associated with a lower risk of osteoporosis than unfractionated heparin.

Conclusion

Systemic anticoagulation with heparin, followed by a course of warfarin therapy constitutes the current standard of care for DVT. While limiting the potential problems of propagation, this therapy does little to address the fundamental pathologic changes that take place within the venous system that lead to deterioration of valve function. Thrombolytic therapy is an attractive option in that it enables restoration of patency, reduction of thrombus load, and mainly, venous valve preservation. While long-term data is unavailable, the potential benefit of preventing postthrombotic syndrome, which can occur months to years after an acute thrombotic event, is extremely attractive. Vascular surgeons should be aware of these newer treatment alternatives to help prevent the long-term sequelae of venous thrombosis.

References

1 Wakefield TW, Greenfield LJ. Diagnostic approaches and surgical treatment of deep-venous thrombosis and pulmonary embolism. *Hematol Oncol Clin North Am* 1993; 7:1251–67.

2 Anderson FA, Jr., Wheeler HB, Goldberg RJ, et al. A population-based perspective of the hospital incidence and case-fatality rates of deep vein thrombosis and pulmonary embolism. The Worcester DVT study. *Arch Intern Med* 1991; **151**:933–38.

3 Nordstrom M, Lindblad B, Bergqvist D, Kjellstrom T. A prospective study of the incidence of deep-vein thrombosis within a defined urban population. *J Intern Med* 1992; **232**:155–60.

4 Silverstein MD, Heit JA, Mohr DN, Petterson TM, O'Fallon WM, Melton LJ, 3rd. Trends in the incidence of deep-vein thrombosis and pulmonary embolism: a 25-year population-based study. *Arch Intern Med* 1998; **158**:585–93.

5 Bates SM, Ginsberg JS. Clinical practice. Treatment of deep-vein thrombosis. *N Engl J Med* 2004; **351**:268–77.

6 Stamatakis JD, Kakkar VV, Sagar S, Lawrence D, Nairn D, Bentley PG. Femoral vein thrombosis and total hip replacement. *Br Med J* 1977; **2**:223–25.

7 Moser KM, LeMoine JR. Is embolic risk conditioned by location of deep-venous thrombosis? *Ann Intern Med* 1981; **94**:439–44.

8 Lagerstedt CI, Olsson CG, Fagher BO, Oqvist BW, Albrechtsson U. Need for long-term anticoagulant treatment in symptomatic calf-vein thrombosis. *Lancet* 1985; **2**:515–18.

9 Moser KM, Fedullo PF, LitteJohn JK, Crawford R. Frequent asymptomatic pulmonary embolism in patients with deep-venous thrombosis. *JAMA* 1994; **271**:223–25.

10 Galle C, Papazyan JP, Miron MJ, Slosman D, Bounameaux H, Perrier A. Prediction of pulmonary embolism extent by clinical findings, D-dimer level and deep-vein thrombosis shown by ultrasound. *Thromb Haemost* 2001; **86**:1156–60.

11 Anand SS. Comparison of 3 and 6 months of oral anticoagulant therapy after a first episode of proximal deep-vein thrombosis or pulmonary embolism and comparison of 6 and 12 weeks of therapy after isolated calf deep-vein thrombosis. *Vasc Med* 2001; **6**:269–70.

12 Franchini M. Thrombotic complications in patients with hereditary bleeding disorders. *Thromb Haemost* 2004; **92**:298–304.

13 Buller HR, Agnelli G, Hull RD, Hyers TM, Prins MH, Raskob GE. Antithrombotic therapy for venous thromboembolic disease. *Chest* 2004; **126**:401S–28S.

14 Gordon SG, Franks JJ, Lewis B. Cancer procoagulant A: a factor X activating procoagulant from malignant tissue. *Thromb Res* 1975; **6**:127–37.

15 Hull R, Delmore T, Genton E, *et al.* Warfarin sodium versus low-dose heparin in the long-term treatment of venous thrombosis. *N Engl J Med* 1979; **301**:855–58.

16 Hull R, Delmore T, Carter C, *et al.* Adjusted subcutaneous heparin versus warfarin sodium in the long-term treatment of venous thrombosis. *N Engl J Med* 1982; **306**: 189–94.

17 Gould MK, Dembitzer AD, Doyle RL, Hastie TJ, Garber AM. Low-molecular-weight heparins compared with unfractionated heparin for treatment of acute deep venous thrombosis. A meta-analysis of randomized, controlled trials. *Ann Intern Med* 1999; **130**: 800–9.

18 Hyers TM, Agnelli G, Hull RD, *et al.* Antithrombotic therapy for venous thromboembolic disease. *Chest* 2001; **119**:176S–193S.

19 Mekkes JR, Loots MA, Van Der Wal AC, Bos JD. Causes, investigation and treatment of leg ulceration. *Br J Dermatol* 2003; **148**:388–401.

20 Schainfeld RM. Chronic venous insufficiency. *Curr Treat Options Cardiovasc Med* 2003; **5**:109–119.

21 Berard A, Abenhaim L, Platt R, Kahn SR, Steinmetz O. Risk factors for the first-time development of venous ulcers of the lower limbs: the influence of heredity and physical activity. *Angiology* 2002; **53**:647–57.

22 Ioannou CV, Giannoukas AD, Kostas T, *et al.* Patterns of venous reflux in limbs with venous ulcers. Implications for treatment. *Int Angiol* 2003; **22**:182–87.

23 Kahn SR, Solymoss S, Lamping DL, Abenhaim L. Long-term outcomes after deep-vein thrombosis: postphlebitic syndrome and quality of life. *J Gen Intern Med* 2000; **15**:425–29.

24 Strandness DE, Jr., Langlois Y, Cramer M, Randlett A, Thiele BL. Long-term sequelae of acute venous thrombosis. *JAMA* 1983; **250**:1289–92.

25 Saarinen JP, Domonyi K, Zeitlin R, Salenius JP. Postthrombotic syndrome after isolated calf deep-venous thrombosis: the role of popliteal reflux. *J Vasc Surg* 2002; **36**:959–64.

26 Lacroix P, Aboyans V, Preux PM, Houles MB, Laskar M. Epidemiology of venous insufficiency in an occupational population. *Int Angiol* 2003; **22**:172–76.

27 Meissner MH. Thrombolytic therapy for acute deep-vein thrombosis and the venous registry. *Rev Cardiovasc Med* 2002; **3**:S53–60.

28 Elsharawy M, Elzayat E. Early results of thrombolysis vs anticoagulation in iliofemoral venous thrombosis. A randomised clinical trial. *Eur J Vasc Endovasc Surg* 2002; **24**:209–14.

29 Chang R, Cannon RO, 3rd, Chen CC, *et al.* Daily catheter-directed single dosing of t-PA in treatment of acute deep-venous thrombosis of the lower extremity. *J Vasc Interv Radiol* 2001; **12**:247–52.

30 Cho JS, Martelli E, Mozes G, Miller VM, Gloviczki P. Effects of thrombolysis and venous thrombectomy on valvular competence, thrombogenicity, venous wall morphology, and function. *J Vasc Surg* 1998; **28**:787–99.

31 Meissner MH, Caps MT, Zierler BK, Bergelin RO, Manzo RA, Strandness DE, Jr. Deep-venous thrombosis and superficial venous reflux. *J Vasc Surg* 2000; **32**:48–56.

32 Vedantham S, Vesely TM, Parti N, Darcy M, Hovsepian DM, Picus D. Lower extremity venous thrombolysis with adjunctive mechanical thrombectomy. *J Vasc Interv Radiol* 2002; **13**:1001–8.

33 Delomez M, Beregi JP, Willoteaux S, *et al.* Mechanical thrombectomy in patients with deep-venous thrombosis. *Cardiovasc Intervent Radiol* 2001; **24**:42–48.

34 Kasirajan K, Gray B, Ouriel K. Percutaneous AngioJet thrombectomy in the management of extensive deep venous thrombosis. *J Vasc Interv Radiol* 2001; **12**:179–85.

35 Bush RL, Lin PH, Bates JT, Mureebe L, Zhou W, Lumsden AB. Pharmacomechanical thrombectomy for treatment of symptomatic lower extremity deep-venous thrombosis: safety and feasibility study. *J Vasc Surg* 2004; **40**:965–70.

36 McRae SJ, Ginsberg JS. Initial treatment of venous thromboembolism. *Circulation* 2004; **110**:I3–9.

CHAPTER 16

Vascular trauma

Ulises Baltazar, Esteban A. Henao, W. Todd Bohannon,
Michael B. Silva, Jr

The presentation of vascular injury may vary from simple intimal injury to full thickness rupture of the vessel wall. The former may further be complicated by dissection, where blood flow propagates between vessel wall layers, creating a separate, false lumen. The latter can result in extravasation, sometimes contained by the surrounding soft tissue, resulting in pseudoaneurysm. Fistulas between artery and vein may also result. Classically, treatment options for the spectrum of injuries seen in the vascular system have been surgical or medical. Currently, there are numerous endovascular alternatives that have been successfully performed.

The idea of placing intraarterial stents to treat vascular disease is not new. In 1969, Dotter published his experience with a "coil-spring endarterial tube graft."[1] Then in 1991, Becker published a case report describing the percutaneous placement of a balloon-expandable graft in the subclavian artery for life-threatening hemorrhage.[2] Since then, the endovascular field has introduced new methods to safely manage traumatic vascular injuries that can be dangerous to approach and difficult to repair otherwise.

An inherent advantage of the endovascular treatment of trauma is the use of angiography. This allows the delineation of vascular anatomy and its relationship to entry and exit wounds, location of bleeding areas, and adjacent landmarks for the positioning and deployment of catheters, stents, coils, or other therapeutic modalities. It has also been shown that endovascular techniques decrease the blood loss, extent of dissection, and anesthesia requirements.[3] Additionally, standard surgical approaches can be complemented by endovascular adjuncts, such as the occlusion balloon, which can be safely used for proximal and distal control of vessels. Some endovascular solutions are becoming the standard of care, as with embolization techniques in the treatment of pelvic hemorrhage.[4]

Endovascular therapy for traumatic injuries of the vascular tree should be limited to the stable patient. Trauma victims that are unstable or difficult to resuscitate should proceed to the operating theater for further stabilization and definitive intervention. Clinical assessment is essential in evaluating the hard and soft signs of vascular injury that can prompt further evaluation with angiography, and possible endoluminal intervention.

Endovascular techniques in vascular trauma

Preoperative administration of crystalloid and blood products should continue as dictated by the patient's clinical condition, and the surgeon's judgment. Preoperative antibiotics should be administered, especially if endovascular prosthesis insertion is considered. Intravenous heparinization should also be considered, depending on the degree of concomitant injuries or other contraindications to administration.

Prior to initiating any endovascular procedure, one should ensure that the patient is properly situated on an angiography table. Availability and a working knowledge of the loading and deployment of contrast from a power injector is also a prerequisite. The endovascular surgeon should also be familiar with the inventory at his or her institution so that materials may be readily available for deployment during the trauma evaluation. One should also be prepared to convert to the standard open procedure at all times.

Remote vascular access is then obtained, most commonly by percutaneous right or left femoral access. This is described in detail elsewhere in the text. With major pelvic bone trauma or tissue loss at the inguinal access site, the contralateral femoral or left brachial puncture should be performed. In the hypotensive patient, ultrasound guidance or bone landmarks under fluoroscopy can be extremely useful to obtain access. If the femoral vein is punctured, a sheath should be placed to serve as a landmark for arterial puncture as well as an additional line for resuscitation.

The brachial artery can be palpated in the medial aspect of the arm between the fibers of the biceps and triceps muscles. Ideally, a 21-gauge needle is used 3–4 cm above the elbow crease, to cannulate the artery followed by 0.018 in. wire. The wire is extremely flexible; if it is forced in the soft tissue or vasculature, it can coil on itself, potentially causing further injury and delay in definitive therapy. After the lumen is cannulated, the access wire and dilator are removed, and 0.035 in. wire can be inserted. The access sheath is then exchanged for an appropriately sized sheath, and diagnostic angiography of the vascular bed in question is performed.

Endovascular devices in vascular trauma

The most common indication for intraarterial stent placement in traumatic related injuries is arterial dissections.[5] Options include the Wallstent (Boston Scientific), which is a self-expanding stent made of superalloy braided in a tubular mesh configuration, and the Express stent (Boston Scientific), which is a laser cut balloon expandable stainless steel stent. Stents can also include coverings, such as the Wallgraft (Boston Scientific) and Viabahn (WL Gore, Flagstaff, AZ). Both are self-expanding stents covered with Dacron polyester and thin PTFE, respectively. The Viabahn has a nitinol exoskeleton with a pull-string deployment system used in most Gore devices. The pullback deployment mechanism of the Wallgraft is similar to the Wallstent. All these devices are compatible with 0.035 in. wires. Larger diameter stent grafts can be constructed with Palmaz stents (Johnson & Johnson Interventional Systems, Warren, NJ) with thin ePTFE secured with suture made of PTFE or polypropylene. Endovascular tube grafts have been used to treat aortic traumatic injuries. Modular parts from endograft devices commercially available in the United States can potentially be used for short segment injuries to the aortoiliac tree.

Blood vessel obliteration can be achieved with coils, polyvinyl alcohol (PVA), gelfoam or acrylic copolymer spheres, among others commercially available. Coils come in standard size configurations, such as the platinum-based 0.035 in Tornado coils (Cook, Bloomington, IN) or variable size configurations found in the Vortex coil (Boston Scientific) available in 0.018, 0.021, and 0.038 in. diameters. Others, such as the Gianturco or Guglielmi detachable coils are also available. PVA is a semipermanent occlusive agent with a limited potential for recanalization. This particle has the property of expanding up to 15 times its original size when in contact with blood. The precise site of arterial occlusion cannot be seen directly because it is radiolucent, so it is assessed indirectly with analysis of repeated aniographic studies during embolization, requiring increased use of contrast.[6] Gelfoam (Upjohn, Kalamazoo, MI) is a gelatin sponge with a high grade of recanalization. It is useful for temporary control of small, terminal branches. Embospheres and EmboGold (Biosphere Medical Inc, Rockland, MA) are spherical, hydrophilic, microporous beads made of an acrylic co-polymer, which is then crosslinked with gelatin. EmboGold has a radioopaque coating that allows easy visualization with fluoroscopy. They constitute an alternative option to PVA. Other agents have been used in the past, such as autologous blood clots, fat particles and liquid tissue adhesives (isobutyl-2-cyanoacrylate).

Carotid artery trauma

The reported incidence of carotid injuries varies widely, ranging between 0.3 and 20%.[7] Blunt trauma to the carotid occurs at 0.1–0.45%, with mortality rates as high as 20–40%.[8] Penetrating carotid injuries account for about 3% of injuries.[9] Clinical findings that support diagnostic workup include mandibular or facial fractures, C2–C3 fractures, neck contusion or laceration, neck hematoma, and mechanism of injury (deceleration). Penetrating zone II trauma with hard signs, such as bleeding, expanding hematoma, or loss of carotid pulses with acute neurologic deficits mandates immediate surgical exploration without further studies.

Duplex ultrasound can identify dissection as well as pseudoaneurysm. It is operator dependent and zone I or III lesions are difficult to visualize. Any abnormal findings, such as turbulent flow, reduced flow velocity, absence of flow, or presence of an echolucent intraluminal lesion, should lower the threshold for further investigation with angiography. CT angiography has been used for penetrating injuries of the neck with a 75% sensitivity to diagnose

(a) 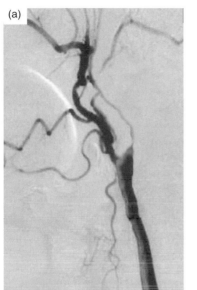 (b)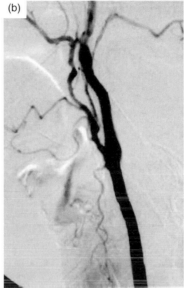

Figure 16.1 Blunt traumatic to the carotid artery. (a) Carotid angiogram demonstrating a dissection originating from the proximal carotid artery. (b) The dissection was successfully treated with a self-expanding stent placement.

venous vascular injury.[10,11] However, digital subtraction angiography is still the gold standard for diagnostic carotid artery injuries and offers the opportunity for therapy. Traumatic carotid lesions amenable to endovascular treatment are intimal dissection, pseudoaneurysm and arteriovenous fistula.[12–15]

Treatment options for carotid dissections with intact distal flow include surgical repair, endovascular stenting, or observation with repeat diagnostic studies 1–2 weeks after the injury. However, systemic heparinization in patients without contraindication is the current standard.[9] Surgical approaches are rarely done. Noncovered stents are usually placed to treat short dissections (Figure 16.1).[16,17] If the site of entry is identified, an attempt at placement can be considered for extended dissections if anticoagulation is contraindicated.

Pseudoaneurysms are usually the result of dissections, and when large, tend to expand and cause compressive symptoms, requiring operation or embolization.[18,19] Surgical intervention can be complex, especially for lesions near the skull base, where temporomandibular joint subluxation or vertical ramus osteotomy may be required to obtain exposure. Covered stents are the prosthesis of choice to exclude pseudoaneurysm. Coils have also been used to treat these lesions and in some cases both have been applied.[18,19] The major risk in treating pseudoaneurysms is distal embolization and stroke. The use of distal protection devices is limited to clinical trials.

Technique

A femoral approach or direct cervical operative exposure can be used as the entry options for carotid endoluminal intervention. A 180 cm starter wire is introduced to the abdominal aorta, followed by placement of a 5 Fr sheath. The wire is advanced to the aortic arch under fluoroscopic guidance where a pigtail catheter is positioned in the ascending aorta. The C-arm is positioned to left anterior oblique (LAO) at 30° for visualizing the tip of the catheter to the midcervical spine. Digital subtraction angiography is performed with the injector set for delivery of 15 mL/s for a total of 30 mL of contrast. The peak opacified image is saved as a landmark in order to selectively cannulate the appropriate ostia. The Simmons 1 or 2 catheter (Boston Scientific) is an excellent tool. These catheters have a long, gentle "hook" form that, at the time of guidewire insertion, is lost. The Simmons catheters can then be reformed against the aortic valve, the subclavian artery, or the iliac artery. Ideally, the wire should be advanced into the left subclavian artery, with the catheter following into the vessel. The wire is then partially removed and the catheter is pushed forward, reforming its original shape.

The other option is to place the catheter in the ascending aorta, partially remove the wire, and rotate the catheter on its own axis in a gentle fashion, allowing it to recover its original shape. All motions are accomplished under fluoroscopy guidance, to help avoid an accidental "knotting" of the catheter. Once the catheter is reformed, gentle movements are performed to bring the tip into the appropriate position in relation to the landmark of the artery in question. Once the catheter "hooks" the vessel ostium, withdrawing motions are applied to advance the catheter. The wire is then advanced gently to access the target artery. Particular care is taken not to advance the wire too distally in the internal carotid artery. It may be helpful to use about 2 cc of contrast at this point to corroborate position.

Carotid angiography is performed with a power injection of 4 cc/s for a total of 7 cc of contrast in arterioposterior (AP) and lateral positions. Additional views (i.e. oblique) may be needed to properly assess the anatomy and extent of injury. The intracranial circulation is also evaluated with AP and lateral views with similar power injector settings. In order to cannulate the left internal carotid, starting from the ostium of the innominate, the catheter is carefully advanced until it disengages the artery. The catheter is then rotated 15° anteriorly until the landmark for the vessel is reached. This technique avoids the need for wire reinsertion. After the wire is carefully advanced, a straight Glide catheter (Boston Scientific) or angle catheter is advanced over the wire, and injection of 3–5 cc of contrast is done to demonstrate the lumen. A stiff Glidewire or Amplatz is then exchanged, and a long sheath is placed prior to any intervention. This maneuver is fundamental in order to prevent accidental loss of access.

From this position in the carotid, any number of modalities can be used to treat a particular lesion. An appropriate bare or covered stent may be deployed. It is a good option to use balloon angioplasty to help "size" the vessel in question to minimize discrepancy in proximal and distal size landing points. Alternatively, a standard or microcatheter may be used, depending on the degree of vessel selectivity, to place coils strategically in the vascular bed to eliminate sources of hemorrhage. Yet another mode is to combine covered stenting and coil deployment in the treatment of large pseudoaneurysms.

Subclavian and axillary arterial injuries

Penetrating injury of the subclavian and axillary arteries is far more common than blunt lesions. Of the 93 cases of subclavian artery injury reported by Graham and associates, only two were related to blunt mechanism.[20,21] Subclavian and axillary arterial injury is blunt in 3% and less than 1% of reported cases, respectively.[20,21] Surgical exploration has been the standard of care, but remains invasive and extensive, with possible approaches including supra and infraclavicular dissections, median sternotomy and, thoracotomy.[22] These difficult anatomical approaches, along with substantial tissue edema, and significant blood loss have contributed to reported mortality rates between 3% and 33%. Absolute indications for angiogram at the initial evaluation are absence of pulses, persistent shock despite resuscitation, and copious intrathoracic bleeding. Relative indications include injury with associated brachial plexus palsy, fractured clavicle and concomitant fracture of the first three ribs, supraclavicular contusion with or without hematoma and soft tissue injury of the neck and upper extremity.[22]

A recent series published by du Toit demonstrated the feasibility of endovascular approaches to subclavian and axillary arterial injuries.[23] Ten patients with penetrating injuries ($N = 9$ from gunshot wounds, $n = 1$ from a stab wound) were treated with stent graft deployment. No deaths, amputations, or procedure-related morbidities were noted, and short-term follow up of 7 months demonstrated no evidence of stenosis or occlusion. Xenos and colleagues recently compared their open versus endovascular experience of subclavian and axillary artery injuries, noting significantly less blood loss and procedure time with the stenting group, and no difference in patency rate between the two groups at 1 year.[24] Long-term patency rates are unknown. However, in a patient who is a poor candidate for general anesthesia or has a poor life expectancy, stent placement is clearly a viable option. Lacerations, intimal flaps, vessel occlusion, pseudoaneurysm, arteriovenous fistulas, and avulsion of branches can be treated with covered stents (Figure 16.2). In those patients who are to undergo an open procedure, endovascular approaches can serve as an adjunct to vascular control, as with balloon occlusion devices.[25]

Technique

The site of injury can be approached remotely, either through femoral or brachial percutaneous access, or brachial cutdown. For a dissection or intimal

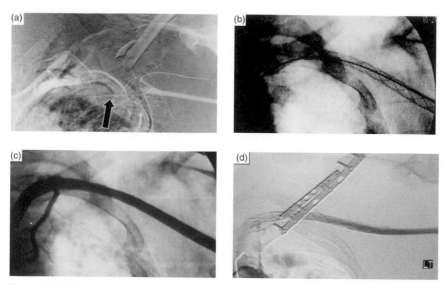

Figure 16.2 Blunt trauma to the shoulder. (a) A severe blunt trauma resulted in a scapulothoracic dissociation with clavicle fracture and subclavian artery transection (arrow). (b) A Wallgraft was used to repair the arterial injury. (c) Angiogram demonstrated subclavian artery patency. (d) The arterial repair was followed by clavicle fixation.

flap, it is imperative to cannulate the true lumen, which can be facilitated through a brachial cut down, as dissections rarely reach the arm. The brachial artery also offers a more direct, less tortuous approach to the repair. It is feasible to gain access from both a femoral and brachial site, and establish continuity in the injured vessel by traversing the defect with a guidewire, and subsequently come across the lesion from the opposite side with a snare device to control the wire. Only select lesions that can be traversed by a guidewire should be approached from an endovascular perspective.

Active bleeding in a stable patient can be treated with covered stents (Figure 16.3). However, this particular anatomic area is subject to possible compression effects between the clavicle and the first rib. There may be a discrepancy as to the degree this has on stents placed in trauma patients versus those that are afflicted with thoracic outlet syndrome or occlusive disease. Probably, the best performance is obtained from a Wallstent or Wallgraft (Boston Scientific). During the deployment of a stent graft, occlusion of side branches can occur, and careful clinical and radiological judgment is basic for these procedures. In the treatment of pseudoaneurysms of the subclavian or axillary artery, active attempts at thrombosis with coils or other embolic means to eliminate flow into the sac may be necessary due to the large collateral circulation. There are also cases in which branch vessels may need to be dealt with individually, such as in penetrating injury of the right internal mammary artery, where coil embolization may be useful selectively.

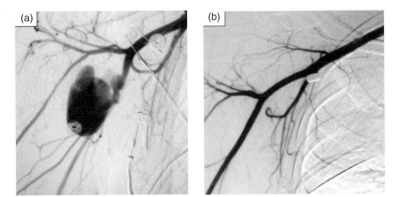

Figure 16.3 Gun shot wound to the subclavian artery. (a) Angiogram demonstrating a large bleeding pseudoaneurysm in the right axillary artery. (b) The injury was successfully treated with a covered stent.

Thoracic aortic injury

Thoracic aortic injury is usually fatal. It is estimated that 80–90% of the victims die at the scene and 30% of survivors die within 6 h.[26,27] Most of the injuries are distal to the left subclavian artery. The ligamentum arteriosum offers a fixed point that can cause distal arterial injury (i.e. transection, tear, or intimal injury). The suspicion should be raised after mechanism of injury, clinical symptoms, and portable chest X-ray. In recent years, software for helical computed tomography has improved the quality of the images. The aortogram remains the gold standard study for diagnosis of thoracic aortic injury, however, sensitivity and specificity for helical computed tomography are 100% and 83% and for digital subtraction angiogram are 92% and 99%, respectively.[28]

For those patients who survive such insult, the standard of care is surgical repair with a prosthetic repair. The mortality for this approach is close to 30–40% and paraplegia between 8% and 14% among other comorbidities.[26,27] The timing of the surgery has been a subject of controversy.[29] While bleeding and occlusion mandates immediate open approach, the contained injury in a patient with multiple major injuries (i.e. head injury, pulmonary contusion, hemodynamically unstable), treatment can be deferred. The medical management is based on beta blockers and agents to reduce afterload. Kasirajan and associates recently published their series of open versus endovascular treatment of acute thoracic aortic trauma.[30] They found that the endovascular group had shorter operative times, less blood requirements, longer ICU length of stay, and lower overall mortality rates when compared with open repair group. Endovascular repair also favors those that are unable to maintain single lung ventilation or those with concomitant injury prohibiting heparinization (Figure 16.4).

Endovascular therapy for thoracic aortic injury has opened new treatment options as well as new debates. Several stent grafts are undergoing clinical

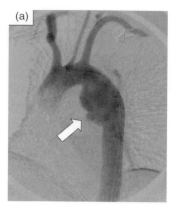 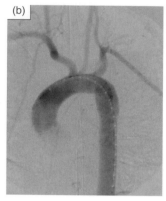

Figure 16.4 Aortic transection due to blunt trauma. (a) Aortogram demonstrating an aortic transection distal to the left subclavian artery (arrow). (b) A stent graft was used, which successfully repair the aortic transection.

investigations in the United States, including the Gore TAG thoracic endo-prosthesis (WL Gore, Flagstaff, AZ) and the Talent thoracic stent-graft system (Medtronic, Santa Rosa, CA). Several drawbacks have been proposed for the use of endografts. First, the need for a neck length between 10 and 20 mm is required for a landing zone. In order to achieve this, the left subclavian artery may be covered. Ischemia of the left upper extremity can be prevented or treated with a carotid subclavian bypass. However, subclavian artery exclusion is welltolerated in most individuals. Second, the concern remains regarding proximal fixation and endoleaks. It is difficult to follow the aortic arch contour due to the nonflexible nature of the proximal segment of the stents. The patient is subjected to long-term follow up for endoleaks. Third, the need for controlled, transient hypotension during deployment is the key for a successful and precise placement. This also can result in further comorbidities in an already critical patient. Fourth, there is a need for heparinization. Anticoagulation is recommended when a large delivery device is placed in the vascular system to decrease embolization or occlusion. In a trauma setting, this represents a risk with potential deleterious outcome.

Technique

The procedure is performed under general anesthesia and is important to have full capability to convert into an open procedure if necessary. The standard advanced trauma life support (ATLS) regimen should proceed as necessary, although fluid resuscitation and mean arterial pressure should be tapered, so as not to apply more pressure on the traumatized segment. The pigtail catheter for angiogram can be placed through a brachial or femoral approach. A femoral cut down access is the preferred device entry site. Since the average sheath diameter is 22–24 Fr, it could potentially be helpful to verify the diameter of the external and common iliac arteries and fabricate an iliac conduit with PTFE to accommodate the delivery system if necessary. After reviewing the films, the size of the graft is usually oversized by 10–20%. If exclusion of the left subclavian is anticipated, a carotid subclavian bypass may be constructed. If external compression of the main bronchus is present due to thrombus, this will not be relieved by endograft placement and a bronchial stent may be deployed to alleviate atelectasis. Completion angiogram is obtained through the pigtail catheter and if type I endoleaks are identified, balloon angioplasty or, if unsuccessful, a proximal aortic cuff placement is indicated. If the result is satisfactory the femoral arteriotomy is repaired and incision is closed. The brachial sheath is removed and manual pressure is applied for 20–30 min, always corroborating adequate distal perfusion. Completion helical computed tomography is obtained as baseline study for future follow up.

Aortoiliac and femoral arterial injury

The overall mortality for blunt abdominal aortic injury is 24%.[31] Most of the experience in the endovascular arena is after treatment of infrarenal abdominal aortic aneurysm. Penetrating injuries after gun shot wounds or iatrogenic injuries during catheter-based procedures are the main source of experience for endovascular therapy after trauma (Figure 16.5). The lesions to treat usually are lacerations, pseudoaneurysms, intimal flaps with dissections and arteriovenous fistulas. The traumatic injury of the iliac arteries is usually associated with penetrating injury and in some cases secondary to a pelvic fracture. To treat the latter etiology, an endovascular approach seems ideal since retroperitoneal dissection of the pelvic area could increase bleeding after releasing the tamponade effect from the pelvic fracture. Successful coil embolization controls

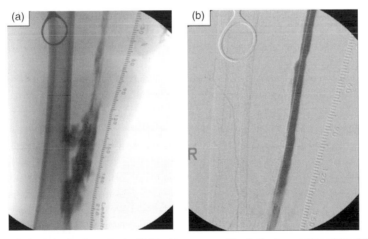

Figure 16.5 Angiogram of a patient with blunt trauma resulting in the transection of the right superficial femoral artery. (a) Contrast extravasation is seen at the site of vessel transection. (b) A covered stent was deployed that successfully restored the artery patency.

internal iliac artery bleeding after pelvic fracture. An unusual etiology is after hip surgery, where the external iliac artery can be damaged.[32]

The femoral artery injuries are usually approached with open operative techniques. Significant deformity, secondary to edema and bleedingm, could be an indication for endovascular treatment. The usual lesions are secondary to penetrating injuries or lacerations secondary to femur fractures. Iatrogenic injuries after the use of thrombectomy catheters or after balloon angioplasty therapy are not uncommon. The lesions can be pseudoaneurysms, lacerations, and arteriovenous fistulas. Surgical treatment is required in bleeding with persistent shock, arterial thrombosis, and compression of neurovascular bundle.

Successful embolization of epigastric branches or the profunda femoral artery can also be accomplished. The use of stents across a joint is typically held in disfavor. In acute situations, when a surgical approach is precluded, endovascular therapy with covered stents opens a new therapeutic option.

Technique

Aortoiliac arterial injury can be accessed via percutaneous or cut down of the common femoral artery. After standard approach is completed, a 5 Fr sheath is introduced under fluoroscopic guidance. A pigtail catheter is introduced to obtain the initial aortogram and pelvic views. Adequate visualization of the internal iliac arteries usually requires anterior oblique views. If the injury to treat is a dissection, cannulation of the true lumen can be a challenge. A contralateral approach or through the brachial artery is chosen in order to access the true lumen and the wire is fed into the femoral arteries. The up and over technique is usually simplified with the use of a contra flush catheter (Boston Scientific).

After the angiogram is completed, the bifurcation is identified. A 0.035 in. starter wire is introduced about 1–3 mm beyond the catheter tip. The catheter is rotated toward the common iliac artery to be cannulated and a gentle, slow withdrawing movement is done until the catheter or wire hooks the orifice of the artery, at which point the wire is advanced into the artery to be treated. If cannulation is difficult, a Bern catheter (Boston Scientific) is typically helpful to direct the wire in the chosen lumen. A Glidewire (Boston Scientific) can also be useful in negotiating difficult anatomy. It can be difficult for a stent graft to go up and over the aortic bifurcation. A cut down on the affected limb will allow the making of an arteriotomy in the common femoral arteries, making possible the manual manipulation of the wire, keeping the cannulation within the true lumen. After this is completed, the stiff end of the wire is advanced into the aorta, an exchange catheter is carefully inserted, the wire is removed, and then reversed, or a super stiff wire is inserted if the device has been selected. For an aortic injury, an aortic stent graft can be deployed to treat the lesion. On some occasions an aortic cuff or "home made" (Palmaz stent with PFTE) stent graft can also be utilized for pseudoaneurysm, arteriovenous fistulas, or lacerations.

For dissections in the iliac system a balloon expandable stent is a good choice. We use the Express stent (Boston Scientific) that has the benefit of controlled deployment, allowing precise placement.

For femoral injuries, the best approach utilizes the standard "up and over" technique. Oblique views may be useful for adequate imaging of the profunda femoris artery. Cannulation of small branches, as in other vascular beds, can be assisted with the use of Glidewires in different calibers, such as the 0.018 and 0.035. in. The correct catheter shape can also facilitate this task. The Renegade Hi-Flo microcatheter (Boston Scientific) is a 0.027 in. system that allows one to cannulate small vessels for embolization.

Abdominal and pelvic artery trauma

Visceral bleeding is the major determinant of mortality during the first 4 h after traumatic injury. Most injuries in an acute-trauma setting are initially found on computed tomography. Hemodynamically unstable patients should proceed directly to the OR for exploration. However, those individuals that are hemodynamically stable and demonstrate active bleeding on computed tomography may benefit from the diagnostic and potentially therapeutic efforts of endovascular evaluation, beginning with angiography.

Splenic injuries are more commonly being treated nonoperatively. Those patients who demonstrate contrast blush and blunt injury when treated with selective embolization have been shown to be successfully hemostatic in 87–95% of cases.[33] The fundamental goal of endovascular embolization is to preserve splenic tissue. Davis and colleagues recently reported their experience with embolization of traumatic pseudoaneurysms of the spleen, with a significant improvement in their nonoperative approach to splenic trauma.[34] Most series resulted in less transfusion requirements and less complications than operative repair.

Liver injury accounts for 15–20% of blunt abdominal injuries.[31,35] Penetrating injuries to the abdomen most frequently affect the liver. Hepatic artery embolization is generally indicated in cases of continued bleeding, and those that remain difficult to resuscitate in the setting of an abnormal tomogram showing hepatic parenchymal extravasation. More high-grade liver injuries are being treated with catheter-directed embolization, resulting in fewer blood transfusions and reduced open operative intervention.[36]

Traumatic injury to the pelvis accounts for 6–8% of all trauma deaths. Pelvic arterial rupture is associated with a 50–75% mortality rate.[37,38] Most bleeding, however, occurs from disruption of the sacral venous plexus. The level of instability often mandates external fixation of the pelvis to minimize hemorrhage. Bleeding from lateral compression, vertical shear, and combined injury mechanisms are often associated with arterial trauma. Open surgical intervention of zone III retroperitoneal hematoma is not indicated, but can be a major source of blood loss. Most bleeding stops after fixation, unless it is from an arterial source, at which point in the workup the patient should proceed

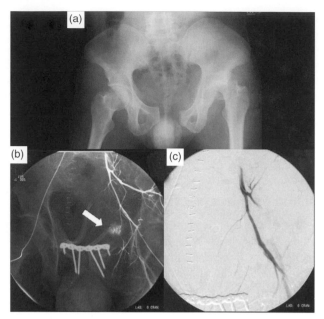

Figure 16.6 Pelvic trauma.(a) A severe blunt trauma to the pelvis caused a massive pelvic hemorrhage and an unstable pelvic fracture. (b) Following pelvic stabilization, angiogram demonstrating a bleeding pelvic arterial branch. (c) The bleeding vessel was successfully treated with coil embolization.

to angiography and possible embolization (Figure 16.6). Matalon and associates have demonstrated an 85–94% success rate in obtaining hemostasis in posttraumatic arterial injuries to the pelvis.[39]

Technique

Contralateral femoral access from the suspected bleeding site of injury is preferred. A 5-French pigtail catheter can then be used to perform abdominal and pelvic angiography to delineate bleeding source(s). A-3 French microcatheter inside a 5-French steerable catheter can then be used to obtain accurate, selective placement for embolization. Liquid and powdered embolizing agents, such as alcohol and gelfoam, respectively, should be avoided due to the risk of nerve damage and distal embolization. Gelfoam pledges soaked in antibiotics combined with coil placement can be used together for safer, optimal hemostatic results.

Conclusion

Trauma to the vascular system presents several challenges to the surgeon, in both diagnosis and treatment. Exposure to central anatomic positions can add time, blood loss, and potential for morbidity and mortality. Although long-term data is still being collected for newer approaches, endovascular techniques show promise in minimizing these potential problems. At the same time, they do not necessarily exclude the possibility of open intervention during the same procedure, or at a separate, possibly more optimal, time. As devices continue to evolve, and techniques continue to be perfected, more indications for endovascular interventions will undoubtedly become accepted. However, treatment based on sound clinical judgment and patient selection will do more to determine the fate of endovascular surgery. Endovascular techniques are already utilized widely in clinical practice and they can provide similar clinical applications in vascular trauma. Vascular surgeons should be familiar with a broad array of endovascular techniques to provide the best treatment for the individual patient, considering anatomic location of injury, concomitant injuries, and overall clinical status to assure the best possible outcomes.

References

1 Dotter CT. Transluminally-placed coilspring endarterial tube grafts. Long-term patency in canine popliteal artery. *Invest Radiol* 1969; 4:329–32.

2 Becker GJ, Benenati JF, Zemel G, *et al.* Percutaneous placement of a balloon-expandable intraluminal graft for life-threatening subclavian arterial hemorrhage. *J Vasc Interv Radiol* 1991; 2:225–29.

3 Parodi JC, Schonholz C, Ferreira LM, Bergan J. Endovascular stent-graft treatment of traumatic arterial lesions. *Ann Vasc Surg* 1999; 13:121 29.

4 Chaufour J, Melki JP, Riche MC, *et al.* Hemorrhagic vascular complications of pelvic fractures. The role of embolization. 9 cases. *Presse Med* 1986; 15:2097–100.

5 McArthur CS, Marin ML. Endovascular therapy for the treatment of arterial trauma. *Mt Sinai J Med* 2004; 71:4–11.

6 Matsumaru Y, Hyodo A, Nose T, Hirano T, Ohashi S. Embolic materials for endovascular treatment of cerebral lesions. *J Biomater Sci Polym Ed* 1997; 8:555–69.

7 Nanda A, Vannemreddy PS, Willis BK, Baskaya MK, Jawahar A. Management of carotid artery injuries: Louisiana State University Shreveport experience. *Surg Neurol* 2003; 59:184–90; discussion 190.

8 Singh RR, Barry MC, Ireland A, Bouchier Hayes D. Current diagnosis and management of blunt internal carotid artery injury. *Eur J Vasc Endovasc Surg* 2004; 27:577–84.

9 Feliciano DV. Management of penetrating injuries to carotid artery. *World J Surg* 2001; 25:1028–35.

10 Munera F, Soto JA, Nunez D. Penetrating injuries of the neck and the increasing role of CTA. *Emerg Radiol* 2004; 10:303–9.

11 LeBlang SD, Nunez DB, Jr. Helical CT of cervical spine and soft tissue injuries of the neck. *Radiol Clin North Am* 1999; 37:515–32, v–vi.

12 ul Haq T, Yaqoob J, Munir K, Usman MU. Endovascular-covered stent treatment of posttraumatic cervical carotid artery pseudoaneurysms. *Australas Radiol* 2004; 48:220–23.

13 Biggs KL, Chiou AC, Hagino RT, Klucznik RP. Endovascular repair of a spontaneous carotid artery dissection with carotid stent and coils. *J Vasc Surg* 2004; 40:170–73.

14 Lo D, Vallee JN, Bitar A, *et al.* Endovascular management of carotid-cavernous fistula combined with ipsilateral internal carotid artery occlusion due to gunshot: contra-lateral arterial approach. *Acta Neurochir (Wien)* 2004; **146**:403–6; discussion 406.

15 Redekop G, Marotta T, Weill A. Treatment of traumatic aneurysms and arteriovenous fistulas of the skull base by using endovascular stents. *J Neurosurg* 2001; **95**:412–19.

16 Kremer C, Mosso M, Georgiadis D, *et al.* Carotid dissection with permanent and transient occlusion or severe stenosis: Long-term outcome. *Neurology* 2003; **60**:271–75.

17 Malek AM, Higashida RT, Phatouros CC, Lempert TE, Meyers PM, Smith WS, *et al.* Endovascular management of extracranial carotid artery dissection achieved using stent angioplasty. *AJNR Am J Neuroradiol* 2000; **21**:1280–92.

18 Bush RL, Lin PH, Najibi S, Dion JE, Smith RB, III. Coil embolization combined with carotid-subclavian bypass for treatment of subclavian artery aneurysm. *J Endovasc Ther* 2002; **9**:308–12.

19 Bush RL, Lin PH, Dodson TF, Dion JE, Lumsden AB. Endoluminal stent placement and coil embolization for the management of carotid artery pseudoaneurysms. *J Endovasc Ther* 2001; **8**:53–61.

20 Graham JM, Mattox KL, Feliciano DV, DeBakey ME. Vascular injuries of the axilla. *Ann Surg* 1982; **195**:232–38.

21 Graham JM, Feliciano DV, Mattox KL, Beall AC, Jr., DeBakey ME. Management of subclavian vascular injuries. *J Trauma* 1980; **20**:537–44.

22 Lin PH, Koffron AJ, Guske PJ, *et al.* Penetrating injuries of the subclavian artery. *Am J Surg* 2003; **185**:580–84.

23 du Toit DF, Leith JG, Strauss DC, Blaszczyk M, Odendaal Jde V, Warren BL. Endovas-cular management of traumatic cervicothoracic arteriovenous fistula. *Br J Surg* 2003; **90**:1516–21.

24 Xenos ES, Freeman M, Stevens S, Cassada D, Pacanowski J, Goldman M. Covered stents for injuries of subclavian and axillary arteries. *J Vasc Surg* 2003; **38**:451–54.

25 Bakhritdinov F, Zufarov MM, Babadzhanov SA. The use of balloon occlusion of subclavian artery defect in patients with traumatic injuries. *Angiol Sosud Khir* 2003; **9**:41–42.

26 Graham JM, Feliciano DV, Mattox KL, Beall AC, Jr. Innominate vascular injury. *J Trauma* 1982; **22**:647–55.

27 Feliciano DV, Mattox KL. Thoracic and vascular injuries. *Compr Ther* 1979; **5**:24–29.

28 Wintermark M, Wicky S, Schnyder P. Imaging of acute traumatic injuries of the thoracic aorta. *Eur Radiol* 2002; **12**:431–42.

29 Fattori R, Napoli G, Lovato L, *et al.* Indications for, timing of, and results of catheter-based treatment of traumatic injury to the aorta. *AJR Am J Roentgenol* 2002; **179**:603–9.

30 Kasirajan K, Heffernan D, Langsfeld M. Acute thoracic aortic trauma: a comparison of endoluminal stent grafts with open repair and nonoperative management. *Ann Vasc Surg* 2003; **17**:589–95.

31 Keller MS. Blunt injury to solid abdominal organs. *Semin Pediatr Surg* 2004; **13**:106–11.

32 Freischlag JA, Sise M, Quinones-Baldrich WJ, Hye RJ, Sedwitz MM. Vascular complica-tions associated with orthopedic procedures. *Surg Gynecol Obstet* 1989; **169**:147–52.

33 Dent D, Alsabrook G, Erickson BA, *et al.* Blunt splenic injuries: high nonoperative management rate can be achieved with selective embolization. *J Trauma* 2004; **56**:1063–7.

34 Davis KA, Fabian TC, Croce MA, *et al.* Improved success in nonoperative management of blunt splenic injuries: embolization of splenic artery pseudoaneurysms. *J Trauma* 1998; **44**:1008–13; discussion 1013–15.

35 Letoublon C, Arvieux C. Nonoperative management of blunt hepatic trauma. *Minerva Anestesiol* 2002; **68**:132–37.

36 Wahl WL, Ahrns KS, Brandt MM, Franklin GA, Taheri PA. The need for early angiographic embolization in blunt liver injuries. *J Trauma* 2002; **52**:1097–101.

37 Hotker U, Rommens PM. Blunt abdominal trauma and severe pelvic rupture. What to do? *Acta Chir Belg* 1997; **97**:65–8.

38 Brown JJ, Greene FL, McMillin RD. Vascular injuries associated with pelvic fractures. *Am Surg* 1984; **50**:150–54.

39 Matalon TS, Athanasoulis CA, Margolies MN, *et al.* Hemorrhage with pelvic fractures: efficacy of transcatheter embolization. *AJR Am J Roentgenol* 1979; **133**:859–64.

CHAPTER 17

Endovascular devices in peripheral interventions

Russell Lam, Mai Pham, Rakesh Safaya

The modern era of peripheral endovascular interventions began with Seldinger's description of percutaneous transfemoral access for guidewire and catheter placement in 1953.[1] A subsequent report in 1964 by Charles T Dotter, who described the first percutanous transluminal angioplasty to recanalize an occluded artery, underscored the importance of endovascular devices in peripheral interventions.[2] Since then, many cardinal works by pioneers including Andreas Gruentzig who performed the first coronary balloon angioplasty and Juan Parodi who performed the first endoluminal abdominal aortic aneurysm (AAA) repair all highlighted the critical role of endoluminal devices in arterial interventions.[3,4] While there are innumerous endovascular catheter-based tools used in peripheral interventions, this chapter provides a broad overview on some of the most commonly used endoluminal devices, including diagnostic catheters, stents, and stent grafts.

Diagnostic catheters

Catheters serve as a conduit that provides an access to a designated vascular structure. Today, catheters are manufactured in a preformed configuration and available in almost any shape. Catheters are constructed from a variety of materials, including nylon, polyethylene, Teflon, and polyurethane. Polyethylene is relatively easy to shape into a given configuration, and it remains a commonly used catheter-based material. Teflon yields a slippery property and can be used to pass through densely adherent vascular environment. Nylon, in contrast, provides increased stiffness and torque-control characteristics. In general, the most commonly used diagnostic catheters are 4 Fr or 5 Fr in diameter. Catheter lengths are usually 65 cm for abdominal or pelvic angiography and 90 cm or longer for thoracic or carotid angiography.

The most defining characteristic of a catheter is its configuration, as shaped by its distal curvature. Some basic catheter configurations are used in almost all cases. In contrast, certain uniquely shaped catheters are designed specifically for a particular arterial vasculature. In order to selectively cannulate a particular vessel, the catheter tip must be angled or curved in such a way to engage the vessel origin. Such catheter tips can be simple or complex, depending on

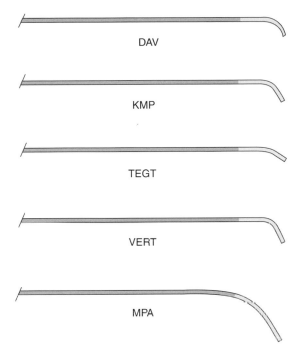

DAV

KMP

TEGT

VERT

MPA

Figure 17.1 Commonly used angled-catheters.

the number of curves configured at the tip. An angled-tip catheter can be used for selecting an angled vessel branch or a bifurcation branch vessel. They are commonly used for upward branch vessels such as cerebral and subclavian arteries. Commonly used angled catheters with a simple curve or hockey-stick shaped tip are illustrated in Figure 17.1. Certain aortic visceral branches, such as the celiac or superior mesenteric artery, have a sharp angled origin, which may be difficult to cannulate. These vessels may require a hook-shaped catheter, which can be reformed in the aorta and then pulled into the orifice of the desired vessel. Examples of these catheters that can be used to cannulate visceral branches include Cobra, Simmons, Inferior Mesenteric Artery (IMA), and Neiman catheters. Cobra catheters have primary and secondary downward-curves that can be pulled into the vessels for catheterization. This catheter can be further configured to C1 and C2 catheters, depending on the angle of the primary curve. Commonly used catheters for visceral and renal vessel catheterization are illustrated in Figure 17.2. For cerebral diagnostic angiography, these catheters typically have double curves. Simmons catheters are configured like a shepherd's hook, whose shapes can be further divided to Simmons 1 (SIM1) and Simmons 2 (SIM2) catheters. These catheters are commonly used for both cerebral and visceral vessel catheterization. Headhunter (HN) catheters have a sharper secondary and tertiary curve, while a JB1 catheter is a similar version of the headhunter catheters. Commonly used catheters for cerebral catheterization are illustrated in Figure 17.3.

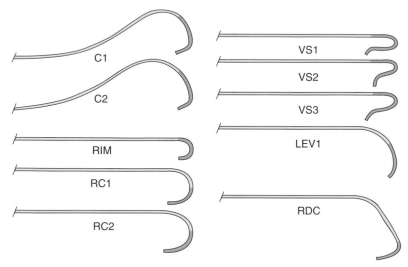

Figure 17.2 Commonly used catheters for visceral or renal angiography.

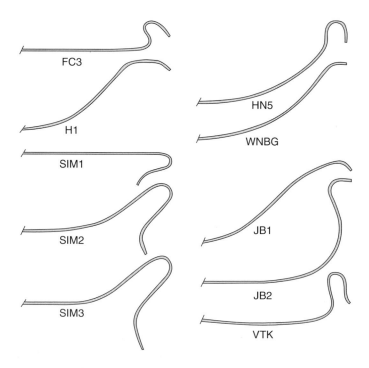

Figure 17.3 Commonly used catheters for cerebral angiography.

Table 17.1 Self-expanding stents.

Company	Device name	Material used	Guidewire system (in.)	Stent diameter (mm)	Stent length (mm)	Delivery system length (cm)
Abbott	Xceed	Nitinol	0.035	5, 6, 7, 8	20, 30, 40, 60, 80	80,120
Abbott	Xpert	Nitinol	0.018	5, 6, 8	20, 30, 40, 60	80, 120
Bard	Luminnex	Nitinol	0.035	6, 7, 8, 9, 10, 12	20, 30, 40,50, 60, 80, 100, 120	80, 130
Bard	Conformexx	Nitinol	0.035	6, 7, 8, 9, 10	20, 30, 40, 60, 80, 100, 120	135
Boston Scientific	Monorail Wallstent	Elgiloy	0.014	6, 8, 10	21, 22, 24, 29, 31, 36, 37	135
Boston Scientific	Wallstent	Elgiloy	0.035	5, 6, 7, 8, 9, 10	18, 20, 23, 24, 34, 35, 36, 38, 39, 40, 42, 45, 46, 47, 49, 52, 55, 59, 60, 61, 66, 67, 69, 80, 90, 94	75, 135
Boston Scientific	Sentinol	Nitinol	0.035	5, 6, 7, 8, 9, 10	21, 40, 60, 80	75, 135
Cook	Zilver	Nitinol	0.035	6, 7, 8, 9, 10	20, 40, 60, 80, 100	80
Cordis	Precise	Nitinol	0.018	5, 6, 7, 8, 9, 10	20, 30, 40	135
Cordis	Smart Control	Nitinol	0.035	6, 7, 8, 9, 10	20, 30, 40, 60, 80, 100	80, 120
Edwards Lifesciences	LifeStent NT	Nitinol	0.014	6, 7, 8	20, 30, 40, 60, 80	75, 120
EV3	Protégé	Nitinol	0.035	6, 7, 8, 9, 10, 12	20, 30, 40, 60, 80	80, 120
Guidant	Absolute	Nitinol	0.035	6, 7, 8, 9, 10, 12	28, 38, 56, 80	80, 120
Medtronic	Bridge SE	Nitinol	0.035	6, 7, 8, 9, 10	20, 40, 60, 80	75, 120

Stents

Endoluminal stents are used to buttress open a vascular lumen. Stents were developed to overcome the limitations of balloon angioplasty namely elastic recoil and dissection. Based on the metal elastic property, stents can be divided into either balloon-expandable or self-expanding categories. Self-expanding

Table 17.2 Balloon-expandable stents.

Company	Device name	Material used	Guidewire system (in)	Stent diameter (mm)	Stent length (mm)	Delivery system length (cm)
Abbott	Wavemax	Stainless Steel	0.035	5, 6, 7, 8, 9, 10, 12	12, 17, 28, 38, 58	75, 135
Boston Scientific	Express LD	Stainless Steel	0.035	5, 6, 7, 8, 9, 10	17, 27, 37, 57	75, 135
Boston Scientific	Express SD	Stainless Steel	0.018	4, 5, 6, 7	15, 19	90, 150
Cordis	Palmaz	Stainless Steel	0.035	4, 5, 6, 7, 8	10, 15, 20, 29, 39	n/a (unmounted)
Cordis	Palmaz Genesis	Stainless Steel	0.035	4, 5, 6, 7, 8, 9, 10	12, 15, 18, 24, 29, 39, 59, 79	80, 135
Edwards Lifesciences	LifeStent LP SDS	Stainless Steel	0.018	4, 5, 6, 7	18, 36, 56	75, 120
Edwards Lifesciences	LifeStent SDS	Stainless Steel	0.035	6, 7, 8, 9, 10	18, 26, 36, 56	75, 120
EV3	Paramount	Stainless Steel	0.035	5, 6, 7, 8	16, 26, 36	75
Guidant	Herculink Plus	Stainless Steel	0.014	4, 5, 6, 7	12, 15, 18	80, 135
Medtronic	Racer	Cobalt	0.035	5, 6, 7	10, 17	75, 120
Medtronic	Bridge Assurant	Stainless Steel	0.035	6, 7, 8, 9, 10	20, 30, 40, 60	80, 130

stents, which can be constructed of stainless steel or nitinol, are delivered in a constraining sheath, which when withdrawn permits the stent to expand to a predetermined diameter. Balloon-expandable stents, which are typically constructed of stainless steel or tantalum materials, are mounted on angioplasty balloon catheters. Once the balloon-mounted stents are delivered to a desired vessel location, the inflation of the angioplasty balloon catheter would result in the expansion of the stent to its desired diameter. Some of the commonly used balloon-expandable stents in the United States are listed in Table 17.1. Examples of commonly used self-expanding stents are listed in Table 17.2.

Vena cava filters

An inferior vena cava (IVC) filters are devices developed to replace surgical ligation or placement of IVC clips to prevent fatal pulmonary embolism (PE). The first filter introduced was the Mobin-Uddin umbrella filter in 1967. Currently there are 10 IVC filters that are approved by the Food and Drug Administration (FDA) (Table 17.4). Among them, there are three temporary or retrievable filters, which are designed for endoluminal retrieval once the need for PE prophylaxis is no longer needed. These temporary filters are Recovery filter (Bard, Tempe, AZ), Gunther Tulip filter (Cook, Bloomington, IN), and OptEase filter (Cordis, Warren, NJ). IVC filters are designed for their physical properties, clot-trapping effectiveness, ability to preserve flow in the IVC, and ease of placement. An overview of these various IVC filter devices is displayed in Table 17.3.

Stent grafts

Since Juan Parodi reported his initial experience of successful endovascular aneurysm repair using a homemade endograft by attaching a Palmaz stent within a Dacron tube,[1] significant advance has taken place in the endograft device technology in the past decade. Numerous stent-graft devices have undergone rigorous clinical trials, which demonstrated both durable and excellent clinical results when compared to open aneurysm operations. Although the Ancure device (Guidant Corporation, Indianapolis, IN) was the first device that received the FDA approval for clinical application in 1999, this device was removed from the market by the manufacturer in October 2003. Presently, there are four approved devices in the United States for infrarenal aortic aneurysm treatment. A brief description of each of these devices is provided below. Features of theses devices compared with other devices that are available outside the United States, are summarized in Table 17.4.

AneuRx

The AneuRx device (Medtronic, Santa Rosa, CA) is a modular device that has an exoskeleton, which is constructed with nitinol frame with woven polyester fabric material (Figure 17.4). The main device and contralateral limb require a 22 Fr and 6 Fr introducer sheaths, respectively. Based on a multicenter clinical study from 1996 to 1999, a total of 1193 patients with infrarenal AAA were treated with the AneuRx device.[5] Long-term primary outcome measures reveal 97% freedom from rupture, 97% freedom from aneurysm-related death, 91% freedom from surgical conversion, and 62% probability of survival at 5 years by Kaplan–Meier analysis. Secondary outcome measures include stent-graft patency in 91%, endoleak in 15%, aneurysm enlargement in 15%, and stent-graft migration in 6% of patients at 5 years.[6] The AneuRx stent-graft system has evolved to a fourth-generation device since completion of the clinical trial with improvements in stent design, fabric material, and delivery system.

Excluder

The Excluder device (WL Gore and Associates, Flagstaff, AZ) is composed of a durable and lower permeability expandable polytetrafluoroethylene (ePTFE) graft with a reinforcing film, an electropolished nitinol stent, and bonding

Table 17.3 IVC filters.

Company	Filter name	Material	Indicated caval diameter (mm)	Maximum deployed length (mm)	Catheter system inner-diameter (Fr)	Approach	Indicated use
Bard	Simon Nitinol Filter	Nitinol	28	38	7	Jugular, Femoral, Antecubital	Permanent
Bard	Recovery Filter	Nitinol	28	41	7	Femoral	Permanent, or Temporary
B Braun/Vena Tech	Vena Tech LP Filter	Phynox Wire	28	43	7	Jugular, Femoral	Permanent
B Braun/Vena Tech	Vena Tech LGM Filter	Phynox Wire	28	38	10	Jugular, Femoral	Permanent
Boston Scientific	Over-the-Sire Greenfield Filter	Stainless Steel	28	50	12	Jugular, Femoral	Permanent
Boston Scientific	Titanium Greenfield Filter	Titanium Alloy	28	50	12	Jugular, Femoral	Permanent
Cook	Bird's Nest Filter	Stainless Steel	40	80	12	Jugular, Femoral	Permanent
Cook	Gunther Tulip Filter	Conichrome	30	50	7	Jugular, Femoral	Permanent, or Temporary
Cordis	TrapEase Filter	Nitinol	30	50	6	Jugular, Femoral, Antecubital	Permanent
Cordis	OptEase Filter	Nitinol	30	54	6	Jugular, Femoral, Antecubital	Permanent, or Temporary

Table 17.4 Endovascular AAA devices.

Company	Device name	Stent material	Graft material	Proximal fixation site	Main body delivery sheath (OD)	Main body diameter (mm)	Main body length (cm)	Iliac limb diameter (mm)	Iliac limb length (cm)
Endologix	Powerlink	Cobalt-Chromium Alloy	ePTFE	Infrarenal or Suprarenal	20 Fr or 22 Fr	25, 28, 34*	8, 10, 12*	16	4, 5.5
Cook	Zenith	Stainless Steel	Woven Polyester	Suprarenal	20 Fr or 23 Fr	22, 24, 26, 28, 30, 32	7.4, 8.8, 10.3, 11.7, 13.2	8, 10, 12, 14, 16, 18, 20, 22, 24	3.7, 5.4, 7.1, 8.8, 10.5, 12.2
Gore	Excluder	Nitinol	ePTFE	Infrarenal or Suprarenal	18 Fr	23, 26, 28.5, 31*	14*, 15*, 16, 17*, 18	12, 14.5, 16, 18, 20	9.5, 10, 11.5, 12, 13.5, 14
Medtronic	AneuRx	Nitinol	Woven Polyester	Infrarenal or Suprarenal	21 Fr	20, 22, 24, 26, 28	13.5, 16.5	12, 13, 14, 15, 16	8.5, 11.5
Medtronic	Talent	Nitinol	Woven Polyester	Suprarenal	22 Fr or 24Fr	24, 26, 28, 30, 32, 34	14, 15.5, 17	8, 10, 12, 14, 16, 18, 20, 22, 24	7.5, 9, 10.5

*Sizes available outside United States

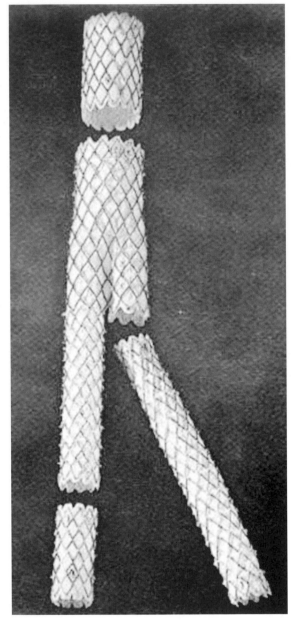

Figure 17.4 The AneurRx stent-graft device.

film for stent to graft attachment (Figure 17.5). The device retains the original reinforcing film, lending strength and durability to the graft wall. The low permeability design employs a microstructure technology that results in significantly reduced graft permeability. The device uses ePTFE tape and other

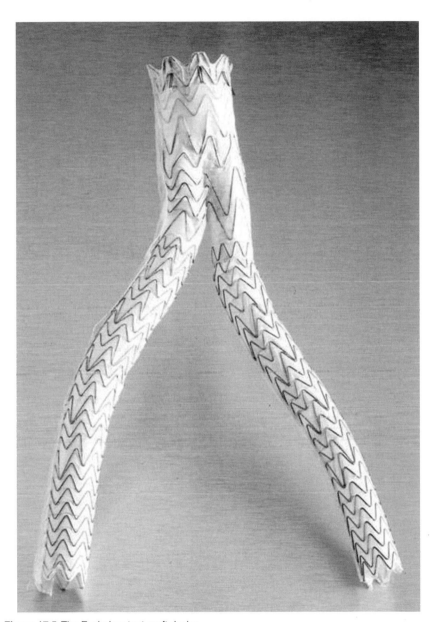

Figure 17.5 The Excluder stent-graft device.

technologies to adhere nitinol rings that vary in the size and shape of the sinusoidal curves, which makes the device quite flexible and deliverable in relatively small catheters. It does have proximal fixation using barbs on the proximal portion of the device. The delivery profile is small, with delivery through an 18-Fr sheath. Clinical data with this device in the US clinical trial

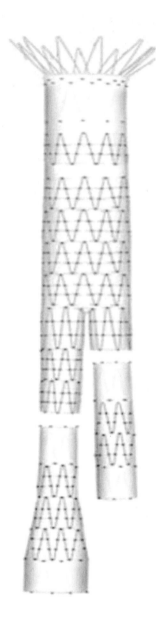

Figure 17.6 The Zenith stent-graft device.

of 235 patients showed there is a significant reduction in length of stay and improvement in return to normal activity.[7] The device-related complications have become extremely low, which translates to high levels of safety. When pivotal study results and adverse events are compared to surgical controls,

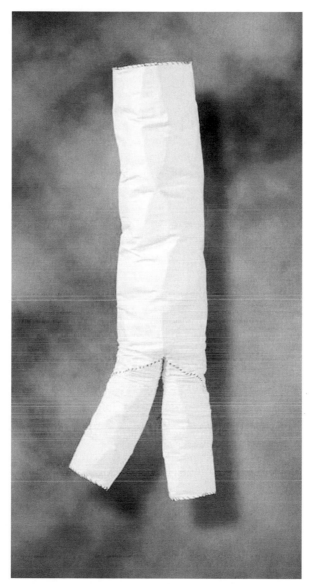

Figure 17.7 The Powerlink stent-graft device.

there is a dramatic reduction in the morbidity in the study group compared to the surgical control group, similar to other device trials.[8]

Zenith

The Zenith device (Cook Inc., Bloomington, IN) is a modular device that has many different anatomic options in terms of sizing (Figure 17.6). The size matrix allows its use in 29-mm-diameter necks, and large-diameter iliac arteries. It utilizes suprarenal attachment, with positive fixation utilizing barbs. Initial clinical data included 200 patients, 80 of who were in the standard-risk trial, and there was also a high-risk component that provided data.[9] A review of 30-day morbidity shows that the number of patients who are free from morbidity with endografts is significantly reduced, compared with the surgical cohort. As with all clinical trials, there was a marked reduction in morbidity in the study group compared to the surgical group, but there was no statistical improvement in mortality. The treatment success was found to be equivalent in both groups. Statistically significant benefits can be seen in all aspects; similarly, the quality-of-life parameters, which are being increasingly measured in clinical trials, and benefits were observed in all important aspects, such as patients getting back to their normal life, and compared favorable to surgical therapy. In terms of aneurysm size, the Zenith device was associated with remarkable aneurysm shrinkage during the course of the trial.[9,10]

Powerlink

The Powerlink device (Endologix, Irvine, CA) received its FDA approval in 2005. It consists of a self-expanding metallic endoskeleton covered with an ePTFE graft (Figure 17.7). It is delivered through one surgically exposed femoral artery, with a contralateral 9 Fr sheath, which can be placed percutaneously. The stented endoskeleton main body is constructed as a single continuous wire woven into a double spine without sutures or welds. The stented portion is constructed of a cobalt–chromium alloy. The endoskeleton is covered with a graft material made from ePTFE. It is a one-piece bifurcated design. The graft material is sutured to the endoskeleton only at the ends of the device. The delivery sheath has a 21 Fr outer diameter and a long, tapered tip. A large multicenter trial was conducted that compared 192 endovascular patients who where treated with the Powerlink device and 66 surgical patients who underwent open repair.[11] This study found significantly reduced hospital length of stay, operative time, procedural-related adverse events, and gastrointestinal complications in the endovascular group when compared to the surgical cohort. At the time of the first-month CT scan, endoleaks were noted in 25 patients, yielding a 30-day endoleak rate of 22.7%.[11] Type II endoleaks predominated, and there were no type III or IV endoleaks. There were no ruptures, graft fabric defects, or wire fractures. Significant reduction in mean AAA diameter and volume was noted at every follow-up interval. Increase in AAA diameter was noted in only 1.5% of patients at 24 months.[11,12]

References

1 Seldinger SI. Catheter replacement of the needle in percutaneous arteriography; a new technique. *Acta Radiol* 1953; **39**:368–76.

2 Dotter CT, Judkins MP. Transluminal treatment of orteriosclerotic obstruction. Description of a new technic and a preliminary report of its application. *Circulation* 1964; **30**:654–70.

3 Gruntzig A, Hopff H. [Percutaneous recanalization after chronic arterial occlusion with a new dilator-catheter (modification of the Dotter technique) (author's transl)]. *Dtsch Med Wochenschr* 1974; **99**:2502–10, 2511.

4 Parodi JC, Palmaz JC, Barone HD. Transfemoral intraluminal graft implantation for abdominal aortic aneurysms. *Ann Vasc Surg* 1991; **5**:491–99.

5 Zarins CK. The US AneuRx clinical trial: 6-year clinical update 2002. *J Vasc Surg* 2003; **37**:904–8.

6 Zarins CK, Bloch DA, Crabtree T, Matsumoto AH, White RA, Fogarty TJ. Aneurysm enlargement following endovascular aneurysm repair: AneuRx clinical trial. *J Vasc Surg* 2004; **39**:109–17.

7 Matsumura JS, Brewster DC, Makaroun MS, Naftel DC. A multicenter controlled clinical trial of open versus endovascular treatment of abdominal aortic aneurysm. *J Vasc Surg* 2003; **37**:262–71.

8 Matsumura JS, Katzen BT, Hollier LH, Dake MD. Update on the bifurcated EXCLUDER endoprosthesis: phase I results. *J Vasc Surg* 2001; **33**:S150–53.

9 Greenberg RK, Lawrence-Brown M, Bhandari G *et al.* An update of the Zenith endovascular graft for abdominal aortic aneurysms: initial implantation and mid-term follow-up data. *J Vasc Surg* 2001; **33**:S157–64.

10 Greenberg RK, Chuter TA, Sternbergh WC, 3rd, Fearnot NE. Zenith AAA endovascular graft: intermediate-term results of the US multicenter trial. *J Vasc Surg* 2004; **39**:1209–18.

11 Carpenter JP. Midterm results of the multicenter trial of the powerlink bifurcated system for endovascular aortic aneurysm repair. *J Vasc Surg* 2004; **40**:849–59.

12 Carpenter JP. Multicenter trial of the PowerLink bifurcated system for endovascular aortic aneurysm repair. *J Vasc Surg* 2002; **36**:1129–37.

Index